CLINICAL MANUAL
OF PEDIATRIC
ANESTHESIA

CLINICAL MANUAL
OF PEDIATRIC
ANESTHESIA

Editors

Deborah K. Rasch, M.D.

Associate Professor
Department of Pediatrics and Anesthesiology
University of Texas Health Science Center
San Antonio, Texas

Dawn E. Webster, M.D.

Assistant Professor
Department of Anesthesiology
University of Texas Health Science Center
San Antonio, Texas

McGraw-Hill, Inc.
Health Professions Division

New York   St. Louis   San Francisco   Auckland
Bogotá   Caracas   Lisbon   London   Madrid
Mexico City   Milan   Montreal   New Delhi
Paris   San Juan   Singapore   Sydney   Tokyo   Toronto

CLINICAL MANUAL OF PEDIATRIC ANESTHESIA

1234567890   DOC DOC   9876543

ISBN 0-07-051119-5

This book was set in Times Roman by Compset, Inc.
The editors were Michael J. Houston and
Mariapaz Ramos Englis;
the production supervisor was Clare Stanley;
the project supervision was by Edelsack Zucker
Editorial Service;
the cover designer was Marsha Cohen/Parallelogram.
R.R. Donnelley & Sons Company was printer and binder.

Library of Congress Cataloging-in-Publication Data

Clinical manual of pediatric anesthesia / edited by Deborah K.
  Rasch, Dawn E. Webster,
      p.   cm.
    Includes bibliographical references and index.
    ISBN 0-07-051119-5
    1. Pediatric anesthesia—Handbooks, manuals, etc.
I. Rasch, Deborah K.   II. Webster, Dawn E.   [DNLM:
1. Anesthesia—in infancy & childhood.   WO 440 C641 1993]
RD139.C55   1993
617.9′6798—dc20
DNLM/DLC
for Library of Congress   93-13511
                                                              CIP

This book is printed on acid-free paper.

This handbook is dedicated to the residents of the Department of Anesthesiology at the University of Texas Health Science Center at San Antonio for whom it was originally prepared.

Contents

PART V: PEDIATRIC TRANSPLANTATION (ANESTHETIC AND SURGICAL CONCERNS)

Contributors

Numbers in brackets refer to the contributors' chapters.

Amy C. Benedikt, M.D. [19]
Instructor
Department of Anesthesiology
University of Texas Health Science Center
San Antonio, Texas

Christopher A. Bracken, M.D., Ph.D. [30]
Assistant Professor
Department of Anesthesiology
University of Texas Health Science Center
San Antonio, Texas

Lois L. Bready, M.D. [15, 16]
Professor
Department of Anesthesiology
University of Texas Health Science Center
San Antonio, Texas

John H. Calhoon, M.D. [27]
Assistant Professor
Department of Thoracic & Cardiovascular Surgery
Chief, Pediatric Cardiac Surgery
University of Texas Health Science Center
San Antonio, Texas

Bonny Carter, M.D. [9]
Assistant Professor
Department of Anesthesiology
University of Texas Health Science Center
San Antonio, Texas

C. Y. Jennifer Chan, Pharm.D. [3]
Clinical Assistant Professor
Department of Pharmacology
University of Texas Health Science Center
San Antonio, Texas

Ewell A. Clarke, M.D. [5]
Associate Professor of Radiology
Department of Radiology
University of Texas Health Science Center
San Antonio, Texas

Ralph F. Erian, M.D., F.R.C.P.(C) [28]
Associate Professor and Director of Critical Care Medicine
Department of Anesthesiology
University of Texas Health Science Center
San Antonio, Texas

Alice Gong, M.D. [21]
Assistant Professor
Department of Pediatrics, Division of Neonatology
University of Texas Health Science Center
San Antonio, Texas

Frederick L. Grover, M.D. [27]
Head
Division of Cardiothoracic Surgery
Veterans Affairs Medical Center
Denver, Colorado

Mary Ann Gurkowski, M.D. [4, 7, 20, 29]
Assistant Professor
Department of Anesthesiology
University of Texas Health Science Center
San Antonio, Texas

Chantal R. Harrison, M.D. [17]
Associate Professor
Department of Pathology
University of Texas Health Science Center
San Antonio, Texas

Kelly Gordon Knape, M.D. [11]
Assistant Professor and Director of Obstetrical Anesthesia
Department of Anesthesiology
University of Texas Health Science Center
San Antonio, Texas

Scott E. LeBard, M.D. [31]
Instructor in Anesthesiology
Mayo Medical School
Senior Associate Consultant in Anesthesiology and
    Pediatric Critical Care
Mayo Clinic
Rochester, Minnesota

Laura Loftis, M.D. [13]
Instructor
Department of Pediatrics
University of Texas Health Science Center
San Antonio, Texas

Kim Lopez, M.D. [2]
Instructor
Department of Pediatrics
University of Texas Health Science Center
San Antonio, Texas

Michelle Moro, M.D. [18]
Instructor
Department of Anesthesiology
University of Texas Health Science Center
San Antonio, Texas

Joseph J. Naples, M.D. [27]
Professor and Director of Anesthesiology
Medical Center Hospital
Department of Anesthesiology
University of Texas Health Science Center
San Antonio, Texas

Deborah A. Nicholas, M.D. [22]
Director of Anesthesiology Services
Greenville Unit
Shriner's Crippled Children's Hospital
Greenville, South Carolina

Allen D. Noorily, M.D. [23]
Assistant Professor
Department of Otolaryngology
University of Texas Health Science Center
San Antonio, Texas

Susan H. Noorily, M.D. [14, 23]
Assistant Professor
Department of Anesthesiology
University of Texas Health Science Center
San Antonio, Texas

Myung K. Park, M.D. [6]
Professor of Pediatrics and Head
Division of Cardiology
University of Texas Health Science Center
San Antonio, Texas

Mary Dale Peterson, M.D. [26]
Associate Professor
Department of Anesthesiology
University of Texas Medical Branch at Galveston
Chief, Department of Anesthesiology
Driscoll Children's Hospital
Corpus Christi, Texas

Trevor G. Pollard, M.D. [13, 14]
Clinical Professor
Department of Anesthesiology
University of Texas Health Science Center
San Antonio, Texas

Rajam S. Ramamurthy, M.D. [20]
Professor
Department of Pediatrics, Division of Neonatology
University of Texas Health Science Center
San Antonio, Texas

Deborah K. Rasch, M.D. [7, 9, 10, 14, 15, 19, 20, 21, 25, 26, 27, 28, 29]
Associate Professor and Director of Pediatric Anesthesia
Department of Pediatrics and Anesthesiology
University of Texas Health Science Center
San Antonio, Texas

James Rogers, M.D. [18]
Assistant Professor
Department of Anesthesiology
Division of Pain Management
University of Texas Health Science Center
San Antonio, Texas

Paul M. Seib, M.D. [25]
Chief of Pediatric Cardiology
Department of Pediatrics
Wilford Hall USAF Medical Center
San Antonio, Texas

Dawn E. Webster, M.D. [1, 2, 8, 12, 21]
Assistant Professor
Department of Anesthesiology
University of Texas Health Science Center
San Antonio, Texas

Alan D. Zablocki, M.D. [24]
Clinical Associate Professor
Department of Anesthesiology
University of Texas Health Science Center
San Antonio, Texas

Preface

The opportunity to care for children in the operating room or critical care setting can be a very rewarding experience, but it can also be very anxiety-provoking, especially for residents in anesthesia training or for anesthesiologists who only occasionally care for pediatric patients. With this in mind, we compiled the materials in this handbook to provide a quick reference for clinically relevant information as well as the basic theory behind the safe administration of pediatric anesthesia. This includes a series of very comprehensive chapters written by non-anesthesiologists who relate their experience with pediatric diseases. Interpretation of the pediatric ECG is written by a well-known authority, Dr. Myung Park. Dr. Park, who has published a large volume of literature in pediatric cardiology, describes a very systematic approach to a difficult topic. Another chapter, "Approach to the Pediatric Chest X-Ray," contains valuable information about radiographic findings that are usually normal in children but would be interpreted as abnormal in the adult. This is a chapter in which almost everyone who cares for pediatric patients in the perioperative period can find useful guidelines for identifying disease states. Chapter 17 provides a rational approach to transfusion therapy in the pediatric patient and describes the differences between available blood components.

The chapters on neonatal emergencies, pediatric and neonatal resuscitation, and the pediatric trauma patient are equally comprehensive and contain very current subject matter regarding the management of these urgent situations. Specialty anesthesia is also discussed with special attention to pediatric cardiac malformations and their anesthetic management, as well as pediatric transplantation.

We acknowledge that there are many acceptable methods of practice in any situation, and have attempted to present a variety of these, including a brief discussion of advantages and disadvantages where appropriate. We hope this text will assist the anesthesiologist in the management of the pediatric patient and stimulate interest to pursue each topic in more detail elsewhere in the literature.

Acknowledgments

We would like to acknowledge the hard work and dedication of Ms. Annette Harris and Mr. Michael Bohme in the preparation of this manuscript.

Part I

General Pediatric Anesthesia

CHAPTER 1

Preparation for Pediatric Anesthesia (Pearls and Pitfalls)

Dawn E. Webster

Providing anesthetic care for the infant or child is fun, reward-ing, and challenging. The anesthesiologist or anesthesia resi-dent who does not work in a children's hospital but cares for children in a predominantly adult environment faces an addi-tional challenge when preparing the room, equipment, and themselves for the experience. The preoperative evaluation and preparation of the patient is covered in Chap. 4 of this hand-book. This chapter will focus on preparation of the room and the selection of equipment and will review some of the most basic aspects of pediatric anesthesia. These subjects will all be covered in more detail elsewhere in this handbook.

PEARLS AND PITFALLS IN PEDIATRIC ANESTHESIA

The anesthesiologist dealing with infants is walking through a minefield of various potential complications and bad outcomes, some of which are preventable and some, regardless of effort, non preventable (page 569).

Frederic A. Berry*

Anesthetic care of the pediatric patient differs in many ways from that of the adult. The following is a brief summary of some of the most essential facts in pediatric anesthesia. These little

*Berry F: Anesthesia complications occurring primarily in the very young, in Benumof J, Saidman L (eds): *Anesthesia and Perioperative Complications*. Chicago, Mosby Year Book, 1992, pp 548–571. Quoted with permission.

"pearls and pitfalls" are presented in the form of the mnemonic ABCDEF:

A: Apnea.

B: Bradycardia, bubbles, breath sounds, blood volume.

C: Cold.

D: Disbelief of monitors.

E: Extubation, equipment, emotional development.

F: Fluids.

A: Apnea

The child who becomes apneic or has an obstruction at any time desaturates and becomes hypercarbic more rapidly than the adult. Airway management of the pediatric patient must be impeccable because there is little room for error. Evaluation of the airway may be difficult in the infant or uncooperative child. Standard guidelines for recognizing the difficult airway have not been validated in pediatric patients. The presence of a cleft lip or palate, a history of pharyngeal incompetence or subglottic stenosis, or certain disease entities (Hurler syndrome, Pierre Robin syndrome, or Treacher Collins syndrome) should alert the anesthesiologist to possible airway difficulties. Even the normal child has anatomic differences from the adult that favor obstruction (see Chap. 2). The child with an upper respiratory infection is also at increased risk for airway complications during the perioperative period (see Chap. 4).

B: Bradycardia

Cardiac output is rate dependent in infants. Bradycardia is serious because it results in a decrease in cardiac output. If a child becomes bradycardic, we must first address the adequacy of ventilation and rule out hypoxia. Other causes of bradycardia include vagal stimulation, anaphylaxis, and drugs.

B: Bubbles

Bubbles in the intravenous fluids are to be avoided because many children have a probe patent foramen ovale, putting them at risk for a paradoxic air embolus. Children with congenital heart disease and known intracardiac communication are at the greatest risk for this. A frequent site of bubble introduction is the three-way stopcock and the injection ports.

Bubbles should be eliminated from all intravenous tubing, and the tubing should contain a bubble trap. When drugs are administered, care should be taken not to introduce air. One way to accomplish this is to draw slightly more drug into the syringe than you plan to administer, make sure the syringe has no air bubbles, and when injecting the drug into a stopcock, fill the stopcock to the brim (either from your syringe or the intravenous line) before connecting the syringe. A bubble that finds its way into the intravenous tubing can be removed at the site of the T connector or, in some cases, may be retrieved using a long spinal needle. As always, prevention is preferable to cure!

B: Breath Sounds

Breath sounds in the small infant may be transmitted far and wide from the site of actual air exchange. This may make evaluation of endotracheal tube placement difficult. If doubt exists about whether the endotracheal tube has actually been placed in the trachea, direct visualization of the tube through the cords or presence of a CO_2 tracing are reliable. Breath sounds, particularly in the very small infant, are not. Pneumothorax and endobronchial intubation may also be difficult to diagnose because of misleading, transmitted breath sounds. The best places to evaluate breath sounds are the axilla and upper lung fields. The presence of chest wall motion should be ascertained in conjunction with the evaluation of breath sounds.

B: Blood Volume

Blood loss in the pediatric patient is calculated as the percent of total blood volume. The practitioner who infrequently anesthetizes children must realize that what may be an insignificant amount of blood loss in the adult may comprise a large percent of blood volume in the infant or small child.

C: Cold

A cold room results in a cold child. Hypothermia can result in delayed awakening, prolonged action of muscle relaxants, and postoperative shivering. Attention to creating a warm operating room environment and the use of other warming devices (as discussed in the equipment section of this chapter) will help to maintain temperature homeostasis.

D: Disbelief of Monitors

The physiologic status of the infant and child under anesthesia can change rapidly. If a monitor gives a value that you are tempted not to believe, BELIEVE IT! Check the child first; then, trouble shoot the monitors.

Although pulse oximetry and capnography have been shown to be helpful in detecting potentially dangerous respiratory events, they are of no use if they are disbelieved, misinterpreted, or turned off.

E: Emotional Development

The emotional development of the pediatric patient is an important factor in perioperative care. The choice of premedicant and method of administration, the type of induction, and the type of postoperative analgesia will all be influenced by the patient's emotional and intellectual development. Fear of separation from parents, fear of needles, and the anxiety created by strange surroundings all contribute to making a trip to the operating room an overwhelming experience. Children who are "repeat" visitors may have varied reactions to their surroundings, depending on their initial experience. Knowledge and understanding of this important aspect of pediatric anesthesia will improve patient safety and greatly contribute to the comfort of the child and the parents. This subject is discussed in greater detail in Chap. 4.

E: Extubation

Accidental extubation can easily occur in the infant because the infant trachea is very short (5-cm long in the neonate). Whenever an infant or small child is repositioned or moved in the slightest, the position of the endotracheal tube should be reevaluated. For the same reason, accidental endobronchial intubation can occur just as easily.

The timing of extubation is very important in infants and children. Although there are times when we could argue in favor of deep extubation, awake extubation is usually prudent and justifiable. The pros and cons of awake and deep extubation, as well as the technique for each of these, are discussed more thoroughly in Chap. 7. Presuming an awake extubation is desired, the adult criteria are not useful in infants because babies will not open their eyes or do anything else on command. Signs of "awakeness" and muscle strength in an infant must be evaluated without the cooperation of the patient. Signs of awakeness include spontaneous eye opening, purposeful movement, and grimacing as though crying. Muscle strength may be evaluated clinically by seeing that the infant can raise both legs 90° perpendicular to the operating room table. If there is doubt about the readiness for extubation, the patient should remain intubated and ventilated as long as necessary.

E: Equipment

It is difficult or impossible to "make do" with the wrong size of equipment in the pediatric patient. Preparation must be made beforehand to have a selection of all necessary equipment in appropriate sizes. This is discussed further in the remainder of this chapter.

F: Fluids

The problem of not recognizing significant amounts of blood loss in the pediatric patient has already been discussed. Other problems with intraoperative and postoperative fluid replacement include inappropriate intravenous administration equipment, which could lead to accidental overhydration, and concern about glucose requirements during surgery. Proper calculation of fluid needs and correct equipment for volume administration are essential. Chap. 9 covers fluid management in the pediatric surgical patient in more detail, and the basic guidelines are covered.

PREPARATION OF THE ROOM

The anesthesia machine should be checked as usual. A machine that can deliver air, oxygen, and nitrous oxide is advantageous, particularly in the ex-premature infant in whom retinopathy of prematurity is a consideration or in a patient for whom nitrous oxide is contraindicated. A Pediatric Circle System or a nonrebreathing circuit (Bain or Jackson Rees) apparatus should be in place and checked for leaks. The advantage of the Jackson Rees is that it has no valves to obstruct exhalation, but it requires high flows, is cumbersome, and can be difficult to scavenge. The Pediatric Circuit does not cause increased resistance to ventilation if the valves are working properly; however, in small infants, pulmonary compliance may be difficult to assess using this circuit because of the compressability of the gases within the tubing. The appropriate-sized bag for either circuit can be estimated by the following formula:

$$70 \times \text{weight in kg} = \text{mL bag size (round up to the nearest 0.5 L)}$$

Monitors

Standard intraoperative monitoring for the pediatric patient includes continuous electrocardiography (ECG), intermittent blood pressure, esophageal or precordial stethoscopes, in-line inspired oxygen analysis, end-tidal CO_2, temperature, and pulse oximetry.

Monitors should have child-sized apparatus to work properly. For example, the blood pressure cuff should be two-thirds the length of the upper arm, and infant-sized pulse oximeter probes are available. Small ECG pads are available for use in very small infants, and pediatric-sized esophageal stethoscopes, precordial stethoscopes, and temperature probes are available.

Automatic, noninvasive blood pressure monitoring is desirable, but the device used should have the capability of correctly measuring parameters in the infant or child. In some cases, a neonatal Dinamap may be necessary. Some devices require a knob in the back to be adjusted to the patient's age group. A Doppler probe and manual blood pressure manometer can also be used.

The pulse oximeter reading may be disturbed by excessive movement of the child and by the presence of heating lights. A towel over the extremity with the pulse oximeter probe is often necessary when infrared interference is encountered. The probe should be demonstrated to be working adequately before induction begins, and the alarms should be turned on. End-tidal CO_2 is the most reliable monitor for the verification of the proper placement of the endotracheal tube. The monitor should be attached before induction, and the alarms turned on. The absence of end-tidal CO_2 should be cause for immediate reevaluation of the placement of the endotracheal tube by direct vision or for bag–mask ventilation. The continued absence of end-tidal CO_2 after confirmation of the placement of the endotracheal tube should prompt an evaluation for low cardiac output or bronchospasm. If these are absent, the monitor should be checked and, if necessary, a portable end-tidal CO_2 device attached.

Temperature monitoring may be tympanic, oropharyngeal, esophageal, axillary, skin, or rectal. Temperatures taken from the lower third of the esophagus and from the external auditory canal correlate most closely with the core temperature. Skin and axillary temperatures generally do not correlate well with the core temperature and may be unreliable in detecting rapid increases in temperature. Rectal temperature may be influenced by many factors, which may make it unreliable. If tympanic temperature is monitored, a probe designed specifically for that site should be used and should be placed gently to avoid damage to the tympanic membrane. Esophageal temperature probes should be placed at the correct depth because too high placement will reflect the temperature of inspired gases. An esophageal temperature probe or stethoscope is not recommended in pediatric tracheostomy cases, in which identification of the trachea may depend in part on palpation of the rigid tube (presumably endotracheal) in the trachea.

Room Temperature

Room temperature is the most important factor in keeping an infant or child warm during anesthesia. The room must be

Table 1-1   Age and Room Temperature Guidelines

AGE	TEMPERATURE
Newborn	80°F
Newborn–6 months	78°F
6 months–2 years	76°F

warmed slowly or high humidity may contaminate sterile equipment. The guidelines for room temperature are shown in Table 1-1.

Other equipment that should be present in the room to help maintain the child's temperature include a functioning warming blanket, overhead heating lamps for infants, a heated humidifier or in-line humidifying device (in-line humidifiers are not approved for use in infants weighing less than 10 kg), and a head cap.

Warming blankets are most useful in infants under 10 kg. The blanket should be set at no higher than 40°C and should be covered with a sheet so that no part of the infant's skin makes contact. Warming lights should be kept approximately 36 in. from the skin of an infant to prevent burns. (This may differ depending on the manufacturer; check their instructions.) If a heated humidifier is in the anesthesia circuit, it should have a servo-control mechanism so that it does not become overheated. The anesthesia circuit should be checked after the humidifier is in place because improper placement may result in hypoventilation. Hot fluid from the humidifier should not be allowed to come into contact with the patient's trachea because thermal damage may result.

AIRWAY EQUIPMENT

Minimal airway equipment for the infant and child with a "normal" airway includes masks, oral airways, tongue blades, laryngoscope blades and handles, endotracheal tubes, and suction devices.

Masks should be sized so that the top of the mask covers the bridge of the nose; the bottom should contact the cleft in the chin. Clear masks seem to be accepted more easily than black masks by most children. The application of a scent (e.g., bubblegum or strawberry) to the inner part of the mask may render it even more acceptable. Figure 1-1 illustrates appropriate mask selection.

Oral airways should be placed using a tongue blade or laryngoscope blade to pull the tongue forward. Improper placement

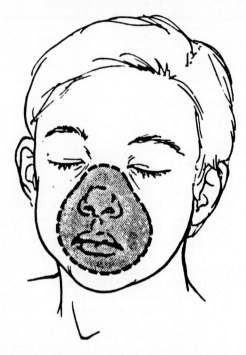

Figure 1-1 Proper mask fit in the pediatric patient. The mask should extend from the bridge of the nose to the cleft of the chin. Used with permission. *Textbook of Pediatric Advanced Life Support,* 1988. Copyright © American Heart Association.

or incorrect size can contribute to airway trauma and can worsen airway obstruction. When the flanged end of the oral airway is held at the incisors with the curve running parallel with the roof of the mouth, the tip of the airway should reach the angle of the jaw. This is illustrated in Fig. 7-1. The practice of putting an airway in backward and twisting it in position, as

Table 1-2   Laryngoscope Blade Choice

Premature infant	Miller 0
Newborn–2 years	Miller 1
2–6 years	Miller 2, WisHippel 1.5
6–12 years	Miller 2, MacIntosh 2

Table 1-3   Endotracheal Tube and Suction Catheter Guidelines

ENDOTRACHEAL TUBE SIZE	MAXIMUM SUCTION CATHETER SIZE
2.0	#5 Fr
2.5	#6 Fr
3.0, 3.5	#8 Fr
4	#10 Fr

frequently done in adults, will frequently result in improper positioning and may contribute to an unexpected adenoidectomy as well!

A selection of laryngoscope blades should be available. Table 1-2 may aid in the selection of the appropriate-sized blade.

The endotracheal tube size can be chosen in many ways. The size that approximates the diameter of the tip of the little finger, the size that approximates the size of the nares, or the use of a formula are easy guidelines. The formula used most frequently at our institution is:

$$(16 + \text{age in years})/4 = \text{Internal diameter of endotracheal tube}$$

One-half size above and below whatever is chosen is also made available to account for individual variation among patients.

Stylets should be fitted to the tube in such a way that the tip does not protrude from the Murphy eye or the end of the endotracheal tube. Take care that the size of stylet is small enough to be easily withdrawn from the endotracheal tube after it is in place.

The suction apparatus should be functional, and a pediatric Yankauer hard tip suction and soft suction catheters should be available. If endotracheal suction is needed, the guidelines in Table 1-3 may help prevent permanent obstruction of the endotracheal tube from a suction catheter that was too large.

INTRAVENOUS ACCESS

Considerations for intravenous access are twofold: (1) what fluids are needed and (2) how they are best administered. Fluid needs intraoperatively and a discussion of glucose needs are included in Chap. 9. In general, the older infant and child do not require intraoperative glucose and may have an isoosmotic, nonglucose-containing solution for maintenance. Maintenance fluids may be calculated by the 4–2–1 rule (Table 1-4).

Table 1-4   4–2–1 Rule

WEIGHT	INTRAVENOUS FLUID RATE
10 kg	4 mL/kg/h
11–20 kg	40 + 2 mL/kg/h for every 1 kg weight over 10 kg
> 20 kg	60 + 1 mL/kg/h for every 1 kg weight over 20 kg

Adapted from Firestone L, Leibowitz P: *Clinical Anesthesia Procedures of the Massachusetts General Hospital.* Boston, Little Brown, 1988, p. 398.

The premature infant or neonate usually gets a glucose-containing solution (dextrose 10% in water) at a maintenance rate, with other replacement needs (third-space losses and blood loss) replaced with a nonglucose-containing crystalloid, colloid, or blood, depending on the case and the patient.

The correct equipment is helpful to make sure that a small child does not accidentally receive more or less fluid than intended. Infusion pumps are frequently used for infants less than 5 kg, and 150-mL burettes for older infants. T connectors are often used to administer drugs with minimal dead space, and therefore, there is a reduced need for extra volume to "flush" in the drug. If the T connector is out of reach, low-volume extension tubing can be attached, which will allow drug administration with as little as 0.3 mL of a normal saline flush.

Achievement of intravenous access can sometimes be a challenge in small, chubby infants or children who have had multiple intravenous attempts in the past. If a vein cannot be cannulated after inhalational induction with halothane, a cut down or central venous cannulation may be needed. Emergency drugs that might be needed before IV access can be attained include: (1) succinylcholine, which can be given intramuscularly (4 mg/kg) or sublingually and (2) atropine, which can be given intramuscularly (0.02 mg/kg) or down the endotracheal tube.

Some resuscitation drugs can also be placed down the endotracheal tube if needed before the line is in place, for example, lidocaine, epinephrine, atropine, and naloxone. This will be discussed more thoroughly in Chap. 20.

DRUGS

Drugs for pediatric anesthesia are prepared on a weight basis. The most frequent error in pediatric drug dosing is to err by a factor of 10. There are many satisfactory techniques for the induction and maintenance of anesthesia in the pediatric patient. Some of these are discussed in Chap. 6. An appendix of drug doses commonly used in pediatric patients is found at the end of Chapter 3. It is wise to have drugs that may need to be given urgently, including atropine and succinylcholine (if not contraindicated), drawn up in unit doses before induction begins. It is difficult to calculate accurately when a child has gone into laryngospasm and stress levels are high.

BIBLIOGRAPHY

Cohen M, Cameron C: Should you cancel the operation when a child has an upper respiratory tract infection? *Anesth Analg* 1991; 72:282–288.

Coté CJ, Rolf N, Lui LMP, et al: A single-blind study of combined pulse oximetry and capnography in children. *Anesthesiology* 1991; 74:980–987.

Dedrick DF, Coté CJ: Pediatric equipment, in Ryan JF, Coté C, Todres ID, Coudsouzian N (eds): *A Practice of Anesthesia for Infants and Children.* New York, Grune and Stratton, 1986, pp 271–288.

Epstein RA: Humidification during positive pressure ventilation in infants. *Anesthesiology* 1971; 35:532–536.

Fisher DM: Anesthesia equipment for pediatrics, in Gregory G (ed): *Pediatric Anesthesia.* Vol. I. New York, Churchill Livingstone, 1989.

Nilsson K: Maintenance and monitoring of body temperature in infants and children. *Paediatr Anaesth* 1991; 1:13–20.

Pounder DR, Blackstock MB, Steward MB: Tracheal extubation in children: Halothane versus isoflurane, anesthetized versus awake. *Anesthesiology* 1991; 74:653–655.

Tiret L, Nivoche Y, Hatton F, et al: Complications related to anaesthesia in infants and children: A prospective survey of 40240 anaesthetics. *Br J Anaesth* 1988; 61:263–269.

CHAPTER 2

Neonatal and Infant Anatomy and Physiology

Dawn E. Webster
Kim Lopez

The neonatal period is defined as the first 28 days of extrauterine life. This is a period of rapid change and development as the neonate continues the process of adaptation to extrauterine life. A knowledge of the unique anatomic and physiologic characteristics of the neonate is critical to the proper conduct of anesthesia. A review of these unique characteristics with implications for anesthetic management and decision making are discussed.

CARDIOVASCULAR SYSTEM

Fetal Circulation

The fetal circulation is unique and characterized by a series of four shunts, which include the placenta, ductus venosus, foramen ovale, and ductus arteriosis (see Chap. 26, Fig. 26-1).

Blood is carried from the placenta, a low-resistance organ, where it is oxygenated by the umbilical vein (pO$_2$, 30–35 mmHg) through the ductus venosus to the inferior vena cava (IVC)(pO$_2$, 24 mmHg). This oxygenated blood mixes with the desaturated blood from the lower extremities and is carried by the IVC to the right atrium. The right atrium also receives blood from the superior vena cava, which drains the upper body. Most right atrial blood enters the right ventricle and main pulmonary artery where it is shunted to the descending aorta through the ductus arteriosus because of the high resistance provided by the lungs. The remainder of right atrial blood is shunted through the patent foramen ovale to the left atrium, left ventricle, and then to the ascending aorta, providing the primary supply to the brain and coronary circulation.

Circulatory Changes After Birth

The circulatory changes after birth include:

1. Elimination of placental blood flow. With clamping of the umbilical vessels, there is an increase in systemic vascular resistance and closure of the ductus venosus because of elimination of blood flow through this shunt.

2. An increase in pulmonary blood flow. With the initiation of breathing, there is an increase in alveolar oxygen tension and increased oxygen saturation with a vasodilatory effect resulting in an 80 percent decrease in pulmonary vascular resistance (PVR). A further fall in PVR occurs during the following 6 to 8 weeks. Sympathetic stimulation, α-adrenergic agents, hypoxia, and acidosis cause pulmonary arterioles to constrict and prevent or delay the fall in PVR.

3. Functional closure of the foramen ovale. The change in circulatory pattern results in pressure alterations with the left atrial pressure exceeding the right atrial pressure and functionally closing the foramen ovale.

4. Closure of the ductus arteriosus. Functional closure occurs at 10 to 15 h of life with anatomic closure 2 to 3 weeks later. The ductus will close in response to an increase in oxygen saturation, an increase in pH, and withdrawal of placental prostaglandins. The sensitivity of the ductal tissue to each of these is related to gestational age, with increasing sensitivity occurring with increasing age.

Cardiac Output

Cardiac output (CO) is the volume of blood pumped by each of the ventricles per minute. In the fetus, however, the ventricles are not in series, and the amount of blood pumped by each ventricle is not identical. Therefore, the term combined ventricular output is used. With birth, left ventricular output doubles and right ventricular output increases 1.5-fold so that each ventricle pumps the same amount of blood in series. The overall CO increases to meet the increased tissue oxygen demands with O_2 consumption increasing from 7 mL/min/kg to 18 mL/min/kg. The CO for the neonate, as for the adult, is described by the Frank Starling mechanism:

$$CO = SV \times HR$$

where SV = stroke volume and HR = heart rate.

For the neonate, however, SV is relatively fixed. Only 30 percent of fetal cardiac muscle is contractile mass compared with 60 percent in the adult. As a result, it is less compliant and less capable of adjusting SV in response to demands for increased CO. The HR is the variable used by the neonate to adjust CO. The newborn HR is 110 to 150 beats/min and decreases gradually with age (Table 2-1). In the neonate, the parasympathetic innervation of the heart is complete; however, sympathetic innervation is lacking, thus predisposing the neonate to bradycardia.

Electrocardiographic (ECG) tracings in the neonate reflect the right ventricular dominance established in utero. In the first week of life, healthy neonates may have an ECG axis of up to +180°. By 3 to 6 months, the adult ratio of ventricular size is achieved, and the axis is no more than +90°. Sinus arrhythmia is very common in infants and children. The ECG may show slight changes in P wave shape, the PR intervals are normal, and the P–P intervals increase at the end of expiration. Occasionally, the variation in rate can be marked enough to cause other arrhythmias to be suspected. Junctional beats may occur when the sinus rate becomes slow enough that the atrioventricular junction takes over. Sinus arrhythmia is exaggerated during convalescence from a febrile illness and by drugs that increase vagal tone. It is frequently seen in the premature infant with apneic spells. It is abolished by exercise and by atropine. Occasionally, premature atrial contractions or premature ventricular beats may be seen in otherwise normal pediatric patients. However, if arrhythmias other than sinus arrhythmia occur in childhood or infancy, they warrant investigation.

Blood pressure in the healthy term neonate (Table 2-2) will be about 60/35 mmHg. It may be 10 to 15 mmHg higher if the cord is clamped late or stripped, but this elevation should normalize within 4 h. Early clamping of the cord (<30/s) may result in a decrease in blood volume of up to 30 percent. The infant

Table 2-1 Heart Rate
(in Beats/Minute)

AGE	RANGE
Newborn	110–150
1–11 months	80–150
2 years	85–125
4	75–115
6	65–100
8	60–110

Table 2-2 Normal Blood Pressure

| | BLOOD PRESSURE (mmHg) | |
AGE	Systolic	Diastolic
Preterm 750 g	44 (33)	24
1000 g	49 (34.5)	26
Full term	60 (45)	35
3–10 days	70–75 (50)	40
6 months	95 (55)	45
4 years	98	57
6 years	110	60
8 years	112	60
12 years	115	65
16 years	120	65

( ) = mean arterial blood pressure.

From Steward DJ: *Manual of Pediatric Anesthesia*. New York, Churchill Livingstone, 1990, p 24.

has a very limited ability to adapt to changes in intravascular blood volume because of inefficient control of capacitance vessels and immature baroreceptors. Under general anesthesia, any baroreceptor response that may have been present is abolished. Research has proved that changes in arterial blood pressure in the newborn are directly proportional to the degree of hypovolemia present. Please refer to Table 2-3 for blood volumes for specific ages.

The cardiovascular response to hypoxia in the neonate is bradycardia with pulmonary and systemic vasoconstriction. Given that HR is the primary determinant of CO for the neonate, CO will decrease. Right to left shunting may occur as ductal tissue responds to the hypoxia or pulmonary artery pressure exceeds systemic pressure.

Table 2-3 Blood Volume Related to Age and Sex

AGE AND SEX	BLOOD VOLUME (mL/kg)
Premature infant	90–100
Newborn	80–90
3 months–1 year	70–80
> 1 year	70
Adult man	60
Adult woman	55

Oxygen Delivery

Oxygen delivery to tissues, the major purpose of the cardio-vascular system, may be adversely affected by anemia. Values for blood volume, hematocrit, and hemoglobin vary from infant to infant, depending on the time of cord clamping. After 1 week of life, the hematocrit level starts to fall from a normal of about 60 percent to a low of 29 to 33 percent at 3 months of age (Table 2-4). This occurs through many mechanisms. First, immediately before birth, there is an unusually high level of erythropoiesis, resulting in a high proportion of young red blood cells at birth. These cells die at about 6 to 8 weeks, with a resultant fall in hematocrit. Second, in the first few days of life, red blood cell production falls to very low levels and remains low for 2 to 3 months. The bone marrow is virtually devoid of red blood cell precursors at this time. Third, erythropoietin levels, high in the fetus and neonate, are barely detectable in the blood by the end of the first week of life. When the hemoglobin level falls to 10 to 11 g/dL at age 2 to 3 months, erythropoietin production is stimulated (Erythropoietin is produced at hemoglobin concentrations of 10 to 11 g/dL in adults also.) The bone marrow responds, and gradually, this anemia is resolved. Transfused red blood cells survive a similar length of time in both newborns and adults. A hemoglobin of less than 12 g/dL constitutes anemia in the newborn. Transfusion therapy may be indicated if the patient requires oxygen therapy or experiences apnea. The premature infant will have an earlier and greater fall in hemoglobin levels. (Seven to 8 g/dL is not uncommon in the less than 1500-g preemie.) They start life with lower hemoglobin, have less iron stores, and require a slightly lower hemoglobin level before erythropoietin production is stimulated. This early anemia is often followed by a late anemia secondary to nutritional deficiency. Transfusion of red blood cells in premature infants has been reported to increase the risk of retinopathy of prematurity. Despite this relative anemia, oxygen delivery is actually improved at 2 to 3 months of age. By this time, most of the hemoglobin is Hgb A; at birth, 90 percent was Hgb F. Fetal hemoglobin binds only weakly with 2,3 diphosphoglycerate (2,3

Table 2-4 Normal Hematocrit According to Age

AGE	HEMATOCRIT
Premature infant	45
Newborn	54
3 months	33
1 year	38

DPG), despite adequate levels of the substance. The 2,3 DPG competes with oxygen for binding on hemoglobin, and a relative lack of 2,3 DPG causes a leftward shift of the oxygen dissociation curve. As the infant gets older and begins to produce Hgb A, 2,3 DPG levels also increase. If CO and venous oxygen saturation remain constant, the amount of oxygen unloaded at peripheral tissues increases constantly to four to five volumes percent by 8 to 11 months of age, despite the development of physiologic anemia. This is because of the compensatory increase in the amount of 2,3 DPG during the time of lowest hemoglobin values.

THE RESPIRATORY SYSTEM

Anatomy

Anatomically, infants have a large head, a short neck, and a large tongue in a small mouth. They have a fat, flat, wide face, which makes a mask fit difficult. They have narrow, easily blocked nasal passages (unfortunately, because they are obligate nose breathers!). The larynx is at C4, rather than at C5 as in the adult (Fig. 2-1). It is also more anterior. The epiglottis is floppy, U shaped, and projects posteriorly at a 45° angle, often requiring lifting with the tip of a straight laryngoscope blade to allow visualization of the glottis (Fig. 2-2). The narrowest part of the airway is at the level of cricoid cartilage, just below the vocal cords. In the adult, the narrowest area is at the vocal cords themselves. The lining of the airway at the cricoid cartilage is pseudostratified, ciliated epithelium, which is loosely bound to areolar tissue. Trauma easily results in edema. The trachea is short, only about 5 cm in the newborn, leaving little margin for error regarding the depth of an endotracheal tube. The tracheal cartilages are easily collapsed by a stray finger or instrument or even by vigorous respiratory efforts against an obstructed airway. The ribs are horizontal, not yet having developed the more vertical angle associated with improved action of the intercostal muscles. Because of these anatomic differences, ventilation is largely diaphragm dependent. In addition, the ribs and cartilage of the newborn are much more pliable than those of older infants; so negative pressure within the thorax results in a greater degree of chest wall collapse and even more inefficient ventilation. Abdominal viscera, which are bulky in infants, can easily impede diaphragmatic breathing, especially if the stomach is distended. The lungs have not completed development at birth, although the basic formation of cartilaginous airways is complete. Alveolarization, which extends centrally, continues until approximately 3 years of age, with alveoli increasing in number from about 25 million to several hundred million.

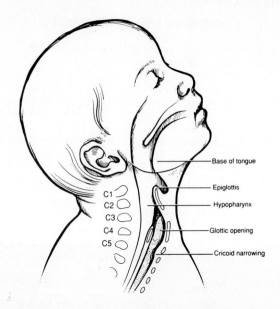

Figure 2-1 Airway anatomy of an infant—the glottic opening is at C4 rather than at C5 as in the adult. The narrowest part of the infant airway is subglottic at the level of the cricoid ring.

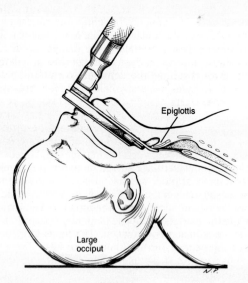

Figure 2-2 Intubation of the infant may require lifting of the epiglottis with the end of a straight laryngoscope blade.

Surfactant

Surfactant stabilizes alveoli to prevent collapse and decreases the inspiratory force required for expansion of the lungs. It is produced by type II pneumocytes, beginning at age 22 weeks and peaking at 36 weeks. After birth, many things can depress the biochemical pathways for surfactant production, for example, hypoxia, hyperoxia, acidosis, and hypothermia. These must be corrected quickly. Lack of surfactant results in alveolar collapse, maldistribution of ventilation, impaired gas exchange, decreased compliance, and increased risk of pneumothorax. *Pneumothorax is more common in the neonatal period than at any other age.* Surfactant is available and may be delivered via an endotracheal tube followed by positive pressure ventilation in the delivery room prophylactically or soon after birth. Rescue surfactant is administered routinely to prevent respiratory distress syndrome in the premature infant.

Control of Ventilation

Control of ventilation is well developed in the term neonate. Because infants have a high metabolic rate, ventilation relative to body mass for any given pCO_2 is greater than in adults. A respiratory rate of 37 breaths/min has been calculated to be the most efficient in the newborn. At this rate, a minimum of muscle energy is used to overcome the elastic recoil of the lungs and chest wall and the resistance to airflow. Term infants require 1 percent of their metabolic energy to maintain ventilation, provided the lungs are normal. The oxygen cost of ventilation is 0.5 mL/0.5 L of ventilation. In the premature infant, the oxygen cost is higher, 0.9 mL/0.5 L. The ventilatory response to inspired CO_2 is proportionately similar to that for adults. The response of the premature infant to inspired CO_2 is less. By contrast with older infants and adults, hypoxia depresses the ventilatory response to CO_2 in the newborn. The premature infant and the newborn are prone to respiratory fatigue because they have lesser amounts of type I (resistant) fibers in the diaphragm. Rapid eye movement (REM) sleep is associated with increased diaphragmatic activity and inhibition of intercostal muscle activity. Because preterm infants spend 50 to 60 percent of their time in REM sleep, they are further prone to diaphragmatic fatigue. Table 2-5 compares the development of type I ventilatory muscles. The ventilatory response to hypoxia in infants is modified by gestational and postnatal age, sleep state, and body temperature. It is summarized in Table 2-6.

Apnea

Apneic episodes in the neonate must be carefully evaluated. Preterm and some term infants may display periodic breathing.

Table 2-5   Development of Type I (Marathon) Ventilatory
Muscles: Percentage of Type I Muscles

	PREMATURE	NEWBORN	AGE AT MATURITY
Diaphragm	10%	25%	8 months (55%)
Intercostal	20%	46%	2 months (65%)

This is defined as apnea lasting 5 to 10 s, alternating with rapid ventilation. It is not serious and usually is gone by 6 weeks of age. It results from incoordination of the feedback loops controlling ventilation. Serious apneic episodes are usually accompanied by bradycardia and last greater than 20 s. The causes are thought to be ventilatory muscle fatigue and impaired chemoreceptor response to hypoxemia. The treatment is stimulation, which will usually abort these episodes, and possibly bag and mask ventilation. Continuous positive airway pressure may be employed to increase the reflex activity of the lung and chest wall. Aminophylline or caffeine may be used to increase central stimulation of respiration. These latter two therapies are directed at reducing the number of apneic attacks and are primarily reserved for apneic episodes secondary to apnea of prematurity.

Lung Volumes and Capacities

On a milliliter per kilogram basis, tidal volume, functional residual capacity, dead space, and change in volume per time are about the same for infants as for adults. Oxygen consumption is two to three times higher in the infant, and because tidal volume is about the same as in the adult, the respiratory rate must be two to three times faster, which it is. This means that resting alveolar ventilation is two to three times greater, making the ratio of alveolar ventilation to functional residual capacity 5:1 in the neonate, where it is only 1.5:1 in the adult. Thus, FRC is a less effective buffer for the neonate. Therefore, a lower oxygen reserve is available when the airway becomes obstructed, resulting in the quick development of hypoxia and subsequent bradycardia. A comparison of adult and infant respiratory variables is listed in Table 2-7. The closing volume is relatively large in the neonate and encroaches on the tidal volume in a manner similar to that seen in elderly people. Atelectasis and hypoxia develop more easily than in the adult. The hypoxia that may develop actually depresses the infant's respiration further, as opposed to the more mature response of tachypnea in the face

Table 2-6 Ventilatory Responses to Hypoxia

AGE	TEMPERATURE	RESPONSE TO HYPOXIA
< 1 week preterm and full term	Normothermic	Biphasic response: brief period of hyperpnea, thought to be caused by central effects of hypoxia on cortex and medulla followed by respiratory depression.
< 1 week	Hypothermic	Ventilatory depression without initial hyperpnea.
> 1 week	Normothermic	Hyperpnea because of maturity of chemoreceptor function. Arousal response to sleep hypoxia present.

Table 2-7   Respiratory Variables in the Infant and Adult

VARIABLE	INFANT	ADULT
Respiratory frequency	30–50	12–16
TV (mL/kg)	6–8	7
Dead space (mL/kg)	2–2.5	2.2
Alveolar ventilation	100–150	60
FRC (mL/kg)	27–30	30
O_2 consumption (mL/kg/min)	6–8	3

TV = tidal volume; FRC = functional residual capacity.

of hypoxia. Finally, although the FRC is similar in value between the neonate and adult, the infant has such a compliant chest wall that it provides no protection for the FRC. As a result, the FRC can be easily lost during inefficient or compromised chest wall motion from obstruction or external compression.

CENTRAL NERVOUS SYSTEM

The infant has an immature central nervous system. The nerve fibers are incompletely myelinated, and the cerebral cortex continues to gain cells throughout the first years of life. Muscle tone and reflexes are also different. Pain perception is present, but infants are not as adept at localizing their pain as are older children. Children actually have a lower pain threshold than adults. The infant skull is less rigid than that of the adult, and expansive suture lines and open fontanelles can help accommodate an increase in intracranial pressure. Neonatal cerebrovascular autoregulation is impaired, especially in the ill or premature infant, making blood flow very pressure dependent. Premature infants have extremely fragile cerebral vessels, especially in the germinal matrix overlying the caudate nucleus. Hence, there is a high incidence of intraventricular hemorrhage.

THE NEUROMUSCULAR SYSTEM

The structural and functional development of the neuromuscular system is also incomplete at birth. The conduction velocity of the motor nerves increases throughout gestation as myelination of nerve fibers occurs. Conversion of myotubules to mature muscle fibers takes place in the latter part of intrauterine life and in the first several weeks after birth. Some slow-contracting muscles are converted to fast contracting (i.e., in the hand), and the diaphragm and intercostal muscles increase the percentage of slow muscle fibers in the first months of life. Synaptic transmission is slow at birth, and the rate at which acetylcholine is made available for release during repetitive nerve stimulation is limited in the infant. This reduced margin of safety of neurotransmission is demonstrable between infants and adults. After 50-Hz tetany, newborns all show a fade in the twitch height. This does not occur in adults. Infants less than 36 weeks of postconceptual age show the most pronounced fade. The train-of-four ratio and degree of posttetanic facilitation do increase with age, suggesting that the immediately available stores of acetylcholine and the enhanced mobilization and synthesis seen with tetanic stimulation are less in the neonate than in the older infant or child. The sensitivity of the postjunctional cholinergic receptor to acetylcholine may vary with age. Even when allowance is made for differences in the volume of distribution and for the type and concentration of anesthesia, infants appear relatively resistant to succinylcholine and relatively sensitive to nondepolarizing neuromuscular relaxants.

THE AUTONOMIC NERVOUS SYSTEM

Infants are highly vagotonic and have a tendency to develop bradycardia with minor vagal stimulation. This is exacerbated by the presence of hypoxia. An arbitrary definition of bradycardia in the first month of life is a heart rate less than 110 beats/min. Bradycardia during anesthesia may have one of three causes: hypoxia, vagal stimulation, or volatile anesthetics. Therefore, procedures such as laryngoscopy, mesenteric traction by surgeons, and eye operations are particularly apt to produce bradycardia in younger infants.

THE RENAL SYSTEM

By 34 weeks of gestation (about 2000 g), glomerulogenesis is complete. In the newborn, the renin–angiotensin–aldosterone system is intact. During the first week of life, the infant is an obligate sodium loser because the distal tubule cannot efficiently reabsorb sodium, even in the face of sodium loss. In the first 48 hours of life, the infant is unable to concentrate or dilute urine, but over the next few days, the glomerular filtration rate increases. The ability to concentrate and dilute urine also increases. At 1 month of age, renal function is about 70 to 80 percent of normal adult function (see Chap. 9).

BIBLIOGRAPHY

Brett C: Cardiovascular physiology in pediatrics, in Gregory GA (ed): *Pediatric Anesthesia*. Vol. 1. New York, Churchill Livingstone, 1983, pp 25–62.

McCallum WD: Fetal cardiac anatomy and vascular dynamics. *Clin Obstet Gynecol* 1981; 24:837–849.

Pang LM, Mellins RB: Neonatal cardiorespiratory physiology. *Anesthesiology* 1975;43:171–196.

Phelan PD, Williams HE: Ventilatory studies in healthy infants. *Pediatr Res* 1969; 3:425–432.

Rudolph AM: *Pediatrics*. East Norwalk, CT, Appleton & Lange, 1987.

Ryan JF, Todres ID, Coté CJ, Goudsouzian N: Muscle relaxants in children, in *A Practice of Anesthesia for Infants and Children*. Orlando, FL, Grune & Stratton, 1986.

Ryan JF, Todres ID, Coté CJ, Goudsouzian N: The pediatric airway, in *A Practice of Anesthesia for Infants and Children*. Orlando, FL, Grune & Stratton, 1986, pp 35–58.

Steward DJ: *Manual of Pediatric Anesthesia*. New York: Churchill Livingstone, 1990.

Wilson TG: Some observations on the anatomy of the infantile larynx. *Acta Otolaryngol* 1953; 43:95–99.

CHAPTER 3

Pediatric Pharmacology

C. Y. Jennifer Chan

Pharmacokinetics describes the absorption, distribution, metabolism, and elimination of a drug. These variables determine the relationship between the administered dose and the concentration achieved. *Pharmacodynamics* describes the effects of an administered drug in relation to the concentration achieved at the site of action. This chapter describes maturational changes that influence a drug's disposition and the pharmacodynamic responses of pediatric patients to administered drugs. *Pharmacokinetic differences* include changes in absorption (inhalation uptake), protein binding, vascular volume, metabolism, and elimination. These pharmacokinetic variations along with anatomic differences have an impact on the pharmacodynamic responses observed in pediatric patients.

Understanding the physiologic changes that affect a patient's response to medication and a knowledge of the drug interactions that can occur with anesthetic agents may prevent or minimize the development of adverse drug reactions. The adverse effects of individual agents will not be discussed. However, the management of the most severe form of reaction, anaphylaxis, will be described.

PHARMACOKINETICS

Absorption

The factors that influence gastrointestinal absorption include gastric pH, gastric emptying time, intestinal transit time, gastrointestinal enzyme activity, and the physiochemical properties of the administered agents. In newborns and neonates, the absorption of drugs from the gastrointestinal tract may be erratic and slow. A similar effect was also reported for drugs administered by the intramuscular route because of the smaller muscle mass, reduced muscular blood flow, and decreased capacity of muscle contraction in such infants.

Uptake of Inhalation Anesthetics

The rise of the alveolar partial pressure to reach equilibrium with the inspired anesthetic pressure depends on the rate of delivery to and the uptake from the lung. The factors that contribute to the rate of delivery are the inspired concentration, alveolar ventilation, and functional residual capacity. The uptake of inhalation anesthetics from the alveoli depends on the cardiac output, blood and tissue solubility, and alveolar-to-venous partial pressure gradient. More rapid uptake in infants and children has been reported for halothane, isoflurane, and enflurane.

The factors that contribute to the more rapid uptake include: (1) a greater alveolar ventilation, (2) a higher cardiac output and greater distribution of cardiac output to the vessel-rich organs, (3) a lower blood solubility secondary to lower albumin and globulin concentrations, and (4) lower tissue solubilities as a result of greater water and decreased protein and lipid contents. These differences between pediatric patients and adults enhance the anesthetic partial pressure equilibrium between the alveoli and tissues, thus increasing the rate of rise of alveolar-to-inspired anesthetic partial pressures.

Distribution

The volume of distribution determines the concentration achieved in the plasma and, thus, the concentration delivered to the site of action. The distribution of a drug is influenced by several age-dependent factors, which include blood flow, body composition, and protein binding. The effect of these maturational changes depends on the physiochemical properties of the drug. For instance, a change of protein binding will have a more significant impact on drugs that are highly protein bound.

The blood flow to the organs varies with age. In neonates and infants, the total body water (predominantly extracellular water) is significantly larger than in adults. Such differences in body composition occur during the first 12 months of life. In this age group, an increase in the volume of distribution results in a larger dose (per kilogram) to achieve the same final serum concentration, especially for drugs that are water soluble. Because of the increased extracellular compartment, drugs that are distributed through this compartment (such as neuromuscular blocking agents) may require a higher dose (in milligrams per kilogram) to produce a similar response. The fat composition is also different in pediatric patients. In full-term neonates, adipose tissue constitutes 12 to 16 percent of the body weight, and it increases rapidly during the first year of life. There is an overall lower fat composition in children than in adults. Adipose tissues serve as a reservoir for the deposition of lipid-soluble medications. A decrease in the percentage of body fat allows a more rapid redistribution from the storage sites to the serum.

All drugs are bound to plasma proteins to a certain extent. Drugs that are bound to protein do not cross cellular membranes to produce a desired or adverse effect. On the other hand, unbound drug in the plasma is available for distribution to the tissues and elimination from the body. Therefore, an increase in the unbound fraction of a drug increases the volume of distribution and the pharmacologic effect. In neonates, the protein binding of drugs is reduced because of their lower plasma albumin, α_1-acid glycoprotein, and globulin concentrations and increased free fatty acid and unconjugated bilirubin. Albumin, α_1-acid glycoprotein, and globulin concentrations approach the adult value by 1 year of age. The free fatty acid and bilirubin are normalized during early infancy.

Metabolism

The primary site of metabolism is the liver, involving metabolic reactions termed Phase I and Phase II. Phase I reactions (oxidation, reduction, hydroxylation, and hydrolysis) depend on enzymatic systems (e.g., cytochrome P-450) and produce metabolites that can be active or inactive. Phase II reactions (glucuronidation, sulfation, acetylation, and amino acid conjugation) require adenosine triphosphate and usually produce inactive products. Medications that suppress or induce these enzyme systems can depress or enhance the rate of metabolism.

The maturation of these metabolic pathways varies among individual infants and is very complex. In general, the drug biotransformation of most drugs is decreased in neonates. Their enzyme activities for Phase I reactions are 50 to 70 percent of adult values, but they rapidly mature to reach values similar to or in excess of adult values by 6 months of age. The hepatic enzyme activities continue to be elevated for the first 2 years of life; then they gradually decrease with age and reach adult values at puberty. These changes are significant for drugs that are eliminated through the cytochrome P-450 system because there is a change from an initial risk of overdose in neonates to a potential of underdose in infants. The maturation of Phase II reactions is not fully understood. In neonates, conjugation by glucuronic acid is decreased more significantly than by sulfate or an amino acid. Therefore, unlike adults, sulfation is more important than glucuronidation in drug metabolism (e.g., morphine) in this age group. Maturation does not occur at the same time. For instance, conjugation by an amino acid reaches adult values at 6 months of life, whereas 2 to 4 years are required for glucuronidation pathways to mature. Conjugation by sulfate matures rapidly in neonates. During the newborn period, the metabolism of morphine is decreased. By 1 to 2 months of age, maturation of the sulfation pathway results in a clearance of morphine that approaches adult values. The clearance rates of morphine in newborns, children, and adults have been reported to be 6 mL/kg/min, 20 mL/kg/min, and 11.5 mL/kg/min, respectively.

Inhalation anesthetics are primarily excreted by the lung through exhalation. The rate of washout is related to blood/gas solubility, alveolar ventilation, and cardiac output. The excretion of inhaled anesthetic is more rapid in infants. A small percentage of absorbed inhaled anesthetics undergo biotransformation by the liver. Hepatic dysfunction and hepatitis have been associated with toxic metabolites produced during the biotransformation of halothane and enflurane. In addition, decreased renal function has been associated with the formation of inorganic fluoride (enflurane and methoxyflurane), which blocks the tubular active resorption in the loops of Henle. The hepatic metabolism of inhaled anesthetic is less in neonates and infants because of their decreased enzymatic activities, lower fat composition, and more rapid washout.

Renal Excretion

The kidney is responsible for the elimination of water-soluble drugs or metabolites. Similar to hepatic function, the renal excretion of medications in neonates is decreased. At birth, the glomerular filtration rate (GFR) is 2 to 4 mL/min for full-term neonates. It increases dramatically after the first week of life and approaches adult values by 3 to 5 months of life. In addition to the GFR, tubular reabsorption and secretion are also important in determining the elimination of drugs, and these two functions mature at a slower and different rate. Beyond the neonatal period, the clearance of renally excreted drugs may be higher than in older children and adults partly because of the relative maturation of the GFR and tubular secretion in relation to the tubular reabsorption. This increased renal clearance together with larger volume of distribution explain why larger than adult doses (in milligrams per kilogram) are used for drugs such as aminoglycosides.

PHARMACODYNAMICS

The differences in response to administered drugs between pediatric and adult patients are related to the pharmacokinetic differences discussed earlier and to anatomic differences. Drug distribution is altered because of the increased percentage of body water and extracellular fluid. This contributes to a larger dose required for some drugs (e.g., gentamicin and succinylcholine) to produce the desired concentrations at the site of action (thus, the desired effects) in infants and children. In addition, children have a higher percentage of muscle and a lower percentage of fat than do adults. Therefore, higher doses (in milligrams per kilogram) of neuromuscular blocking agents may be needed to produce paralysis in children who have greater muscle mass (per kilogram). Newborns have decreased renal and hepatic function, resulting in accumulation of drugs after repeated doses. However, some of these functions can improve rapidly and even exceed adult value. In fact, data suggest that children have greater clearance of many hepatic or renally eliminated drugs and require more frequent repeated doses (e.g., tubocurarine).

Other than a decreased ability to eliminate drugs, newborns and neonates also have an immature blood–brain barrier (BBB). The decreased protein binding in this age group results in more unbound drug available to cross the more permeable BBB to reach and accumulate in the central nervous system. These factors contribute to the increased sedative and respiratory depressant effects of benzodiazepines, barbiturates, and narcotics than that in adults. Neuromuscular transmission is also immature at birth until about 2 months of age. In addition, the diaphragm of a newborn contains a lower amount of slow fibers (Type I), which are more sensitive to nondepolarizing agents. The percentage of slow fibers increases, and the volume of extracellular fluid decreases, to adult values during the first year of life. Therefore, the response to muscle relaxants is different in adults and pediatric patients, and variability of action can be noted among neonates, infants, and children. The degree of the age-dependent dose–response relationship varies with different muscle relaxants.

The inhaled anesthetic requirement, as measured by the minimal alveolar concentration (MAC), has been reported to be higher in infants and children than in adolescents and adults. However, MAC is lower in neonates than in infants. The causes of these differences are unclear.

In general, neonates and infants are more susceptible to the side effects of the drugs used in anesthesia. On the other hand, hepatitis caused by halothane is rare in children. Similarly, inorganic fluoride-induced renal failure is uncommon in pediatric patients receiving inhaled anesthesia with enflurane or methoxyflurane. This observation has been explained by the impaired hepatic metabolism, and thus decreased toxic substance formation, in children. The hypothesis was challenged by Wark and co-workers, who reported no differences in the metabolism of halothane in six children. However, the ages of those children were all greater than 14 months, an age group with mature

Table 3-1   Drug Interactions in Anesthesia

DRUGS	EFFECT
Alcohol	Potential for hypovolemia (additive hypotensive effect) Acute ingestion: enzyme inhibitor, possible decreased hepatic metabolism and hence increased effect Chronic ingestion: enzyme inducer, possible increased hepatic metabolism Additive CNS depressant effect
Aminoglycosides (gentamicin, amikacin, tobramycin)	Cause muscle weakness by acetylcholine release, prolong and enhance effects of neuromuscular blocking agents Neuromuscular blockade by aminoglycoside may not respond to acetylcholinesterase inhibitors
Antihypertensive Agents	Additive hypotensive effects Halothane, fentanyl (with nitrous oxide), and propofol may decrease metabolism of propranolol
Benzodiazepines	Additive respiratory depression Decreased MAC needed for halothane May increase half-life of ketamine
Cimetidine	Enzyme inhibitor, inhibits elimination of drugs that are metabolized by the cytochrome P-450 system (e.g., benzodiazepines, opioids, various anesthetics)
Digoxin	Additive bradycardia
Diuretics	Potential for hypovolemia (additive hypotensive effect) Potential for hypokalemia (increased risk for arrhythmia)
Erythromycin	Inhibit metabolism of alfentanil, increases risk of respiratory depression May inhibit metabolism of other medications that require hepatic elimination
Fentanyl	Halothane decreases clearance of fentanyl and increases fentanyl serum concentration

32

Table 3-1 *(Continued)*

DRUGS	EFFECT
Isoniazid	Enzyme inducer, may decrease effects of drugs that are hepatically eliminated, may increase fluorination of inhaled anesthetics
Ketamine	Halothane decreases clearance of ketamine in plasma and brain and increases duration of ketamine-induced ataxia
Lidocaine	Halothane may decrease clearance of lidocaine
MAO Inhibitor	Potentiate anesthetic and narcotic effects Orthostatic hypotension—more sensitive to vasodilation by anesthetic agents Ephedrine (indirect-acting sympathomimetic) can produce acute hypertensive crisis Meperidine can cause hypertensive crisis, convulsions, and coma
Phenytoin	Inhalation anesthetic may displace phenytoin from albumin. Increased unbound phenytoin level may result in acute toxicity
Theophylline	Potential for increased cardiac arrhythmias (decreased elimination) leading to increased serum concentrations Increased myocardial sensitivity to arrhythmogenic actions of halothane
Tricyclic Antidepressant	Potential for seizure activity (enflurane) Potential for exacerbation of cardiac conduction abnormalities
Verapamil	Halothane, isoflurane, and enflurance increase verapamil concentration and potentiate its effects on conduction, blood pressure, and contractility

CNS = central nervous system; MAC = maximum alveolar concentration; MAO = monoamine oxidase

Phase I metabolism. Other proposed explanations include decreased storage sites because of lower fat composition and higher excretion by exhalation.

Pharmacokinetics and pharmacodynamics of a drug may be affected by concurrent medication administration. Interactions of drugs in anesthesia are described in Table 3-1.

MANAGEMENT OF ANAPHYLACTIC REACTIONS

Anaphylaxis is an acute allergic reaction that is potentially life threatening. It is initiated by mast cell degranulation, releasing histamine, which causes flushing, urticaria, angioedema, hypotension, and other reactions (e.g., bronchospasm and shock) that can lead to death.

Causes

Anaphylaxis can be triggered by a variety of immunologic or nonimmunologic responses. The following are causes that may be encountered by anesthesiologists:

1. *Drug Induced*
   Antibiotics, especially penicillins and cephalosporins, are common causes of anaphylaxis. Therefore, obtaining an accurate history of allergies is important. A rapid infusion of vancomycin can cause "red-man" syndrome (flushing and hypotension), and phenytoin can result in a marked cardiac depressant effect, leading to severe hypotension. Such effects are not hypersensitivity reactions and can be avoided by using a slow infusion rate. The administration of β-lactam cephalosporins (e.g., cefazolin and cefotetan) should be monitored carefully in patients with a history of allergy to penicillin because of the potential of cross-reaction.

2. *Blood Transfusion*
   Mismatched blood transfusions are rare. However, persons who are IgA deficient will react to IgA in administered blood products. Hypotension may also result when citrated blood products are administered rapidly in infants because of binding of ionized calcium by citrate buffer. Calcium chloride 10 to 20 mg/kg IV will treat this problem.

3. *Diagnostic Agents*
   Hyperosmolarity of contrast media may be the cause of mast cell degranulation. Although the incidence rates are lower, isoosmolar contrast media has also been associated with anaphylaxis. Persons with a history of reactions to contrast media carry a higher risk of a second

reaction and should be premedicated with diphenhydramine, H_2-blockers, and steroids if they must undergo contrast studies.

4. *Latex Sensitivity*

An increasing incidence of intraoperative anaphylaxis to latex has been reported in recent years. In one report, all six children who developed intraoperative anaphylaxis had a history of allergic reactions to latex material.

Management

The following list describes the management sequence.

1. Remove the cause.
2. Secure the airway and administer oxygen.
3. Provide fluid replacement: crystalloid or colloid. A large volume may be required.
4. Administer IV or SQ epinephrine to stop mast cell degranulation and cause vasoconstriction (α effect) and bronchodilation (β effect). In children, a dose of 0.01 mg/kg (up to 0.5 mL of 1:1000) is given q 5 to 15 min. If the response is inadequate, may consider continuous infusion (initial dose, 0.1 to 0.3 μg/kg/min and titrate). In patients receiving β-blockers, their condition may worsen with epinephrine because of unopposed α stimulation.
5. Administer corticosteroids: hydrocortisone 5 to 10 mg/kg/dose IV q 6 h or methylprednisolone 0.5 to 1 mg/kg/dose IV q 6 h.
6. Provide antihistamines: H_1 blocker, e.g., diphenhydramine or hydroxyzine 0.5 to 1 mg/kg/dose (up to 50 mg) IV q 6 h and H_2 blocker, e.g., cimetidine 5 mg/kg/dose IV (up to 300 mg) q 6 h or ranitidine 0.5 mg/kg/dose IV (up to 50 mg) then 0.5 mg/kg/dose IV q 6 to 8 h (up to 50 mg q 8 h).
7. Provide other medications such as bronchodilators (aminophylline or β-agonist nebulizer) and other vasopressors, e.g., dopamine, norepinephrine, isoproterenol.

CONCLUSION

The physiologic changes that occur during maturation and the pharmacokinetic alterations in pediatric patients contribute to the differences in the pharmacodynamic responses observed in this patient population. Understanding the altered responses helps in designing the optimal drug regimen when dealing with pediatric patients of various ages. Close monitoring and obtaining an accurate medication and allergy history are important to minimize the adverse effects.

Drug Dosages

DRUG	ROUTE	DOSE
A. Resuscitation Drugs		
Adenosine	IV	100 μg/kg rapid IV bolus, incremental doses 100 μg/kg q 2 min to a max of 300 μg/kg
Atropine	IV	0.01 mg/kg/dose (minimum, 0.1 mg/dose)
Calcium chloride	IV	10 to 20 mg/kg
Calcium gluconate	IV	50 to 100 mg/kg
Epinephrine	IV	0.01 mg/kg (0.1 mg/kg via ETT)
Lidocaine	IV	1 mg/kg
Sodium bicarbonate	IV	1–2 mEq/kg
B. Common Preoperative, Perioperative, and Postoperative Drugs		
Analgesia (also see Narcotics)		
Acetaminophen	PO/PR	10 to 15 mg/kg
Acetaminophen with codeine	PO	0.5 to 1 mg/kg/dose of codeine (each 5 mL of elixir contains 12 mg codeine)
Ketorolac	IV, IM	Safety and efficacy have not been established in pediatric patients. Doses of 0.5 and 0.9 mg/kg IV have been reported in the literature.

Antibiotics

Ampicillin	IV	<7 days: 50 to 100 mg/kg/day (q 12 h)
		>7 days: 100 to 200 mg/kg/day (q 6 to 8 h)
Cefazolin	IV	50 to 100 mg/kg/day (q 6 to 8 h)
Cefoxitin	IV	80 to 160 mg/kg/day (q 6 to 8 h)
Ceftazidime	IV	<7 days: 50 to 100 mg/kg/day (q 12 h)
		>7 days: 100 to 150 mg/kg/day (q 8 h)
Ceftriaxone	IV	50 to 100 mg/kg/day (q 12 to 24 h)
Cefuroxime	IV	100 to 150 mg/kg/day (q 6 to 8 h)
Cephalothin	IV	75 to 125 mg/kg/day (q 6 h)
Clindamycin	IV	<7 days: 15 to 20 mg/kg/day (q 8 h)
		>7 days: 20 to 40 mg/kg/day (q 6 to 8 h)
Gentamicin	IV	<7 days: 5 mg/kg/day (q 12 h)
		>7 days: 6 to 7.5 mg/kg/day (q 8 h)
Oxacillin	IV	100 to 200 mg/kg/day (q 6 h)
Penicillin	IV	100,000 to 200,000 units/kg/day (q 6 h)
Ticarcillin/clavulanate	IV	200 to 300 mg/kg/day (q 6 h)
Vancomycin	IV	<7 days: 20 to 30 mg/kg/day (q 12 h)
		>7 days: 30 to 45 mg/kg/day (q 8 h)

Anticholinergics

Atropine	IV	0.01 to 0.02 mg/kg (minimum, 0.1 mg/dose)
Glycopyrrolate	IM	0.02 to 0.04 mg/kg
	IV/IM	0.005 mg/kg, 0.01 mg/kg
Scopolamine	IM	0.1 mg/kg

(Continued)

Drug Dosages (*Continued*)

DRUG	ROUTE	DOSE
Anticoagulants and Hemostatic Agents		
Aminocaproic Acid	IV	100 mg/kg bolus then 15 to 30 mg/kg/h or 100 mg/kg q 6 h
Cryoprecipitate	IV	4 units/10 kg ↑ fibrinogen level by 100 mg/dL
Desmopressin	IV	0.2 to 0.4 μg/kg
Fresh-frozen plasma	IV	15 to 20 mL/kg ↑ all factors by 25 percent
Platelets	IV	0.2 units/kg ↑ count by 100,000
Protamine	IV	1 mg neutralized ≈ 100 units heparin (maximum, 50 mg; not to exceed 5 mg/min)
Vitamin K	IV/IM/SQ	1 to 5 mg/dose
Anticonvulsants		
Diazepam	IV	0.2 to 0.5 mg/kg
Lorazepam	IV/IM	0.05 to 0.1 mg/kg
Phenobarbital	IV	Loading dose 15 to 20 mg/kg, then 5 to 6 mg/kg/day (qd or bid)
Phenytoin	IV	Loading dose 15 to 20 mg/kg over 30 min; maintenance dose: 5 mg/kg/day (q 8 h)
Antidysrhythmics		
Bretylium	IV	5 to 10 mg/kg to maximum of 30 mg/kg
Digoxin	IV	Loading dose: 30 μg/kg total (in 3 to 4

		divided doses, 6 to 8 h apart)
	PO	Loading dose: 40 μg/kg total (in 3 to 4 divided doses, 6 to 8 h apart)
Lidocaine	IV bolus	1 mg/kg, may repeat q 5 to 10 min
	IV infusion	20 to 50 μg/kg/min
Phenytoin	IV	2 to 4 mg/kg over 5 min
Verapamil	IV	0.1 to 0.2 mg/kg (extreme caution in infants <1 year old)
Antihistamines (H_1 Blocker)		
Diphenhydramine	IV/PO/IM	0.5 to 1 mg/kg/dose
Hydroxyzine	IV/PO/IM	0.5 to 1 mg/kg/dose
β-Blockers		
Esmolol	IV infusion	0.5 mg/kg/min for 2 min then 0.025 to 0.1 mg/kg/min
Labetalol	IV	0.25 mg/kg
Propranolol	IV	0.01 to 0.1 mg/kg (arrhythmias), maximum, 1 mg/dose
Bronchodilators		
Albuterol	Aerosol	0.1 to 0.15 mg/kg
Aminophylline (1 mg aminophylline = 0.8 mg theophylline)	IV bolus	6 mg/kg (for patient receiving theophylline product; each 1 mg/kg of theophylline bolus increases levels by 2 mg/L)

(Continued)

Drug Dosages (*Continued*)

DRUG	ROUTE	DOSE
	IV infusion	4 to 6 mo: 0.4 to 0.5 mg/kg/h
		6 to 9 mo: 0.6 to 0.8 mg/kg/h
		9 to 12 mo: 0.8 to 0.9 mg/kg/h
		1 to 9 yr: 1 mg/kg/h
		9 to 12 yr: 0.7 to 0.8 mg/kg/h
		12 to 16 yr: 0.6 to 0.7 mg/kg/h
		Adjust based on liver function, concurrent medications, signs of toxicity, and levels
Isoproterenol	IV infusion	Initial: 0.1 µg/kg/min titrate to effect or toxicity (heart rate > 180 beats/min, arrhythmia); maximum dose: 1.5 µg/kg/min
Terbutaline	SQ	0.01 mg/kg up to 0.4 mg/dose
	Aerosol	0.1 mg/kg (up to 10 mg)
	IV infusion	0.1 to 0.4 µg/kg/min
Diuretics		
Furosemide	IV	0.5 to 1 mg/kg
	IV infusion	0.2 mg/kg (minimum, 1 mg) bolus then 0.1 mg/kg/h, double q 2 h to maximum of 0.4 mg/kg/h
Mannitol	IV	0.25 to 1 g/kg

H₂-Blocker

Cimetidine	IV/PO	20 to 40 mg/kg/day (q 6 h)
Ranitidine	IV	1 to 2 mg/kg/day (q 6 to 8 h)
	PO	2 to 4 mg/kg/day (q 12 h)

Induction Agents

Diprivan	IV	2 to 3 mg/kg
Ketamine	IV	1 to 2 mg/kg
	IM	5 to 7 mg/kg
Methohexital	IV	2 to 3 mg/kg
Thiopental	IV	3 to 6 mg/kg

Inotropes

Amrinone	IV bolus	0.75 mg/kg
	IV infusion	5 to 10 µg/kg/min
Dobutamine	IV infusion	1 to 20 µg/kg/min
Dopamine	IV infusion	1 to 20 µg/kg/min
Epinephrine	IV infusion	0.1 to 1 µg/kg/min
Isoproterenol	IV infusion	0.1 to 1 µg/kg/min
Phenylephrine	IV infusion	1 to 10 µg/kg/min
Norepinephrine	IV infusion	0.1 to 1 µg/kg/min

Muscle Relaxants

Atracurium	IV	0.2 to 0.5 mg/kg
Pancuronium	IV	0.04 to 0.15 mg/kg
Succinylcholine	IV	1 to 2 mg/kg
	IM	2.5 to 4 mg/kg
Tubocurarine	IV/IM	0.3 to 0.6 mg/kg
Vecuronium	IV	0.04 to 0.2 mg/kg

(Continued)

41

Drug Dosages (*Continued*)

DRUG	ROUTE	DOSE
Narcotic Antagonists		
Naloxone	IV	0.1 mg/kg/dose (up to 2 mg/dose)
Narcotics		
Codeine	IM/PO	0.5 to 1 mg/kg
Meperidine	IV	0.5 to 1 mg/kg
	IM	1 to 1.5 mg/kg
Morphine	IV	0.05 to 0.1 mg/kg
	IV infusion	0.05 to 0.1 mg/kg/h
Sulfantanil	IM	0.1 to 0.2 mg/kg
Fentanyl	IV	10 to 25 μg/kg
	IV	1 to 2 μg/kg
Reversal Agents		
Edrophonium	IV	0.5 to 1 mg/kg
Neostigmine	IV	0.05 to 0.07 mg/kg
Pyridostigmine	IV	0.2 mg/kg
Sedatives		
Chloral hydrate	PO/PR	15 to 50 mg/kg/dose
Diazepam	IV	0.05 to 0.2 mg/kg/dose
	PO	0.1 to 0.5 mg/kg/dose
Hydroxyzine	IV/IM	0.5 to 1.0 mg/kg/dose
Lorazepam	IV/IM	0.05 to 0.1 mg/kg (maximum, 4 mg/dose)
Midazolam	IV	0.01 to 0.02 mg/kg
	IM	0.08 mg/kg
	Intranasal	0.2 to 0.3 mg/kg
	PO	0.3 to 0.5 mg/kg

Steroids

Dexamethasone	IV	0.5 to 1 mg/kg/dose (q 6 h if needed)
Hydrocortisone	IV	5 to 10 mg/kg/dose (q 6 h if needed)
Prednisolone	IV	1 to 2 mg/kg/day (q 6 h if needed)

Vasodilators

Diazoxide	IV	1 to 3 mg/kg (up to 150 mg)
Hydralazine	IV/IM	0.1 to 0.3 mg/kg
Nitroglycerin	IV infusion	1 to 20 µg/kg/min
Nitroprusside	IV infusion	0.5 to 10 µg/kg/min
Phentolamine	IV bolus	5 to 100 µg/kg
	IV infusion	1 to 7 µg/kg/min
Tolazoline	IV bolus	1 to 2 mg/kg
	IV infusion	1 to 2 mg/kg/h
Trimethaphan	IV	50 to 150 µg/kg/min

Miscellaneous

Dantrolene	IV (prevention)	2.5 mg/kg IV day of surgery
	IV (treatment)	2 to 3 mg/kg repeat as needed up to 10 mg/kg then 4 to 8 mg/kg/day (q 6 h)
Glucagon	IV	0.1 mg/kg (up to 1 mg/dose)
Glucose	IV	0.5 to 1 g/kg
Insulin	IV infusion	0.05 to 0.1 unit/kg
		0.1 unit/kg/h
Prostaglandin E$_1$	IV infusion	0.05 to 1 µg/kg/min

IV = intravenous; PO = oral; PR = rectal; IM = intramuscular; SQ = subcutaneous.

BIBLIOGRAPHY

Pharmacokinetics and Pharmacodynamics

Besunder JB, Reed MD, Blumer JL: Principles of drug biodisposition in the neonate: A critical evaluation of the pharmacokinetic-pharmacodynamic interface (Part I). *Clin Pharmacokinet* 1988; 14:189–216.

Besunder JB, Reed MD, Blumer JL: Principles of drug biodisposition in the neonate: A critical evaluation of the pharmacokinetic-pharmacodynamic interface (Part II). *Clin Pharmacokinet* 1988; 14:261–286.

Cook DR, Fischer CG: Neuromuscular blocking effects of succinylcholine in infants and children. *Anesthesiology* 1975; 42:662–665.

Gregory GA, Eger EI, Munson ES: The relationship between age and halothane requirement in man. *Anesthesiology* 1969; 30:488–491.

Kearns GL, Reed MD: Clinical pharmacokinetics in infants and children: A reappraisal. *Clin Pharmacokinet* 1989; 17(suppl 1):29–67.

Kenna JG, Neuberger J, Mieli-Vergani G, et al: Halothane hepatitis in children. *BMJ* 1987; 294:1209–1211.

Lerman J, Robinson S, Willis MM, et al: Anesthetic requirements for halothane in young children 0–1 months and 1–6 months of age. *Anesthesiology* 1983; 59:421–424.

Lerman J: Pharmacokinetics and pharmacodynamics of inhalational anesthetics in infants and children. *Anesthesiol Clin North Am* 1991; 9:763–779.

Lynn AM, Slattery JT: Morphine pharmacokinetics in early infancy. *Anesthesiology* 1987; 66:136–139.

Marshall BE, Wollman H: General anesthetics, in Gilman AG, Goodman LS, Rall TW, et al (eds): *Goodman and Gilman's The Pharmacological Basis of Therapeutics,* ed. 7. New York, Macmillan, 1985, pp 276–301.

Meretoja OA: Neuromuscular blocking agents in pediatric patients: Influence of age on the response. *Anaesth Intensive Care* 1990; 18:440–448.

Morselli PL: Clinical pharmacology of the perinatal period and early infancy. *Clin Pharmacokinet* 1989; 17(suppl 1):13–28.

Salanitre E, Rackow H: The pulmonary exchange of nitrous oxide and halothane in infants and children. *Anesthesiology* 1969; 30:388–394.

Stewart CF, Hampton EM: Effect of maturation on drug disposition in pediatric patients. *Clin Pharm* 1987; 6:548–564.

Stoelting RK, Peterson C: Methoxyflurane anesthesia in pediatric patients: Evaluation of anesthetic metabolism and renal function. *Anesthesiology* 1975; 42:26–29.

Vandenberghe H, MacLeod S, Chinyanga H, et al: Pharmacokinetics of intravenous morphine in balanced anesthesia: Studies in children. *Drug Metab Rev* 1983; 14:887–903.

Wark H, Earl J, Chau DD, et al: Halothane metabolism in children. *Br J of Anaesth* 1990; 64:474–481.

Drug Interactions

Bartkowski RR, Goldberg ME, Larijani GM, et al: Inhibition of alfentanil metabolism by erythromycin. *Clin Pharmacol Ther* 1989; 46:99–102.

Bentley JB, Glass S, Gandolfi AJ: The influence of halothane on lidocaine pharmacokinetics in man. *Anesthesiology* 1983; 59:A246.

Borel JD, Bentley JB, Nenad RE, et al: The influence of halothane on fentanyl pharmacokinetics. *Anesthesiology* 1982; 57:A239.

Chelly JE, Hysing ES, Abernethy DR, et al: Effects of inhalational anesthetics on verapamil pharmacokinetics in dogs. *Anesthesiology* 1986; 65:266–271.

Chelly JE, Hysing ES, Hill DS, et al: Cardiovascular effects of and interaction between calcium channel blocking drugs and anesthetics in chronically instrumented dogs vs. role of pharmacokinetics and the autonomic nervous system in the interactions between verapamil and inhalational anesthetics. *Anesthesiology* 1987; 67:320–325.

Chelly JE, Rogers K, Hysing ES, et al: Cardiovascular effect of and interaction between calcium blocking drugs and anesthetics in chronically instrumented dogs: I. Verapamil and halothane. *Anesthesiology* 1986; 64:560–567.

Dale O, Nilsen OG: Displacement of some basic drugs from human serum proteins by enflurane, halothane and their major metabolites. *Br J Anaesth* 1984; 56:535–542.

Gordon L, Wood AJJ, Koshakji RP, et al: Acute effects of halothane anesthesia on arterial and venous concentrations of propranolol in the dog. *Anesthesiology* 1987; 67:225–230.

Hiller A, Olkkola KT, Isohanni P, et al: Unconsciousness associated with midazolam and erythromycin. *Br J Anaesth* 1990; 65:826–828.

Mazze RI, Woodruff RE, Heerdt ME: Isoniazid-induced enflurane defluorination in humans. *Anesthesiology* 1982; 57:5–8.

Mazze RI: Metabolism of the inhaled anesthetics: Implications of enzyme induction. *Br J Anaesth* 1984; 56:27S–41S.

Merin R: Calcium channel blocking drugs and anesthetics: Is the drug interaction beneficial or detrimental? *Anesthesiology* 1987; 66:111–113.

Mouton-Perry S, Whelan E, Shay S, et al: The effect of intravenous anaesthesia with propofol on drug distribution and metabolism in the dog. *Br J Anaesth* 1991; 66:66–72.

Nakatsu K: Anesthetics and theophylline metabolism. *Anesth analg* 1985; 64:460–461.

Reilly CS, Merrell J, Wood AJJ, et al: Comparison of the effects of isoflurane and fentanyl–nitrous oxide–atracurium anaesthesia on propranolol disposition in dogs. *Br J Anaesth* 1988; 60:791–796.

Reilly CS, Wood AJJ, Koshaki R, et al: The effect of halothane on drug disposition: Contribution of changes in intrinsic drug metabolizing capacity and hepatic blood flow. *Anesthesiology* 1985; 63:70–76.

Somogyi A, Muirhead M. Pharmacokinetic interactions of cimetidine 1987. *Clin Pharmacokinet* 1987; 12:321–366.

Stack CG, Rogers P, Linter SPK: Monoamine oxidase inhibitors and anaesthesia: A review. *Br J Anaesth* 1988; 60:222–227.

Tosone SR, Reves JG, Kissin I, et al: Hemodynamic response to nifedipine in dogs anesthetized with halothane. *Anesth Analg* 1983; 62:903–908.

White PF, Johnston RR, Pudwill CR: Interaction of ketamine and halothane in rats. *Anesthesiology* 1975; 42:179–186.

White PF, Marietta MP, Pudwill CR, et al: Effects of halothane anesthesia on the biodisposition of ketamine in rats. *J Pharmacol Exp Ther* 1976; 196:545–555.

Wood M, Whelan E, Shay S, et al: Acute effect of halothane on drug distribution. *Anesthesiology* 1989; 71:A259.

Anaphylaxis

Atkinson TP, Kaliner MA: Anaphylaxis. *Med Clin North Am* 1992; 76:841–855.

Gold M, Swartz JS, Braude BM, et al: Intraoperative anaphylaxis: An association with latex sensitivity. *J Allergy Clin Immunol* 1991; 87:662–666.

Kaliner MA: Calling a halt to anaphylaxis. *Emerg Med* 1989; 16:51–58.

Nguyen DH, Burns MW, Shapiro GG, et al: Intraoperative cardiovascular collapse secondary to latex allergy. *J Urol* 1991; 146:571–574.

CHAPTER 4

Preoperative Evaluation

Mary Ann Gurkowski

Preoperative evaluation of the child is a complex area and should be approached in an unhurried fashion. A detailed medical history, surgical history, medication list, family history, physical examination, and chart review are essential for understanding the child's medical and surgical problems. The gathering of information pertaining to previous medical and surgical history is sometimes difficult, especially if the child has had multiple hospitalizations. However, perhaps even more important, is the emotional state of the child and parents. Surgery, no matter how minor the procedure, is a major disruption to the lives of both the patient and parents. Our goal as anesthesiologists should be to exhibit a reassuring, comfortable environment. Honesty with the child and parents is also extremely important, and the older the child, the more they should be included in the discussion of the anesthetic plan.

The preoperative form included in this chapter (Fig. 4-1) may be followed as a guideline for questioning the child's parents so that important information is sought in a systematic fashion. All of these factors must be considered and integrated to prepare for the anesthetic management of each child on an individual basis. A review of the chart is necessary even for healthy outpatients because the parent may not remember all of the child's medical history.

PREOPERATIVE TEACHING

Preoperative teaching is an effective way to reduce anxiety in both the parent and child. In 1977, Leigh and colleagues[1] and others reported lower anxiety levels in patients given preoperative reassurance versus a group given no support, presumably by removing the fear of the unknown and replacing this fear with knowledge of what is to be expected. This teaching can begin hours to days before the scheduled surgery. Some hospitals have well-established preoperative teaching programs that

PRE-OP EVALUATION   ANESTHESIA RECORD - PART TWO

HISTORY

| AGE | POP GP | SEX | THIN | AVERAGE |
| | | | MOD OBESE | OBESE |

Medical
Surgical
Allergies - Allergy to what & type of RXN
Medications - Amount and time including non-prescription
Previous Anesthetics - (Include CX's)
Weight _____ Height _____
(Kg)

Family Hx ANES _____
1. High Fevers
2. Muscle Cramps
3. Bleeding hx

INFORMED CONSENT □
TELEPHONE CONSENT □

PROBLEMS include reason for surgery (i.e. RIH)
1
2
3
4
5

ASA CLASS   I   II   III   IV   V   E

HEAD and NECK

Airway problems - include congenital abnormalities
Teeth - loose, chipped, missing, protuberant
TM Joint - range of motion
Cervical Spine - range of motion
Trachea - midline or deviated, tracheostomy
Micrognathia -
Macroglossia -
Cleft lip/palate -

P.E.

_____
THERAPEUTIC APPROACH

1 GETA { IV induction
2 Mask { Inhalation induction
3 Regional - include plan for post-op pain if indicated
4
5

CNS

Sensorium - active, lethargic, irritable
Spine   IVH - Grade -
Sonogram (most recent) -   Retinopathy of Prematurity -
Seizures -   Neuromuscular DS -

1 Fontanel - sunken, flat, bulging
2 Sundowning of eyes
3 Muscular function or atrophy

RECOVERY ROOM   ADMIT TIME _____

RESPIRATION

X-ray - chest, trachea, heart, mediastinum
Asthma -   Apnea -
Broncho pulmonary dysplasia or -
Intubation - Past or present, ett size, how long
URI - How recent, sx (fever
           WBC
           sputum - color)

Rate -
Rales -
Ronchi -
Wheezing -
Stridor -
Retractions (what type) -
Hoarseness -
Apnea/cyanosis with feeding or sleeping -

BP _____ P _____ R _____
Temperature _____

Respiratory status
1 Spont. Resp.
   Natural airway ____ Face tent ____ L/M
   Endotracheal tube ____ Briggs ____ L/M
2 Controlled or assist resp.

CARDIOVASCULAR

CHF -
Congenital anomolies
Cynotic vs acynotic
EKG
HTN -
Rheumatic fever
Exertion tolerance - squatting

Rate
Murmurs
Other cardiac sounds -
Skin turgor -
Cyanosis -

B.P _____ PULSE _____

Ventilator _____ VT _____ f _____

Type _____

Inspiratory force _____
FVC _____

Drugs _____

G.I. - Last feeding/meal, readiness to eat

Hepatitis   Diabetes
Diarrhea } How long
Jaundice

Edge of liver & spleen -
Abdominal distention -

POST OPERATIVE CONDITION

Comments:
   Arrival time, stability of vital signs, adequacy of ventilation, alertness, pain control, undue agitation, or N/V, complications.
Report given to: _____

G.U.
UTI -   Renal DS -

Urine output -

Birth HX - SVD or C-section   Gestation Age.
Complications - i.e. intubation, ventilation

Birthweight
Apgar   Hospital Stay

OB

Teenage Girls LMP
      Poss. Pregnancy

LAB DATA   Hb _____ Hct _____ Gluc _____ Bun _____ Cr _____
URINE   Sugar _____ Acetone _____
        Protein _____ Sp. Gr _____
ELECTROLYTES   Na+ _____ K+ _____ Cl- _____
BLOOD   PaO$_2$ _____ PaCO$_2$ _____ pH _____
GASES   B.E _____ FiO$_2$ _____
       PT _____ PTT _____ Platelets

Hematologic   Lines where & size
Anemia   UAC
Sickle Cell   UVC
Easy Bruising   PIV's where & size
           Central lines
           Art. Line

_____ M.D

Discharge time _____

Condition (circle)
     Good   Fair   Poor

          MD
_____ CRNA
          RN

Figure 4-1   Preoperative evaluation form.

allow the children and their parents to visit the outpatient area, operating room, and recovery room. If such a program does not exist, teaching can begin the evening before or the morning of surgery. A book or video tape can be made using pictures to explain the various events that will take place. A parent or volunteer can review this material with the child and make sure they understand what is about to transpire. It also helps to show the child the equipment (e.g., mask, pulse oximeter probe, and blood pressure cuff) to be used for induction. Preoperative teaching can be just as effective as administration of an anxiolytic agent before surgery.

INFORMED CONSENT

It is necessary that the anesthetic plan with its risks and benefits be presented in a clear, easily understood fashion to the parents and that notation of such information be made in the preoperative note. During this explanation, reference should be made to the anesthesiologist's careful monitoring of parameters, such as temperature (heating blanket and warmed room), heart rate and breath sounds (electrocardiogram and stethoscope), blood pressure, urine output (in selected cases, a urinary catheter may be inserted), and the amount of oxygen in the blood (pulse oximeter). It is important to talk to the child, if they are at an age of understanding (usually ≥ age 2 years), about what the monitors look like and the plan for induction. The details should not be recited in a cold and technical manner but with dialogue that responds to the parents' and child's questions and concerns. The child can be told that there will be no unexpected surprises and that nothing will hurt provided there is no plan to start an intravenous line while awake. Most importantly, never lie to a child. If the plan is to start an intravenous line before induction, tell the child that it will hurt some, but the hurt won't last long. Small children need reassurance that they will not awaken during surgery, but that they will awaken at the end of the surgery, at which time their parents will be waiting for them. Remember that children take things literally. The phrase "I am going to put you to sleep" can be frightening to some children because they have had a pet "put to sleep." The phrase "you are going to have a pleasant nap" may be less anxiety provoking.

The discussion of risks should be done out of earshot of the child to prevent unnecessary anxiety. The parents have a right to know about the possible complications of an anesthetic, and the physician has an obligation to explain those risks that are associated with a particular anesthetic choice. Exactly how much detail to include in the discussion depends on a number of variables, but the important issue is to provide the family with an understanding of the potential risks without producing undue anxiety. The general risks that should probably be discussed with all parents include possible pulmonary problems (croup, atelectasis, pneumonia, aspiration, and prolonged ventilation), postoperative nausea and vomiting, sore throat, and the possibility of tooth loss or damage, especially if the child has any loose teeth. Possible cardiovascular problems (arrhythmias, hypotension, and arrest) and allergic reactions to the drugs probably do not need to be discussed with every family because the benefit of such information that might be imparted is far outweighed by the anxiety it produces. However, if preexisting cardiovascular disease is present or a medication is to be used that has a higher incidence of reaction (i.e., dye injection, protamine, or vancomycin), these risks may be appropriate for discussion. In selected cases, the need for a blood transfusion and the associated risks thereof should be discussed. The risks for planned regional procedures, such as an epidural, caudal catheter, or single-injection caudal, should also be explained. These risks include infection, bleeding, failure of the block, spinal tap, headache, nerve injury, localized bruising, and transient muscle weakness. Other procedures needing an explanation of risks include axillary block, subarachnoid block, and central line placement. The parents should be assured that the procedures done after induction will not be felt by the child. Also, an explanation of what may happen postoperatively, including the necessity for a recovery room stay, possible nausea/vomiting, drowsiness, and disassociation, should also be told to the parents.

It is also important to inform the parents that their child should not eat or drink anything, including water, after the predesignated time. Explain that this is important to help prevent the child from serious pulmonary illness should vomiting occur. Remember to use simple terminology; the term NPO means nothing to the ordinary parent!

There may be times when the parents will not be present for preoperative questioning after a child has been admitted to the pediatric ward. An effort must be made to contact them by phone. This will be important when documenting informed consent. If the parents cannot be contacted the night before surgery, document these attempts and plan to talk to them in the anesthesia holding area the following morning.

PREOPERATIVE NOTE

The preoperative note should be brief but complete. It should state the surgery to be performed, the anesthetic plan, American Society of Anesthesiologists classification, pertinent positive and negative findings in the history and physical examination, and a statement of informed consent. The informed consent statement should list the risks explained and that the parent understands and gives consent. There is usually no need to fill out a separate consent form other than the one obtained for the surgery unless your institution has specific requirements. It may be wise to have the parents initial the part of the consent form pertaining to anesthesia and blood products so as to avoid any miscommunication if a transfusion becomes necessary.

PREOPERATIVE ORDERS

The preoperative orders should include the statement "anesthesia preop orders." This will let the surgeons know at a glance that the child has been seen. The orders should *always* include nothing by mouth (NPO) orders. Laboratory tests, if not already ordered, need to be requested. The preoperative orders may or may not include the timing and dose for administration of a preoperative or chronically taken medication.

Fasting Guidelines

Several authors[2–8] have looked at varying preoperative fasting times compared with gastric pH, gastric volume, and blood glucose concentrations in children before elective operations.

There has always been a concern about prolonged preoperative fasting and the risk of hypoglycemia. Studies by Jensen and associates[2] and Redfern and colleagues[3] both concluded that children older than 1 year of age could be fasted overnight with a minimal risk of hypoglycemia.

These recent studies have changed our professional opinions about fasting guidelines for children. Traditionally, concern about aspiration of gastric contents has led to recommendations for prolonged preoperative fasting. Newer studies have shown that, in children younger than 1 year of age, the administration of clear liquids 3 to 4 h preoperatively did not increase gastric volume or lower the gastric pH. Clear liquids include water, sugar water, apple juice, or breast milk but not cow's milk or formula. There is approximately a 5 percent incidence of increased gastric volume with either of the latter two liquids.[4,5]

Aspiration, although more common in children than adults, is still rare. The incidence in a large European and American pediatric population has been cited as 1:10,000 and 10:10,000 respectively, with very low morbidity related to the aspiration.[9] With this in mind, routine aspiration prophylaxis is probably not indicated in the child with no risk factors for aspiration. Risk factors include a recent meal, mechanical or functional obstruction to digestion, gastroesophageal junction dysfunction, previous esophageal surgery, obesity, head injury, neurologic damage, incoordination of swallowing and respiration, depressed level of consciousness, and the presence of a tracheostomy.

Prolonged preoperative fasting has also created a problem in infants and small children with regard to patient comfort and safety. The sensation of thirst is lessened in children older than

1 year of age and adolescents who were allowed clear liquid intake up until 2 h before surgery.[9,10] Although there are no studies comparing hypovolemia versus preoperative fasting, many anesthesiologists believe that the relative hypovolemia created from prolonged fluid restriction contributes to the hypotension sometimes seen during induction. It appears that the younger the child is and the more prolonged the fasting period, the greater the degree of hypovolemia that occurs and, therefore, hypotension. A comparison of our standard, more conservative, NPO guidelines compared with recent studies is listed in Table 4-1.

Currently, there is still controversy regarding the optimum NPO period in children. Caution must be taken that the parents understand the definition of clear liquids being Kool-Aid, water, Gatorade, or similar juices. This excludes orange juice, caffeine-containing beverages, and formula.

Premedication

Preoperative medications that are commonly administered either alone or in combination include sedatives, anxiolytics, anticholinergics, H_2-blockers, metoclopramide, and nonparticulate antacids. The purpose of a sedative or anxiolytic agent is to relieve anxiety, fear of separation, and pain and to allow a safer, smoother induction of anesthesia. The purpose of an anticholinergic agent is to prevent unwanted autonomic vagal reflexes and to block production of excessive secretions. The purpose of a nonparticulate antacid, an H_2-blocker, or metoclopramide is to decrease the risk of aspiration by either lowering gastric volume or raising gastric pH.

The specific needs of the child need to be considered when selecting a premedicant. This should include a knowledge of their previous hospital experiences and a review of old anesthetic records. Knowledge about the child's reaction to previous premedicants and any aftereffects can be useful.

If possible, preoperative medication should be given orally or via the nasal or rectal route (Table 4-2). Intramuscular injections are best avoided because they are painful and frightening to children. Many children remember the intramuscular injection more than they do the pain associated with the operative procedure. If the child is scheduled as the first case of the day, request that the premedication be given at a specified time. This includes the H_2-blocker and metoclopramide. Otherwise, write that the sedative or anxiolytic agent be given on the anesthesiologist's verbal request the next day. At the appropriate time, notify the nurse caring for the child to administer the medication. Writing an order such as "premed to be given on call to

Table 4-1 Standard NPO Guidelines by Age

| | AGES | | | |
	NEWBORN TO 1 YR	1 TO 14 YR	14 TO 19 YR	ADULT
UTHSC guidelines	Regular formula feeds until 5 h preoperatively; clear liquids until 2 h preoperatively	Solids until midnight, clear liquids until 3 h preoperatively	Nothing after midnight	Nothing after midnight
New guidelines based on recent studies	Regular formula feeds, with last feeding being clear liquids 3 h preoperatively[4]	2 mL/kg of clear liquids up to 2 h preoperatively[7]	Unlimited clear liquids until 3 h preoperatively[10]	240 mL of clear liquids 2 h preoperatively[11]

Table 4-2 Suggestions for Anesthetic Premedication

Oral (preferred route)		
Pentobarbital	3 to 4 mg/kg	1 h before induction
Pentobarbital and meperidine	2 mg/kg each	1 h before induction (children > age 5 yr)
Diazepam	0.1 to 0.3 mg/kg	10 min before induction
Midazolam	0.4 to 0.5 mg/kg	1 h before procedure (useful in patients with URI who *must* have surgery)
Atropine	0.02 mg/kg	
Metoclopramide	0.05 to 0.1 mg/kg	30 min before induction
Ranitidine	1 mg/kg	1 h before induction
Intramuscular		
Pentobarbital	2 mg/kg	30 min before induction
Morphine	0.1 mg/kg	30 min before induction
Demerol	2 mg/kg	30 min before induction
Atropine	0.02 mg/kg	30 min before induction
Intranasal (variably tolerated)		
Midazolam	0.2 mg/kg	5 to 10 min before induction
Sufentanil	1.5 to 4 μg/kg	5 to 10 min before induction
Rectal		
Thiopental	40 mg/kg	10 to 15 min before induction
Methohexital	15 mg/kg of 1% or 25 mg/kg of 10%	10 to 15 min before induction

O.R." usually does not allow adequate time for sedation to occur. Sedatives or anxiolytics are rarely needed in children younger than 10 months of age because stranger anxiety does not occur until this age. Children who have had preoperative teaching may also not need sedatives or anxiolytics. Nonparticulate antacids are usually given by the anesthesiologist in the holding area.

Laboratory Tests

The decision to order laboratory work needs to be based on knowledge of the child's medical history, current or recent medication use, and a physical examination. In these times of rising medical costs, the "shotgun" approach to ordering laboratory tests is no longer practical or feasible. Independent of this reasoning, minimizing laboratory tests will minimize the stress felt by the child, because two of their greatest fears are needles and separation.

There is no evidence to support the common practice of hematocrit screening before elective surgery in otherwise healthy children who will be undergoing minor, relatively bloodless surgery (e.g., myringotomy, circumcision, herniorrhaphy, or strabismus repair). Hematocrit testing is probably appropriate in infants, in patients in whom anemia is suspected, in patients with a bleeding disorder or possible hemoglobinopathy, in patients who are acutely or chronically ill, or in those who are having surgery during which significant blood loss or cardiovascular instability may occur. In these patients, no absolute guidelines exist for a minimally acceptable hematocrit. Management depends on the individual case and whether or not it would be better to correct an existing anemia before proceeding.

SPECIFIC COMMON MEDICAL CONCERNS

Upper Respiratory Tract Infection (URI)

Even though URIs often do not prevent school attendance or other daily activities, many anesthesiologists consider them a contraindication to general anesthesia for elective cases. At times, it can be difficult to decide whether or not a child has allergic rhinitis or a URI. In 1987, Tait and Knight[13] published two articles on respiratory tract infections in children. They listed eight signs and symptoms that are useful to identify the child with a URI. These are (1) sore or scratchy throat, (2) sneezing, (3) rhinorrhea, (4) congestion, (5) malaise, (6) nonproductive cough, (7) fever greater than 101°F, and (8) laryngitis.

Usually two or more of these findings together are required to make the diagnosis of a URI.

Children with URIs can present a dilemma for the anesthesiologist. The largest prospective study was done by Cohen and Cameron.[14] They looked at 1283 children with a preoperative URI and 20,876 children without a URI. Their study found that children with a URI were two to seven times more likely to experience respiratory-related adverse events during the intraoperative, recovery room, and postoperative phases of their operative experience. Respiratory events included laryngospasm, bronchospasm, stridor, breath holding, and postoperative croup. In addition, if a child had a URI and had endotracheal anesthesia, the risk of respiratory complications increased 11-fold. These authors' recommendations for children with URI were:

1. There is a need for hospitals to develop discharge criteria for recovery room and day-surgery pediatric patients who have a URI before surgery.
2. For children with asymptomatic or mild URI, the postponement of elective procedures is recommended for children younger than 1 year of age. For children older than 1 and less than 5 years of age, the risk-to-benefit ratio of the surgical procedure must be considered on an individual basis because these children are still at risk for respiratory complications whether or not they had a preoperative respiratory illness. Children older than age 5 years had lower rates of respiratory complications. Therefore, older children with URIs may be at less risk because of anatomically larger airways.
3. Although not a part of this study, it is recommended that children with significant preoperative symptoms of URI should have their surgery postponed. If children with relatively minor URIs are at a high risk for respiratory problems, it is likely that children with greater preoperative problems would be at an even higher risk.

The recommended time before rescheduling surgery for a child with URI is 3 to 6 weeks. Empey and colleagues[15] and others demonstrated that acute viral URIs produced bronchial reactivity that may last for 6 weeks. Of course, there will always be those children who are never completely free of symptoms or seem to have a URI every month. Waiting 3 to 6 weeks in these children is not feasible. It is important in these cases to obtain a detailed history to ascertain an accurate impression of the child's baseline physical status. Ask the parent to describe the child's symptoms when the child is healthiest. Then avoid anesthetizing the child only if the symptoms are clearly "changed from baseline." Also, be sure to inform the parents that their child does have a higher anesthesia risk for pulmonary complications.

Sickle Cell Anemia

Children with sickle cell anemia are at an increased anesthetic and surgical risk because their red blood cells can be stimulated to sickle, therefore creating sludging with vascular occlusive symptoms. The factors that stimulate sickling are a decrease in PaO_2, pH, blood flow, blood volume, and temperature. The sludging that occurs can potentiate vasoocclusion, ischemia, or infarction of the various organs.

Some children require chronic transfusion therapy to minimize their symptoms and prevent further organ damage. Preoperatively, the signs and symptoms of hemochromatosis should be sought. These include pigmentation of the skin, cirrhosis, glycosuria, and hyperglycemia, all of which are secondary to the deposition of hemosiderin. Pulmonary function tests, chest x-ray, electrocardiography, and possibly an echocardiogram should also be performed. These children can develop multiple pulmonary infarctions with resultant cor pulmonale. They can also develop cardiomegaly and high output failure secondary to their chronic anemia. A neurologic examination should be performed to document any evidence of a stroke or residual hemiparesis. Renal function should be documented. Hematuria and an inability to concentrate urine is common. Intravenous hydration should be started before beginning the NPO orders to prevent increased viscosity and red blood cell sludging.

The most important preoperative decision is whether or not to transfuse the child before surgery. This will need to be a combined decision between the surgeon, the anesthesiologist, and the hematologist. The primary purpose of preoperative transfusion is to reduce the blood's viscosity and therefore prevent venous thrombosis and microvascular stasis. In 1976, Murphy and colleagues[16] noted that there were high viscosities in patients with sickle cell anemia and that, when small amounts of normal cells were mixed with hemoglobin S cells, the blood viscosity significantly decreased. Lessin and associates[17] confirmed these results using in vitro test in 1978. Because of these findings, most physicians recommend reducing the hemoglobin S level to less than 40 percent if the decision preoperatively to transfuse has been made.

Cardiac Disease/Noncardiac Surgery

Children with congenital heart disease scheduled for noncardiac surgery need a thorough preoperative evaluation. This should include a history, physical, and recent cardiology evaluation. The type of lesion, severity of the symptoms, and nature of the surgery will determine the preoperative preparation. In the sicker children, avoidance of stress is important to prevent decompensation. In this situation an anxiolytic–sedative combination is very helpful for reducing stress. The anxiolytic agent, most commonly midazolam or diazepam, can be given orally 1 h before surgery. If further sedation is needed, then intramuscular morphine 30 min after oral premedication can be administered. This intramuscular injection will be better tolerated in an amnestic, semisedated patient. Most children with congenital heart disease will need prophylactic antibiotics. Tables 4-3 to 4-7 list the cardiac conditions, the surgical procedures, and the recommended standard prophylactic regimens.[18] Most of these children would benefit from supplemental oxygen during transport to the operating room.

SPECIFIC SURGICAL PROCEDURES

Other preoperative orders are based on the child's condition and the planned surgery. Table 4-8 lists some common pediatric procedures and their specific considerations, which will be covered in greater detail elsewhere in this manual. This table is not exhaustive, but it is intended to demonstrate that, not only the patient's condition, but also the planned surgical procedure and anesthetic technique will somewhat alter the information you need to obtain preoperatively and the discussion you will have with the parents.

Table 4-3 Cardiac Conditions in Which Endocarditis Prophylaxis Recommended

---

Prosthetic cardiac valves, including bioprosthetic and homograft valves

Previous bacterial endocarditis, even in the absence of heart disease

Most congenital cardiac malformations

Rheumatic and other acquired valvular dysfunction, even after valvular surgery

Hypertrophic cardiomyopathy

Mitral valve prolapse with valvular regurgitation

Used with permission. Dajani A, Bisno AL, Chung KJ, et al: Prevention of bacterial endocarditis. Recommendations by the American Heart Association. JAMA 1990; 264(22):2919–2922.

Table 4-4   Endocarditis Prophylaxis in Dental or Surgical Procedures*

Recommended
    Dental procedures known to induce gingival or mucosal
        bleeding, including professional cleaning
    Tonsillectomy and/or adenoidectomy
    Surgical operations that involve intestinal or respiratory
        mucosa
    Bronchoscopy with a rigid bronchoscope
    Sclerotherapy for esophageal varices
    Esophageal dilation
    Gallbladder surgery
    Cystoscopy
    Urethral dilation
    Urethral catheterization if urinary tract infection is present
    Urinary tract surgery if urinary tract infection is present
    Prostatic surgery
    Incision and drainage of infected tissue
    Vaginal hysterectomy
    Vaginal delivery in the presence of infection

Not Recommended
    Dental procedures not likely to induce gingival bleeding, such
        as simple adjustment of orthodontic appliances or fillings
        above the gum line
    Injection of local intraoral anesthetic (except intraligamentary
        injections)
    Shedding of primary teeth
    Tympanotomy tube insertion
    Endotracheal intubation
    Bronchoscopy with a flexible bronchoscope, with or without
        biopsy
    Cardiac catheterization
    Endoscopy with or without gastrointestinal biopsy
    Cesarean section
    In the absence of infection for urethral catheterization,
        dilation and curettage, uncomplicated vaginal delivery,
        therapeutic abortion, sterilization procedures, or insertion
        or removal of intrauterine devices

---

*This table lists selected procedures but is not meant to be all-inclusive. In addition to prophylactic regimens for genitourinary procedures, antibiotic therapy should be directed against the most likely bacterial pathogen. In patients who have prosthetic heart valves, a previous history of endocarditis, or surgically constructed systemic–pulmonary shunts or conduits, physicians may choose to administer prophylactic antibiotics even for low-risk procedures that involve the lower respiratory, genitourinary, or gastrointestinal tracts.

Used with permission. Dajani A, Bisno AL, Chung KJ, et al: Prevention of bacterial endocarditis. Recommendations by the American Heart Association. JAMA 1990; 264(22):2919–2922.

Table 4-5   Recommended Standard Oral Prophylactic Regimen for Dental, Oral, or Upper Respiratory Tract Procedures in Pediatric Patients Who Are at Risk*

DRUG	DOSING REQUIREMENT (ORAL)	
	Initial[†]	Follow-up[‡]
Amoxicillin	50 mg/kg	25 mg/kg
Erythromycin[§] stearate or ethylsuccinate	20 mg/kg	10 mg/kg
Clindamycin[§]	10 mg/kg	5 mg/kg

*Includes those with prosthetic heart valves and other high-risk patients.
[†]Total pediatric dose should not exceed total adult dose. The following weight ranges may also be used for the initial pediatric doses of amoxicillin: < 15 kg, 750 mg; 15 to 30 kg, 1500 mg; and > 30 kg, 3000 mg (full adult dose).
[‡]6 h after initial dose.
[§]In amoxicillin and penicillin allergic patients.

Used with permission. Dajani A, Bisno AL, Chung KJ, et al: Prevention of bacterial endocarditis. Recommendations by the American Heart Association. JAMA 1990; 264(22):2919–2922.

Table 4-6   Recommended Standard Intravenous and Intramuscular Prophylactic Regimen for Dental, Oral, or Upper Respiratory Tract Procedures in Pediatric Patients Who Are at Risk*

DRUG	DOSING REGIMEN*
Standard Regimen	
Ampicillin	50 mg/kg IV or IM 30 min before procedure; then 25 mg/kg IV or IM 6 h after initial dose.
Ampicillin/Amoxicillin/Penicillin-Allergic Patient Regimen	
Clindamycin	10 mg/kg IV 30 min before procedure and 5 mg/kg IV 6 h after initial dose.
High-Risk Regimen	
Ampicillin, gentamicin	Ampicillin 50 mg/kg IV or IM plus gentamicin 2.0 mg/kg 30 min before procedure; repeat one-half the initial dose 8 h after initial dose.

Table 4-6   (*Continued*)

DRUG	DOSING REGIMEN*
Ampicillin/Penicillin-Allergic Patient Regimen	
Vancomycin	20 mg/kg IV over 1 h, starting 1 h before procedure; no repeated dose necessary.

IV = intravenous; IM = intramuscular.
*Total pediatric doses should not exceed total adult doses: ampicillin 2 g, gentamicin 80 mg, vancomycin 1 g, and clindamycin 300 mg.

Used with permission. Dajani A, Bisno AL, Chung KJ, et al: Prevention of bacterial endocarditis. Recommendations by the American Heart Association. JAMA 1990; 264(22):2919–2922.

Table 4-7   Regimens for Genitourinary/ Gastrointestinal Procedures

DRUG	DOSING REGIMEN*
Standard Regimen	
Ampicillin, gentamicin, and amoxicillin	Intravenous or intramuscular administration of ampicillin 50 mg/kg, plus gentamicin 2.0 mg/kg 30 min before procedure, followed by amoxicillin 50 mg/kg orally 6 h after initial dose. Alternatively, the parenteral regimen may be repeated once 8 h after the initial dose.
Ampicillin/Amoxicillin/Penicillin-Allergic Patient Regimen	
Vancomycin and gentamicin	Intravenous administration of vancomycin 20 mg/kg over 1 h plus intravenous or intramuscular administration of gentamicin 2.0 mg/kg 1 h before procedure; may be repeated once 8 h after initial dose.
Alternate Low-Risk Patient Regimen	
Amoxicillin	50 mg/kg orally 1 h before procedure; then 25 mg/kg 6 h after initial dose.

*Total pediatric dose should not exceed total adult doses (see Table 4-6).

Used with permission. Dajani A, Bisno AL, Chung KJ, et al: Prevention of bacterial endocarditis. Recommendations by the American Heart Association. JAMA 1990; 264(22):2919–2922.

Table 4-8   Preoperative Considerations for Specific Operations

SURGICAL PROCEDURE	SPECIFIC PREOPERATIVE CONSIDERATIONS
Cleft lip and palate	Check for associated anomalies, anemia, aspirin intake, and availability of blood products (for palate repairs). These children frequently have upper respiratory tract infections and otitis media and should be evaluated for signs of acute infection.
Strabismus correction	Inform parents of the likelihood of nausea and vomiting postoperatively. Ask about family history or symptoms of malignant hyperthermia.
Extremity surgery	If a regional technique is planned for postoperative pain relief, discuss procedure and risks. Obtain consent for this in addition to consent for intraoperative care.
Laser of vocal cord papillomata	Careful review of prior anesthetic records for history of airway difficulties and for endotracheal tube size. Discuss with the parents the risk of eye, skin, and airway burns.
Dental surgery	Check for a history of heart disease. If antibiotics have been ordered for patients with chronic heart disease, be sure they are given at the correct time preoperatively (Tables 4-3 to 4-6). Many of these children have behavior disorders or retardation, and preoperative sedation may be needed.
Tonsillectomy and adenoidectomy	Check for aspirin use (within 2 weeks), acute infection, and evidence of right heart failure and pulmonary hypertension. Be aware of the possibility that the child may have obstructive sleep apnea, and arrange sleep studies if needed. Check the electrocardiogram and chest x-ray for evidence of right ventricular hypertrophy if history

(Continued)

Table 4-8 *(Continued)*

SURGICAL PROCEDURE	SPECIFIC PREOPERATIVE CONSIDERATIONS
	of obstructive sleep apnea. Inform parents of the likelihood of postoperative nausea and vomiting.
Nasal surgery and excision of polyps	May be associated with cystic fibrosis, chronic asthma, or sinusitis.
Bronchoscopy and laryngoscopy	Carefully evaluate the airway. Rarely, an awake intubation or surgical tracheostomy may be indicated. Inhaled anesthetic with maintenance of spontaneous ventilation is used more often.
Major abdominal procedures	There is a possibility of large blood loss and postoperative ventilation. Ascertain the availability of blood products. Consider caudal or epidural route for postoperative analgesia. Obtain parental consent and discuss with the parents the possible need for transfusion.
Major thoracic surgery	Evaluate pulmonary function, check on arterial blood gases, ensure that adequate blood products are available for transfusion, and avoid respiratory depressants in children with impaired pulmonary function. Inform parents of possible postoperative ventilation. Consider epidural route for postoperative analgesia.
Urologic surgery	Evaluate renal function carefully. If the child has poor renal function check for the presence of a coagulopathy, anemia, acid–base, and fluid–electrolyte abnormalities. Beware of possible cardiopulmonary disease and polypharmacy (including steroids). Check position of shunts or fistulas. Ensure availability of blood products for transfusion (may need washed cells).

(Continued)

Table 4-8 *(Continued)*

SURGICAL PROCEDURE	SPECIFIC PREOPERATIVE CONSIDERATIONS
Orthopedic procedures	Look for history or signs of congenital anomalies and/or neuromuscular diseases. If regional anesthesia is planned for postoperative analgesia, discuss procedure risks with parents. Ascertain availability of blood products and discuss with the parents the possible need for transfusion.

REFERENCES

1. Leigh JM, Walker J, Janaganathan P: Effect of preoperative anesthetic visit on anxiety. *BMJ* 1977; 2:987.
2. Jensen BH, Wernberg M, Andersen M: Preoperative starvation and blood glucose concentrations in children undergoing inpatient and outpatient anaesthesia. *Br J Anaesth* 1982; 54:1071–1074.
3. Redfern N, Addison GM, Meakin G: Blood glucose in anaesthetized children: Comparison of blood glucose concentrations in children fasted for morning and afternoon surgery. *Anaesthesia* 1986; 41:272–275.
4. Van der Walt JH, Carter, JA: The effect of different preoperative feeding regimens on plasma glucose and gastric volume and pH in infancy. *Anaesth Intensive Care* 1986; 14:352–359.
5. Van der Walt JH, Foate JA, Murrell D, et al: A study of preoperative fasting in infants aged less than three months. *Anaesth Intensive Care* 1990; 18:527–531.
6. Aun CS, Panesar NS: Paediatric glucose homeostasis during anaesthesia. *Br J Anaesth* 1990; 64:413–418.
7. Crawford M, Lerman J, Christensen S, et al: Effects of duration of fasting on gastric fluid pH and volume in healthy children. *Anesth Analg* 1990; 71:400–403.
8. Coté CJ: NPO after midnight for children: A reappraisal. *Anesthesiology* 1990; 72:589–592.
9. Tivel L, Nivoche Y, Hattan F, et al: Complications related to anaesthesia in infants and children: A prospective survey of 40,240 anaesthetics. *Br J Anaesth* 1988; 61:263–269.
10. Schreiner MS, Triebwasser A, Keon TP: Oral fluids compared to preoperative fasting in pediatric outpatients. *Anesthesiology* 1990; 72:593–597.
11. Splinter WM, Schaefer JD: Ingestion of clear fluids is safe for adolescents up to 3 h before anaesthesia. *Br J Anaesth* 1991; 66:48–52.

12. Shevde K, Trivedi N: Effects of clear liquids on gastric volume and pH in healthy volunteers. *Anesth Analg* 1991; 72:528–531.
13. Tait AR, Knight PR: Intraoperative respiratory complications in patients with upper respiratory tract infections. *Can J Anaesth* 1987; 34:300–303.
14. Cohen MM, Cameron CB: Should you cancel the operation when a child has an upper respiratory tract infection? *Anesth Analg* 1991; 72:282–288.
15. Empey DW, Laitinen LA, Jacob SL, et al: Mechanisms of bronchial hyperreactivity in normal subjects after upper respiratory tract infection. *Am Rev Respir Dir* 1976; 113:131.
16. Murphy JR, Wengard M, Brereton W: Rheological studies of the HbSS blood: Influence of hematocrit, hypertonicity, separation of cells, deoxygenation, and mixture with normal cells. *J Lab Clin Med* 1976; 87:475.
17. Lessin LS, Kuranstin-Mills J, Klug PP, et al: Determination of rheologically optimal mixtures of AA and SS erythrocytes for transfusion, in Erythrocyte membranes: Recent clinical and experimental advances. *Prog Clin Biol Res* 1978; 20:123.
18. Dajani AS, Bisno AL, Chung KJ, et al: Prevention of bacterial endocarditis. Recommendations by the American Heart Association. *JAMA* 1990; 264(22):2919–2922.

CHAPTER 5

Approach to the Pediatric Chest X-Ray

Ewell A. Clarke

Although routine preoperative chest x-rays are no longer recommended, many children will have had chest films taken for other reasons. It is wise not to overlook this source of potentially valuable information in the preoperative evaluation of the child. Of course, if the history or physical examination raises any suspicion of cardiac or pulmonary disease, frontal and lateral views of the chest should be ordered if no recent ones are available.

Radiographs of infants and children are very different from those of adults, and the disorders affecting the chest also are different. Abnormalities should be discussed with radiologists who have the most experience with pediatric films.

Even for an experienced radiologist, however, a systematic approach to the chest x-ray is necessary to avoid missing important findings. Such an approach is outlined in Table 5-1.

TECHNICAL FACTORS

A film that is too light (underexposed) may give the impression of pulmonary parenchymal disease when there is none. If the film is too dark, pulmonary disease may be obscured. With proper exposure, the intervertebral disk spaces can be seen through the heart, and the pulmonary vascular markings will be visible in the central third of the lung.

Children, being difficult to restrain, produce rotational artifact, and this is a common finding on chest films (Fig. 5-1). The resulting asymmetry of the lung fields and distortion of the cardiac silhouette may lead to errors in diagnosis. The anterior ribs and clavicles should be bilaterally symmetrical compared with the spine.

The degree of inspiration can radically affect the appearance of the chest (Fig. 5-2). Expiration will crowd and accentuate the pulmonary vascular markings and broaden the cardiac silhou-

Table 5-1   Approach to the Pediatric Chest

Technical Factors
    Exposure
    Rotation
    Inspiration
    Artifacts

Neck
    Soft tissues (swelling, gas)
    Tracheal position

Abdomen
    Free air
    Gastric distention
    Bowel gas

Thorax
    Subcutaneous air
    Ribs
    Clavicles
    Spine (scoliosis)

Mediastinum
    Thymus
    Masses
    Trachea (stenosis, foreign body)
    Aorta and main pulmonary artery
    Pneumomediastinum

Heart
    Situs
    Size
    Shape

Diaphragm
    Hernia/eventration
    Elevation/paralysis

Pleura
    Effusion/empyema
    Thickening
    Pneumothorax

Hilar structures
    Adenopathy
    Pulmonary vessels

Lungs
    Inflation/symmetry
    Fissures
    Infiltrates
    Nodules

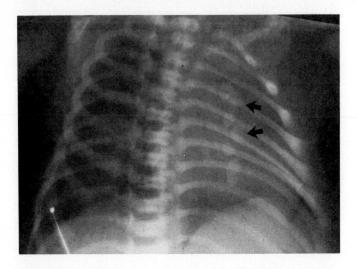

Figure 5-1 Infant rotated to the left. It is impossible to define the cardiac silhouette, and there is asymmetric density of the lungs. The multiple rounded densities in the left hemithorax (arrows) represent the sternal ossification centers.

ette, suggesting cardiac disease or pulmonary edema. Adequate inspiration will place the level of the diaphragm at the eighth rib posteriorly. If the diaphragms are below the 10th posterior rib, reactive airway disease or other cause of air trapping should be considered (Fig. 5-3).

ANCILLARY STRUCTURES

Neck

The tracheal position should be evaluated. There is normal buckling of the trachea to the right at the level of the clavicles in young children (Fig. 5-2A). Any other deviation or narrowing of the trachea should be investigated further (Fig. 5-4). Metallic foreign bodies are occasionally seen in this area and should not be dismissed as artifacts.

Abdomen

Free air will be seen beneath the diaphragm only if the film was taken in the upright position. Infants normally have more bowel gas than do older children and adults, but excessive dilatation of the bowel or stomach may cause respiratory compromise and necessitate decompression.

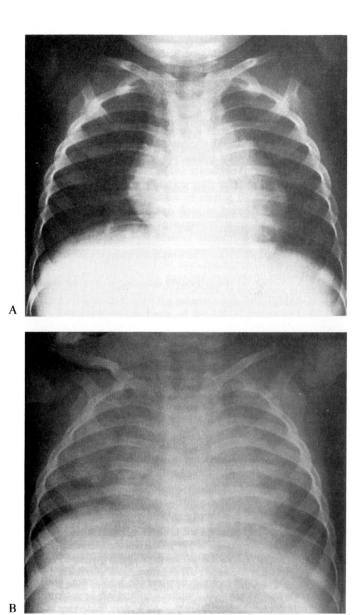

Figure 5-2 Inspiratory (A) and expiratory (B) views of the same infant. The expiratory film in B gives the false impression of cardiomegaly and pulmonary edema. Note normal buckling of trachea to the right at the level of the clavicles.

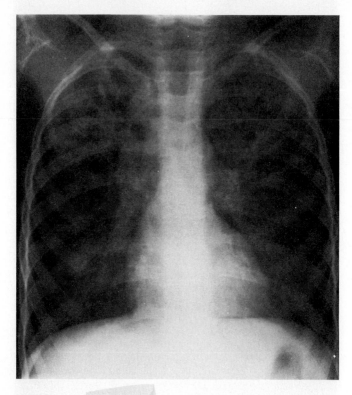

Figure 5-3 Hyperinflation. The diaphragms are at the level of the 11th posterior ribs in this child with cystic fibrosis.

Thorax

Bony structures should be examined for the presence of fractures. With rib fractures, a careful search for pneumothorax should be made. Fractures of the first and second ribs may be associated with great vessel injury and bleeding into the mediastinum or pleural space. The spine should be examined for scoliosis, subluxation, or fracture.

Mediastinum

The thymus is a pleomorphic organ that occupies the anterior mediastinum of young children, and it is most often seen in those younger than age 2 years (Fig. 5-5). It drapes over the heart like a blanket and cannot be separated from it on x-ray unless pneumomediastinum is present. Unlike mediastinal masses, such as abscess or tumor (Fig. 5-6), even a large thymus will not displace the trachea.

The intrathoracic trachea is normally slightly to the right of the midline at the level of the aortic arch. Its diameter should be constant. If it is not, tracheal stenosis, tracheomalacia, or vascular ring may be present. This is another area to look for metallic densities, which may represent foreign bodies in the trachea or esophagus.

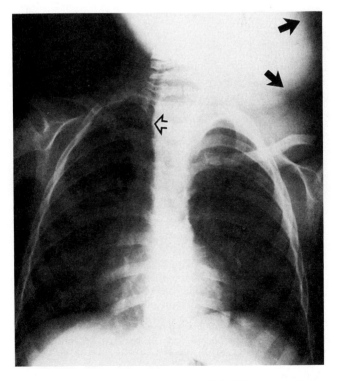

Figure 5-4 Cystic hygroma of the neck (solid arrows). Extension into the superior mediastinum is evident by the rightward displacement of the trachea (open arrow).

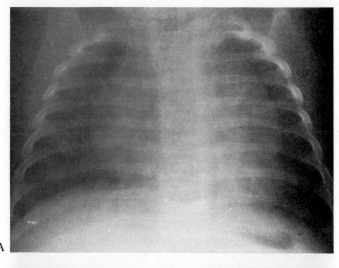

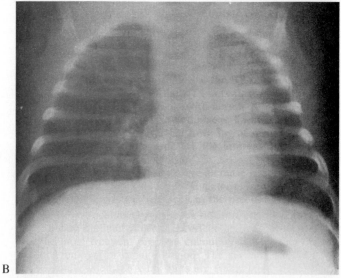

Figure 5-5 Examples of thymic shadows. In A, the thymus drapes down over both sides of the heart, increasing the apparent cardiac size. In B, the left thymic lobe is most prominent.

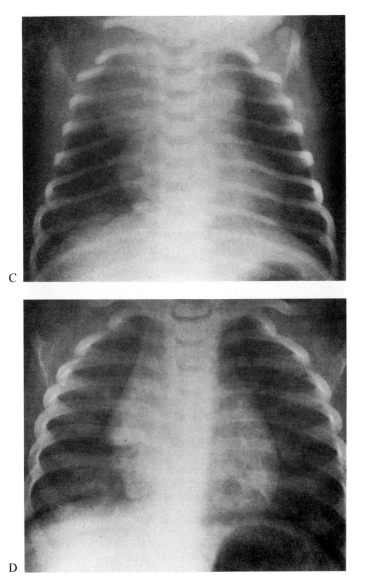

Figure 5-5 (continued) In C, the right lobe predominates. In D, the right lobe resembles the sail of a sailboat, the "sail sign."

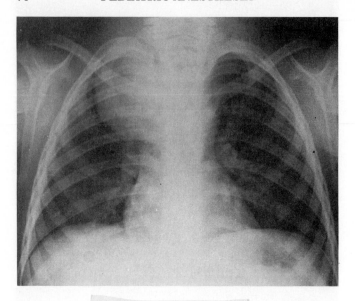

Figure 5-6 Mediastinal abscess extending into the right apex.

HEART

If the apex of the heart is not on the left, a mislabeled film is the most likely diagnosis. If the suspicion of situs inversus remains, correlation with the position of the liver and the stomach on film and on physical examination should be made.

An analysis of cardiac size and shape is more difficult in children. This is especially true in infants in whom the thymus contributes to the apparent cardiac size. Expiratory films and pectus excavatum defects also give the illusion of cardiomegaly (Fig. 5-7). For measurement purposes, a cardiothoracic ratio of 60 percent or less is acceptable before 1 year of age, whereas 50 percent or less is normal for other children. It should be kept in mind that an enlarged cardiac silhouette in a trauma victim may not represent cardiomegaly but rather be a hemopericardium with a risk of cardiac tamponade (see Chaps. 25 and 26 for a discussion of congenital heart disease).

DIAPHRAGM

The dome of the diaphragm is more anterior in children than in adults. If the diaphragms are flattened, air trapping should be suspected (Fig. 5-3). Congenital diaphragmatic hernia usually results in a hemithorax filled with bowel loops (Fig. 20-1). Even-

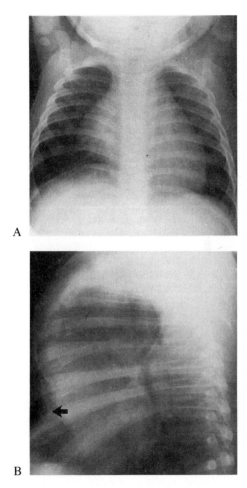

Figure 5-7 Pectus excavatum deformity. The frontal view (A) suggests cardiomegaly, but the lateral view (B) shows that the heart is being compressed and flattened by the sternal defect (arrow).

tration may be congenital or traumatic and may appear simply as an elevated diaphragm.

Elevation of a hemidiaphragm most commonly represents diaphragmatic paralysis (Fig. 5-8). This may be secondary to birth trauma (Erb's palsy). Eventration and paralysis may result in some atelectasis of the adjacent lung, but a large congenital

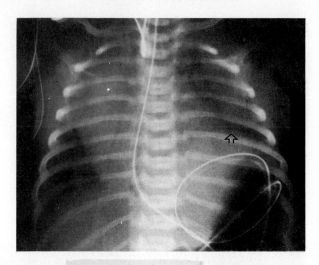

Figure 5-8 Paralyzed left diaphragm (arrow) resulting from birth trauma to the brachial plexus (Erb's palsy). Note the heart and mediastinum displaced to the right in response to the decrease in available room in the left hemithorax.

diaphragmatic hernia usually causes severe pulmonary hypoplasia.

PLEURA AND HILAR REGIONS

The pleural space may contain air, fluid, or scar tissue (pleural thickening). Air leaks in children may result from penetrating injury, asthma, or barotrauma. Air can dissect along vascular bundles and soft tissue planes and appear in the interstitium of the lung, mediastinum, and even in the soft tissues of the neck and thoracic cage (Fig. 5-9). Malposition of the endotracheal or tracheostomy tube should be suspected if any extrapulmonary air is seen. Skin folds may simulate pneumothorax in the neonate (Fig. 5-10).

The most common cause of pleural effusions are pneumonia and congestive heart failure, but pleural fluid may consist of blood, pus, chyle, or transudate. The radiographic presentation varies with the amount of fluid, from minimal blunting of the costophrenic angle to total opacification of the hemithorax (Fig. 5-11).

Prominent hilar shadows may be caused by enlarged hilar nodes, usually secondary to a viral lower respiratory infection (Fig. 5-12). Other causes include tuberculosis (especially if uni-

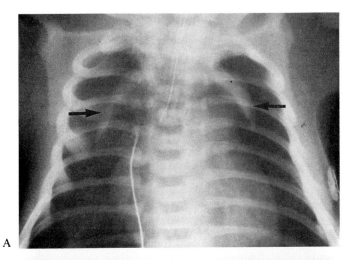

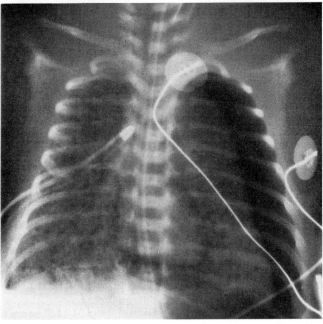

Figure 5-9 Neonatal air leaks. In A, a pneumomediastinum has elevated the thymus (arrows) from the heart. B shows a large left pneumothorax and a pneumopericardium. The heart is quite small, suggesting tamponade. The bubbly appearance of the lungs is the result of pulmonary interstitial emphysema.

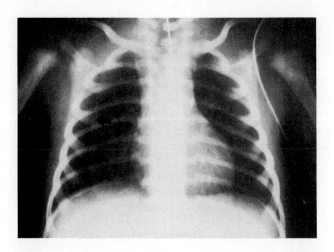

Figure 5-10 Skin fold (arrows) simulating right pneumo-thorax.

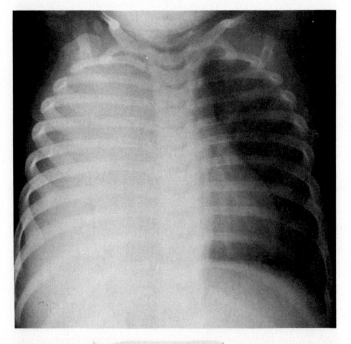

Figure 5-11 Staphylococcal empyema resulting in opacification of the right hemithorax.

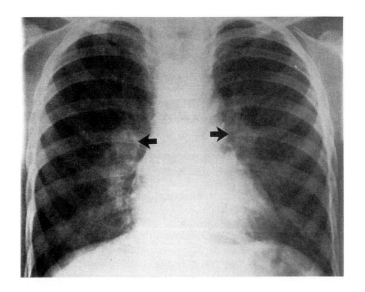

Figure 5-12 Enlargement of hilar nodes (arrows) in a child after measles-induced pneumonia.

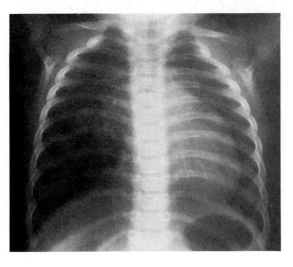

Figure 5-13 Hilar enlargement caused by dilated proximal pulmonary arteries in a child with ventricular septal defect and pulmonary hypertension.

lateral) and enlargement of the pulmonary arteries secondary to pulmonary hypertension (Fig. 5-13).

LUNGS

Evaluation of the pulmonary parenchyma is performed last to avoid overlooking unsuspected disease elsewhere in the chest. The degree of overall inflation has already been addressed. Asymmetric aeration may be secondary to atelectasis or air trapping in one lung or lobe. Unilateral hyperinflation should raise the suspicion of foreign body aspiration, bronchomalacia, or endobronchial lesion (Fig. 5-14). Atelectasis may also occur with foreign body aspiration but is commonly seen in asthma in which mucous plugs obstruct smaller bronchi (Fig. 5-15). Patients with endotracheal tubes commonly have thick secretions and atelectasis from mucous plugging also. Malposition of the endotracheal tube may also cause atelectasis (Fig. 5-16).

Differentiating pulmonary densities caused by atelectasis from consolidation from pneumonia may be difficult. Both pro-

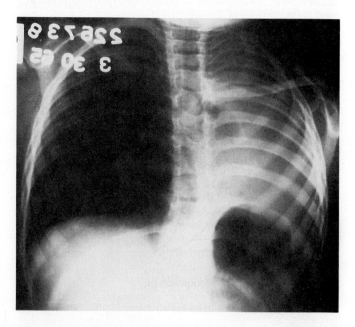

Figure 5-14 Hyperinflation of the right lung caused by a foreign body in the right main bronchus. The heart and mediastinum are markedly displaced to the left.

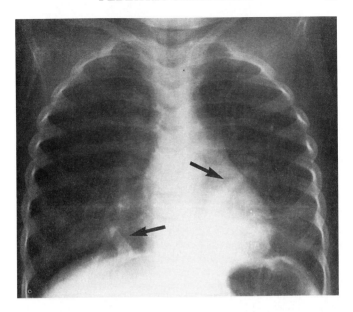

Figure 5-15 Asthmatic patient with wedge-shaped areas of increased density (arrows) representing subsegmental atelectasis ("discoid" atelectasis).

duce densities that conform to the lobes or segments. Both may have air bronchograms, which result from air-filled bronchi surrounded by fluid-filled or collapsed alveoli. Both may produce the "silhouette sign," in which a cardiac border or diaphragm cannot be defined because of increased density of the adjacent lung (Fig. 5-16B). Atelectasis can usually be diagnosed by signs of volume loss, such as a shift of the mediastinum or retraction of fissure lines or diaphragm toward the area of density. However, if the clinical presentation is that of pneumonia, the pulmonary density should not be dismissed as atelectasis.

Pulmonary infiltrates may be classified as interstitial or alveolar. The latter are characteristic of processes that cause alveoli to fill with fluid or pus, such as bacterial pneumonia, hydrocarbon or other aspiration pneumonia, pulmonary edema, pulmonary contusion, and adult respiratory distress syndrome. Alveolar infiltrates may be fluffy and distributed throughout the lung (Fig. 5-17), or they may result in opaque consolidation of a single lobe or segment (Fig. 5-18).

Interstitial infiltrates are characterized by streaky or reticular markings coursing through the lungs or concentrated in the

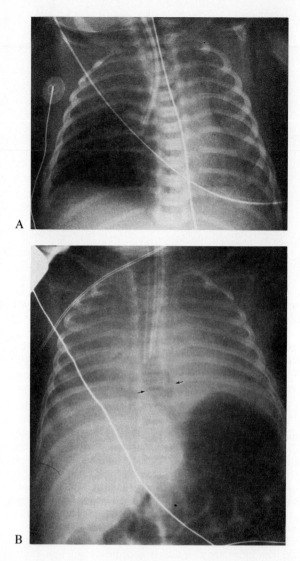

Figure 5-16 Atelectasis caused by malposition of endotracheal tubes. A shows the typical atelectasis of the left lung and right upper lobe seen with right mainstem intubation. B shows generalized pulmonary collapse secondary to esophageal tube placement. Stomach and esophagus (arrows) are dilated.

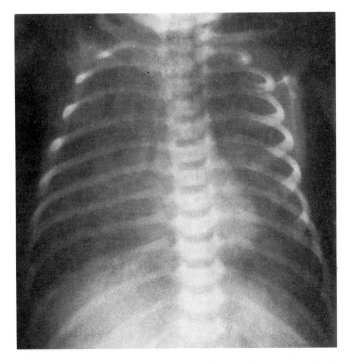

Figure 5-17 Fluffy alveolar-type infiltrate throughout both lungs in a child with bacterial bronchopneumonia.

perihilar regions (Fig. 5-19). This may result in the overall impression that the lungs are somewhat "dirty." Interstitial infiltrates are usually caused by processes that affect both lungs equally, viral processes and asthma being the most common causes. Both may be associated with generalized hyperinflation because of their effect on small airways.

Focal alveolar infiltrates may be missed if certain areas of the lungs are overlooked. Lower lobe pneumonias are commonly missed when they lie behind the cardiac silhouette or diaphragms on the frontal view. A properly exposed film will allow visualization of lung behind these structures; any asymmetric density should be suspect. The lateral view can be helpful in this situation, especially if one important fact is kept in mind, that is, the vertebral bodies should gradually become darker from the upper to the lower thoracic spine (Fig. 5-7B). A lower lobe infiltrate will cause them to become lighter.

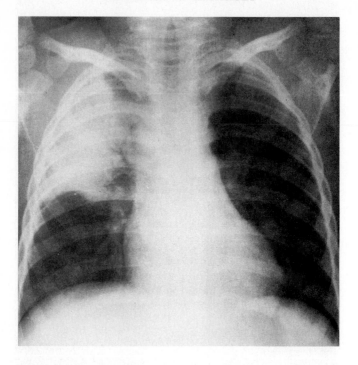

Figure 5-18 Right upper lobe consolidation in a child with pneumococcal pneumonia.

THE NEWBORN CHEST

The differences between the adult and pediatric chest are most pronounced in this age group. For example, lobar pneumonia is almost never seen in the neonate; pneumonia of any cause will involve the entire chest.

Meconium aspiration pneumonitis is, of course, seen only in the neonate. Because meconium is sterile, this begins as a chemical rather than an infectious pneumonitis, but it may become infected later. The radiographic features include a patchy diffuse infiltrate, hyperinflation, and often pneumothorax (Fig. 5-20).

Wet lung disease (transient tachypnea of the newborn) commonly causes respiratory distress in the first 24 h of life. It is not truly a disease but, rather, is a delayed clearing of normal fetal interstitial lung fluid. The radiographic appearance is that of an interstitial infiltrate with possible thickening of the minor

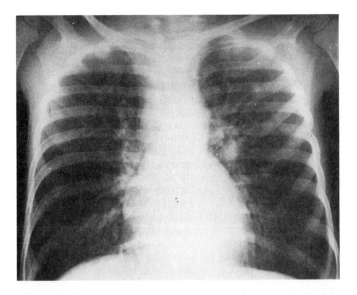

Figure 5-19 Viral pneumonitis. Interstitial markings are increased in the perihilar regions, possibly accompanied by hilar adenopathy.

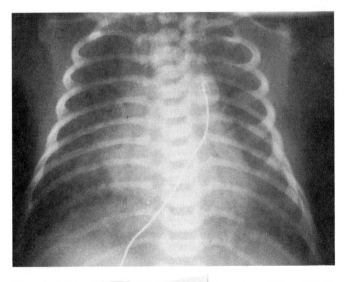

Figure 5-20 Meconium aspiration. There is a diffuse bilateral pulmonary infiltrate in an infant who had meconium in the amniotic fluid at birth.

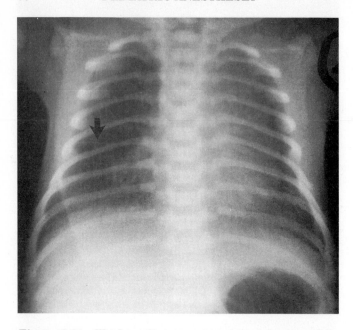

Figure 5-21　Wet lung disease or transient tachypnea of the newborn. Streaky densities radiating from the left hilar region and visualization of the minor fissure (arrow) indicate retained interstitial fluid in this infant at 4 h of age.

fissure on the right (Fig. 5-21). These findings and the symptoms disappear within 24 h as the fluid is cleared.

Hyaline membrane disease (sometimes referred to as respiratory distress syndrome) is seen in small premature infants. It is manifested by a homogeneous haziness of the lungs, often accompanied by prominent air bronchograms secondary to generalized alveolar collapse (Fig. 5-22). The complications of hyaline membrane disease are those associated with high pressure ventilation and high oxygen concentration.

Hyaline membrane disease requiring significant ventilatory support for more than 2 weeks usually results in bronchopulmonary dysplasia (Fig. 5-23). The radiographic appearance is that of a gradually coarsening interstitial infiltrate, which consists of patchy atelectasis and scarring. This is often accompanied by other areas of hyperinflation or cystic change, all secondary to small airway damage. These findings may persist for months or years and may be indistinguishable from the interstitial infiltrates of a viral infection when these children are later seen for wheezing or cough.

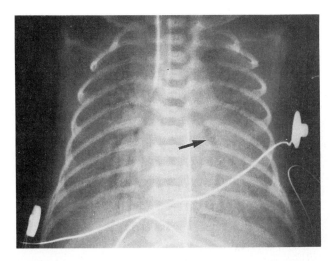

Figure 5-22 Hyaline membrane disease. Note the homogeneous "granular" haze throughout the lungs, with prominent air bronchograms (arrow).

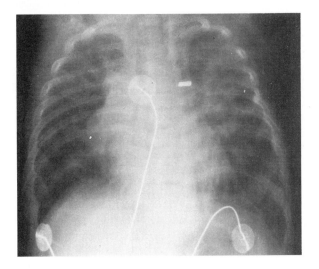

Figure 5-23 Bronchopulmonary dysplasia. Patchy white densities represent areas of chronic atelectasis and fibrosis; the lower lobes are hyperinflated and emphysematous. The ductus arteriosus has been clipped.

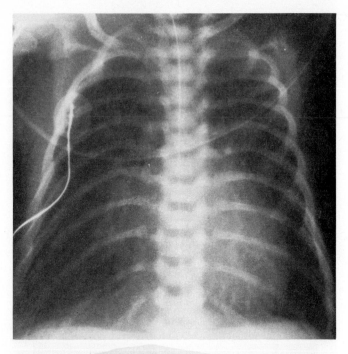

Figure 5-24 Patent ductus arteriosus in a premature infant, manifested by development of cardiomegaly and increased pulmonary vascularity.

The premature infant is also at risk for congestive heart failure secondary to persistent patency of the ductus arteriosus. This is manifested by an enlarging cardiac silhouette followed by indistinctness of the cardiac borders as pulmonary edema increases the density of the adjacent lung (Fig. 5-24).

BIBLIOGRAPHY

Caffey J: *Pediatric X-Ray Diagnosis,* ed 8. Chicago, Year Book Medical Publishers, 1985.

Kirks DR: *Practical Pediatric Imaging.* Boston, Little, Brown, 1984.

Swischuk LE: *Imaging of the Newborn, Infant, and Young Child,* ed 3. Baltimore, Williams & Wilkins, 1989.

CHAPTER 6

Interpretation of Pediatric Electrocardiograms

Myung K. Park

Pediatric electrocardiograms (ECGs) are different from those of the adult in several aspects. We should become familiar with the age-related changes in the cardiogram to interpret pediatric ECGs correctly. A systematic approach to the evaluation of the ECG tracing will be presented with a discussion of the specific abnormalities as they relate to pediatric disease.

AGE-RELATED CHANGES IN ECG

Most of the age-related changes in pediatric ECGs are caused by the right ventricular (RV) dominance seen during the newborn period and infancy. The RV dominance is the result of the fetal circulation and is gradually replaced by the left ventricular (LV) dominance of later childhood and adulthood. The LV/RV ratio is 2.5:1 in the adult; 0.8:1 at birth; 1.5:1 at 1 month of age; and 2.0:1 at 6 months of age. The ECGs of children reflect these age-related anatomic changes. The ECG changes are more rapid during the first half of the first year, and by the age of 3 to 4 years, pediatric ECGs resemble those of the adult.

The following general changes occur with increasing age.

1. The heart rate decreases (Table 6-1).
2. All the durations and intervals (PR interval, QRS duration, and QT interval) increase.
3. The RV dominance of infancy is expressed in the ECG by the following: The QRS axis is more rightward than that in the adult (Table 6-2). The right precordial leads (V4R, V1, and V2) show large R waves and small S waves. The left precordial leads (V5 and V6) show small R waves and deep S waves (Table 6-3). The R/S ratios in the right precordial leads are large, and those in the left precordial leads are small (Table 6-4).

Table 6-1 Normal Resting Heart Rates According to Age

AGE	HEART RATE (BEATS/MIN)
Newborn	110 to 150
2 yr	85 to 125
4 yr	75 to 115
6 yr	65 to 100
> 6 yr	60 to 100

4. The T wave is inverted in V1 in infants and small children, with the exception of the first 3 days after birth. After 5 years of age, the T wave in V1 gradually becomes upright.
5. The ECGs of premature infants, in general, resemble those of full-term newborns, although as a group, they show a little less RV force (or more LV force) than the full-term neonate. (The premature infant has a greater LV/RV ratio than the full-term newborn does.)

ROUTINE INTERPRETATION

The following sequence is one of the many approaches that can be used in routine interpretation of an ECG.

1. Rhythm (sinus or nonsinus), by considering the P axis.
2. Heart rate (atrial and ventricular rates, if different).
3. The QRS axis, the T axis, and the QRS-T angle.
4. Intervals: PR interval, QRS duration, and QT interval.
5. The P wave amplitude and duration.
6. The QRS amplitude and the R/S ratio; also note abnormal Q waves.
7. The ST segment and T wave abnormalities.

Table 6-2 Mean and Range of Normal QRS Axes

AGE	MEAN AXES (RANGE)
1 wk to 1 mo	+110° (+30 to +180)
1 to 3 mo	+70° (+10 to +125)
3 mo to 3 yr	+60° (+10 to +110)
> 3 yr	+60° (+20 to +120)
Adults	+50° (−30 to +105)

Table 6-3 R and S Voltages According to Lead and Age: Mean (and Upper Limits)*

				AGE				
LEAD	0 to 1 mo.	1 to 6 mo.	6 mo to 1 yr	1 to 3 yr	3 to 8 yr	8 to 12 yr	12 to 16 yr	Young Adults
R voltage								
I	4(8)	7(13)	8(16)	8(16)	7(15)	7(15)	6(13)	6(13)
II	6(14)	13(24)	13(27)	13(23)	13(22)	14(24)	14(24)	9(25)
III	8(16)	9(20)	9(20)	9(20)	9(20)	9(24)	9(24)	6(22)
aVR	3(7)	3(6)	3(6)	2(6)	2(5)	2(4)	2(4)	1(4)
aVL	2(7)	4(8)	5(10)	5(10)	3(10)	3(10)	3(12)	3(9)
aVF	7(14)	10(20)	10(16)	8(20)	10(19)	10(20)	11(21)	5(23)
V4R	6(12)	5(10)	4(8)	4(8)	3(8)	3(7)	3(7)	
V1	15(25)	11(20)	10(20)	9(18)	7(18)	6(16)	5(16)	3(14)
V2	21(30)	21(30)	19(28)	16(25)	13(28)	10(22)	9(19)	6(21)
V5	12(30)	17(30)	18(30)	19(36)	21(36)	22(36)	18(33)	12(33)
V6	6(21)	10(20)	13(20)	12(24)	14(24)	14(24)	14(22)	10(21)
S voltage								
I	5(10)	4(9)	4(9)	3(8)	2(8)	2(8)	2(8)	1(6)
V4R	4(9)	4(12)	5(12)	5(12)	5(14)	6(20)	6(20)	
V1	10(20)	7(18)	8(16)	13(27)	14(30)	16(26)	15(24)	10(23)
V2	20(35)	16(30)	17(30)	21(34)	23(38)	23(38)	23(48)	14(36)
V5	9(30)	9(26)	8(20)	6(16)	5(14)	5(17)	5(16)	
V6	4(12)	2(7)	2(6)	2(6)	1(5)	1(4)	1(5)	1(13)

*Voltages are measured in millimeters: 1 mV = 10 mm paper.

Reproduced with permission from Park MK, Guntheroth WG: *How to Read Pediatric ECGs*, ed 3. St. Louis, Mosby Year Book, 1992, p 49.

Table 6-4 R/S Ratio According to Age: Mean, Lower, and Upper Limits of Normal

LEAD	AGE							
	0 to 1 mo	1 to 6 mo	6 mo to 1 yr	1 to 3 yr	3 to 8 yr	8 to 12 yr	12 to 16 yr	Adult
V1								
LLN	0.5	0.3	0.3	0.5	0.1	0.15	0.1	0.0
Mean	1.5	1.5	1.2	0.8	0.65	0.5	0.3	0.3
ULN	19	S=0	6	2	2	1	1	1
V2								
LLN	0.3	0.3	0.3	0.3	0.05	0.1	0.1	0.1
Mean	1	1.2	1	0.8	0.5	0.5	0.5	0.2
ULN	3	4	4	1.5	1.5	1.2	1.2	2.5
V6								
LLN	0.1	1.5	2	3	2.5	4	2.5	2.5
Mean	2	4	6	20	20	20	10	9
ULN	S=0	S=0	S=0	S=0	S=0	S=0	S=0	S=0

LLN = lower limits of normal; ULN = upper limits of normal.

Reproduced with permission from Guntheroth WG: *Pediatric Electrocardiography*. Philadelphia, WB Saunders, 1965.

Rhythm

Sinus rhythm is normal rhythm at any age. Nonsinus rhythm is seen with various forms of arrhythmias, which will be discussed elsewhere. Sinus rhythm has the following characteristics.

1. P waves preceding each QRS complex, with a regular PR interval. (The PR interval may be prolonged as in first-degree atrioventricular block.)
2. Normal P axis (0° to +90°). This produces an upright P wave in leads I and aVF and an inverted P in aVR. (The method of plotting the P axis is the same as that for the QRS axis, which will be discussed subsequently.)

Heart Rate

The heart rate of pediatric patients varies with age, status at the time of ECG recording (awake, sleeping, or crying), and other physical factors, such as fever. The normal resting heart rates (per minute) according to age are shown in Table 6-1. Operationally, tachycardia is present when the heart rate is faster than the ranges of normal for that age, and bradycardia is present when the heart rate is slower than the lower range of normal for that age.

At the usual paper speed of 25 mm/s, 1 mm = 0.04 s, and 5 mm = 0.20 s. The heart rate may be calculated by the following methods.

1. Measure the RR interval (in seconds) and then divide 60 by the RR interval.
2. A quick estimation of the heart rate is possible by inspecting the RR interval in millimeters and using the following relationships: 5 mm = 300/min, 10 mm = 150/min, 15 mm = 100/min, 20 mm = 75/min, and 25 mm = 60/min.
3. Use a convenient ECG ruler.

The QRS and T Axes

The QRS axis, the T axis, and the QRS-T angle are important in the interpretation of an ECG, especially with ventricular hypertrophy and conduction disturbances. In determining the QRS or T axis, we use the hexaxial reference system (Fig. 6-1), which provides information on the left–right and the superior–inferior relationships. A positive (or negative) deflection in an ECG lead implies that the electromotive force is directed to the positive (or negative) lead label for that particular lead. For example, the R wave in lead I represents the leftward force; the S

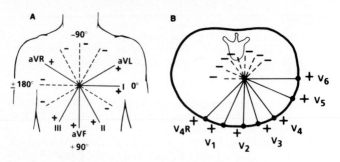

Figure 6-1 Hexaxial reference system (A) and horizontal reference system (B). (Reproduced with permission from Park MK, Guntheroth WG: *How to Read Pediatric ECGs,* ed 3. St. Louis, Mosby Year Book, 1992, p 23.)

wave in lead I, the rightward force; and the S wave in aVF, the superiorly directed force. (The horizontal reference system is not used in determining the axis, but it provides information on the right–left and the anterior–posterior relationships [Fig. 6-1].)

The successive approximation method is a convenient way of determining the QRS axis. (The same approach is used for the P and T axes.)

Step 1. Locate a quadrant, using leads I and aVF (Fig. 6-2).
Step 2. Find a lead with an equiphasic QRS complex. The QRS axis is perpendicular to the lead with an equiphasic QRS complex in the predetermined quadrant.

The normal QRS axis is provided in Table 6-2 with ranges of normal.

The abnormal QRS axis has the following characteristics:

1. Left axis deviation, with the QRS axis less than the lower limits of normal for age, is seen in left ventricular hypertrophy, left bundle branch block (LBBB), or left anterior hemiblock (often called superior QRS axis).
2. Right axis deviation, with the QRS axis greater than the upper limit of normal for age, is seen with right ventricular hypertrophy and right bundle branch block (RBBB).
3. Superior QRS axis (S wave much greater than the R wave in aVF) is seen in endocardial cushion defect and tricuspid atresia.

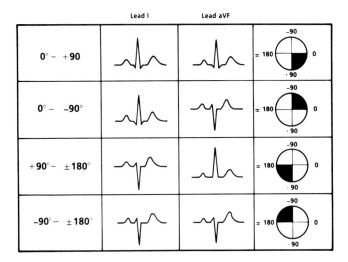

Figure 6-2   Locating quadrants of mean QRS axis from leads I and aVF. (Reproduced with permission from Park MK, Guntheroth WG: *How to Read Pediatric ECGs,* ed 3. St. Louis, Mosby Year Book, 1992, p 13.)

The normal T axis is between 0° to +90°, with the mean of +45°. The abnormal T axis is present when the T wave is inverted in lead I or aVF, usually resulting in a wide QRS-T angle. An abnormal T axis is seen in ventricular hypertrophy with strain, BBB, pericarditis, myocarditis, myocardial ischemia, and intracranial pathology.

The QRS-T angle is the angle formed by the QRS axis and the T axis. Normally the QRS-T angle is usually less than 30°, except in the newborn period. The QRS-T angle of more than 60° may be abnormal and that of more than 90° is certainly abnormal. The abnormal QRS-T angle (> 90°) is seen in severe ventricular hypertrophy with strain, ventricular conduction disturbances, and metabolic or ischemic myocardial dysfunction.

Intervals

The PR interval (measured from the onset of the P wave to the beginning of the QRS complex) has the following characteristics:

1.   The normal PR interval varies with age and heart rate. The older the person is, the slower the heart rate is, and the longer the PR interval is. The mean and upper limits

of normal PR interval according to age and heart rate are presented in Table 6-5.

2. Prolonged PR interval (first-degree atrioventricular block) is seen in myocarditis (viral and rheumatic), congenital heart defects (endocardial cushion defect, atrial septal defect, Ebstein's anomaly), digitalis or quinidine toxicity, hyperkalemia, ischemia or profound hypoxia, and otherwise normal hearts.

3. A short PR interval is seen in Wolff-Parkinson-White (WPW) syndrome, Lown-Ganong-Levine syndrome, or otherwise normal children.

A normal QRS duration is short in the young infant, and it increases with age (Table 6-6). Because the QRS duration increases with a person's age, the definition of ventricular conduction disturbances (such as bundle branch block) should vary with age. A long QRS duration is a characteristic of ventricular conduction disturbances (RBBB, LBBB, WPW syndrome, and intraventricular block), ventricular arrhythmias, and occasionally ventricular hypertrophy.

The QT interval varies only with the heart rate, not with age, except in infancy. Therefore, the QT interval is interpreted in relation to the heart rate (corrected QT interval, QTc). The QTc obtained by the use of Bazett's formula (QT measured/$\sqrt{RR}$ interval) should not exceed 0.44 s, except in infants. A QTc of up to 0.49 s may be normal for the first 6 months of life. Long QT intervals may be seen in hypocalcemia, myocarditis (rheumatic and viral), long QT syndromes (Jervell and Lange-Nielsen syndrome and Romano-Ward syndrome), head injuries or cerebrovascular accidents, diffuse myocardial disease, and drugs (e.g., quinidine and procainamide). Short QT intervals may be seen in hypercalcemia or may be a digitalis effect.

The P Wave

The normal P wave amplitude is less than 3 mm. Abnormally tall P waves are indicative of right atrial hypertrophy. Normal P waves are shorter than 0.09 s in children and 0.07 s in infants less than 12 months of age. Prolonged P waves are seen in left atrial hypertrophy.

THE QRS AMPLITUDE, R/S RATIO, AND ABNORMAL Q WAVES

The QRS amplitude varies with age (see Table 6-3). Large QRS amplitudes are found in ventricular hypertrophy and ventricular conduction disturbances (e.g., BBB and WPW syndrome). Low QRS voltages may be seen in pericarditis, myocarditis, and hypothyroidism, and they are normal in newborns.

Table 6-5 PR Interval with Rate and Age (and Upper Limits of Normal)

RATE	0 to 1 mo	1 to 6 mo	6 mo to 1 yr	1 to 3 yr	3 to 8 yr	8 to 12 yr	12 to 16 yr	Adult
< 60						0.16(0.18)	0.16(0.19)	0.17(0.21)
60 to 80					0.15(0.17)	0.15(0.17)	0.15(0.18)	0.16(0.21)
80 to 100	0.10(0.12)				0.14(0.16)	0.15(0.16)	0.15(0.17)	0.15(0.20)
100 to 120	0.10(0.12)			(0.15)	0.13(0.16)	0.14(0.15)	0.15(0.16)	0.15(0.19)
120 to 140	0.10(0.11)	0.11(0.14)	0.11(0.14)	0.12(0.14)	0.13(0.15)	0.14(0.15)		0.15(0.18)
140 to 160	0.09(0.11)	0.10(0.13)	0.11(0.13)	0.11(0.14)	0.12(0.14)			(0.17)
160 to 180	0.10(0.11)	0.10(0.12)	0.10(0.12)	0.10(0.12)				
> 180	0.09	0.09(0.11)	0.10(0.11)					

Reproduced with permission from Park MK, Guntheroth WG: *How to Read Pediatric ECGs*, ed 3. St. Louis, Mosby Year Book, 1992, p 45.

Table 6-6 QRS Duration: Average (and Upper Limits) for Age

	AGE						
	0 to 1 mo	1 to 6 mo	6 mo to 1 yr	1 to 3 yr	3 to 8 yr	8 to 12 yr	12 to 16 yr	Adult
QRS duration in seconds	0.05(0.07)	0.05(0.07)	0.05(0.07)	0.06(0.07)	0.07(0.08)	0.07(0.09)	0.07(0.10)	0.08(0.10)

Modified and used with permission from Guntheroth WG: *Pediatric Electrocardiography*, Philadelphia, WB Saunders, 1965, p 23.

In infants and children, the R/S ratio is large in V1 and V2 and small in V6 because of the RV dominance seen in this age group. In the adult, the R/S ratio is small in V1 and V2 and is large in V6, reflecting the LV dominance (see Table 6-4 for normal values). Abnormal R/S ratios are seen in ventricular hypertrophy and ventricular conduction disturbances.

The average duration of a normal Q wave is 0.02 s and does not exceed 0.03 s. The maximal Q amplitude in leads aVF, V5, and V6 is usually less than 5 mm in children of any age. It may be as deep as 8 mm in lead III in children younger than 3 years of age. Deep and wide Q waves are seen in myocardial infarction, myocardial fibrosis, and occasionally in hypertrophic cardiomyopathy (QS pattern in V5 and V6). Deep, but not wide, Q waves are seen in association in volume overload lesions (large ventricular septal defect and single ventricle), LV hypertrophy, or combined ventricular hypertrophy.

THE ST SEGMENT AND
T WAVE ABNORMALITIES

A normal ST segment is usually horizontal and isoelectric (at the same level as the PQ and TP segments). In the limb leads, elevation or depression of the ST segment up to 1 mm is not necessarily abnormal. A shift of up to 2 mm is considered normal in V5 and V6. An abnormal ST segment shift may be seen in pericarditis, myocarditis, myocardial ischemia/infarction, severe ventricular hypertrophy (strain), hyperkalemia or hypokalemia, digitalis effects, and intracranial disease.

The normal T wave amplitude in V5 and V6 may be as tall as 11 and 7 mm, respectively, in infants and may be 14 and 9 mm, respectively, in children. Tall, peaked T waves may be seen in hyperkalemia, LV hypertrophy (volume overload type), and cerebrovascular accidents. Flat or low T waves may be seen in normal newborn infants, hypothyroidism, hypokalemia, hyper- or hypoglycemia, pericarditis, myocarditis, myocardial ischemia, and digitalis effects.

ATRIAL HYPERTROPHY

In atrial hypertrophy, abnormalities in the amplitude and/or duration of the P wave are seen.

1. Right atrial hypertrophy: tall P waves (> 3 mm).
2. Left atrial hypertrophy: wide P waves (> 0.10 s in children and > 0.08 s in infants).
3. Combined atrial hypertrophy: a combination of tall and wide P waves.

VENTRICULAR HYPERTROPHY

Ventricular hypertrophy produces abnormalities in one or more of the following areas: QRS axis, QRS voltages, R/S ratio, T axis, and miscellaneous areas.

1. The QRS axis is usually deviated toward the ventricle that is hypertrophied.
2. The QRS voltages increase toward the direction of the respective hypertrophied ventricle.
3. The R/S hypertrophy ratio increases in V1 and V2 and decreases in V6 with RV hypertrophy. With LV hypertrophy, the ratio increases in V6 and decreases in V1 and V2.
4. An abnormal T axis (outside the 0° to +90° quadrant) is seen in severe ventricular hypertrophy with relative ischemia of the hypertrophied myocardium (called "strain" pattern).

Miscellaneous nonspecific changes include: (1) A q wave in V1 is suggestive of RV hypertrophy; (2) an upright T wave in V1 after 3 days of age and in children less than 5 years of age is a sign of probable RV hypertrophy; and (3) deep Q waves (5 mm or greater) or tall T waves in V5 and V6 are signs of LV hypertrophy of the volume overload type.

Criteria for Right Ventricular Hypertrophy

1. Right axis deviation for the patient's age (see Table 6-2).
2. Increased rightward and anterior QRS voltages. R waves in V1, V2, or aVR are greater than the upper limit of normal for patient age (see Table 6-5). The S waves in I and V6 are greater than the upper limit of normal for patient age (see Table 6-3).
3. Abnormal R/S ratio in favor of the RV, in the absence of RBBB (see Table 6-3). The R/S ratio in V1 and V2 is greater than the upper limit of normal (ULN) for age. The R/S ratio in V6 is less than 1 after 1 month of age.
4. Upright T waves in V1 in patients more than 3 days of age (and less than 5 to 6 years), provided the T is upright in V5 and V6.
5. A q wave in V1 (qR or QRS pattern) is suggestive of RV hypertrophy.
6. In the presence of voltage criteria for RV hypertrophy, a wide QRS-T angle with the T axis outside the normal range (usually in the 0° to −90° quadrant) indicates the strain pattern.

RV Hypertrophy in the Newborn

The diagnosis of RV hypertrophy in the newborn is particularly difficult because of the normal dominance of the RV during this period of life. The following clues, however, are helpful in the diagnosis of RVH in newborn infants.

1. Pure R wave (with no S wave) in V1 greater than 10 mm.
2. R in V1 greater than 25 mm or R in aVR greater than 8 mm.
3. A qR pattern in V1 (also seen in 10 percent of healthy newborn infants).
4. Upright T waves in V1 in neonates more than 3 days of age (with upright T in V6) is strongly suggestive of RV hypertrophy.
5. Right axis deviation greater than + 180°.

Criteria for Left Ventricular Hypertrophy

1. Left axis deviation for patient's age (see Table 6-2).
2. QRS voltages in favor of the LV. R waves in I, II, III, aVL, aVF, V5, or V6 greater than the upper limit of normal for age (see Table 6-3). S waves in V1 or V2 greater than the upper limit of normal for age (see Table 6-4)
3. Abnormal R/S ratio in favor of the LV. The R/S ratio in V1 and V2 less than the lower limit of normal for patient's age (see Table 6-4).
4. Q in V5 and V6, 5 mm or greater, coupled with tall symmetric T waves in the same leads (LV volume overload).
5. In the presence of voltage criteria for LV hypertrophy, a wide QRS-T angle with the T axis outside the normal range indicates a strain pattern. This is manifested by inverted T waves in lead I or aVF.

Criteria for Combined Ventricular Hypertrophy

1. Positive voltage criteria for RV and LV hypertrophy (in the absence of BBB or WPW syndrome).
2. Positive voltage criteria for RV or LV hypertrophy and relatively large voltages for the other ventricle.
3. Large equiphasic QRS complexes in two or more of the limb leads and in the midprecordial leads (V2 through V5), called the Katz-Wachtel phenomenon.

VENTRICULAR CONDUCTION DISTURBANCES

Conditions that are grouped under ventricular conduction disturbances have abnormal prolongations of the QRS duration

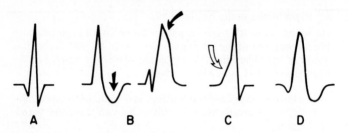

Figure 6-3 Schematic diagram of three types of ventricular conduction disturbances. A, normal QRS complex. B, QRS compexes in right bundle branch block with terminal slurring (black arrows). C, preexcitation with delta wave (open arrow). D, intraventricular block in which the prolongation of the QRS complex is throughout the duration of the QRS complex. (Reproduced with permission from Park MK, Guntheroth WG: *How to Read Pediatric ECGs,* ed 3. St. Louis, Mosby Year Book, 1992, p 76.)

(Fig. 6-3). These conditions include RBBB, LBBB, WPW syndrome, intraventricular block, and an implanted ventricular pacemaker. In BBB (either right or left), the prolongation of QRS duration involves the terminal portion of the QRS complex (terminal slurring). In WPW syndrome, the prolongation is in the initial portion (initial slurring). In intraventricular block, the prolongation is throughout the QRS complex. Note that the normal QRS duration varies with age (see Table 6-6).

Criteria for RBBB

1. Right axis deviation, at least for the terminal portion of the QRS complex.
2. QRS duration longer than the upper limit of normal for the patient's age (see Table 6-6).
3. Terminal slurring of the QRS complex, which is directed to the right and usually, but not always, anteriorly. There are wide and slurred S waves in I, V5, and V6. There is terminal slurring of the QRS complex (with R waves) in aVR, V1, and V2.
4. ST segment shift and T wave inversion are common in adults but not in children.
5. It is unsafe to make a diagnosis of ventricular hypertrophy in the presence of RBBB (or any other ventricular conduction disturbance). Because of the asynchrony of the opposing electromotive forces of each ventricle present in RBBB, a greater manifest potential for both ventricles results.

Although the rsR′ pattern in V1 is unusual in the adult, it is normal in infants and small children provided that the QRS duration is not prolonged, and the voltages of the primary or secondary R waves are not abnormally large.

The two most common examples of the RBBB pattern in pediatric patients are seen in children with atrial septal defect and after open heart surgery involving a right ventriculotomy. In both conditions, the right bundle is usually undamaged. Also, RBBB is associated with Ebstein's anomaly, coarctation of the aorta in infants younger than 6 months, endocardial cushion defect, and otherwise normal children.

Criteria for LBBB (Extremely Rare in Children)

1. Left axis deviation for the patient's age (see Table 6-2).
2. QRS duration longer than the upper limit of normal for age (see Table 6-6).
3. Loss of Q waves in lead I, V5, and V6.
4. The terminal slurring is directed to the left and posteriorly. There are slurred and wide R waves in lead I, aVL, V5, and V6. There are wide S waves in V1 and V2.
5. ST depression and T wave inversion in V4 through V6 are common.
6. QRS voltages may be greater than normal because of the asynchrony of depolarization of each ventricle. Therefore, it is unsafe to make a diagnosis of ventricular hypertrophy in the presence of LBBB.

Intraventricular Block

A prolonged QRS duration is present without the characteristic changes of either RBBB, LBBB, or WPW syndrome. The QRS duration is longer than the upper limit of normal for age and the slurring is throughout the QRS complex. It is associated with metabolic disorders (hyperkalemia), diffuse myocardial disease, severe hypoxia, or drugs (e.g., quinidine and procainamide). Rarely, a prolonged QRS duration may be seen in ventricular hypertrophy.

Criteria for WPW Syndrome

1. A short PR interval, less than the lower limit of normal for the patient's age. (The lower limit of normal of the PR interval according to age is as follows: < 3 years, 0.08 s; 3 to 16 years, 0.10 s; and > 16 years, 0.12 s.)
2. Delta wave (initial slurring of the QRS complex) and wide QRS duration (beyond ULN).

3. The diagnosis of ventricular hypertrophy cannot safely be made.

The WPW syndrome results from an anomalous conduction pathway (bundle of Kent) between the atrium and the ventricle, bypassing the normal delay of conduction in the atrioventricular node. Patients with WPW syndrome are prone to attacks of paroxysmal supraventricular tachycardia.

Two other types of preexcitation are: Lown-Ganong-Levine syndrome, characterized by a short PR interval and a normal QRS duration in patients with episodes of supraventricular tachycardias, and Mahaim-type preexcitation, characterized by a normal PR interval and a long QRS duration with delta wave.

ELECTROLYTE DISTURBANCES

Electrolyte changes can also produce abnormalities in the ECG tracing of otherwise healthy children. The following is a list of potential alterations of the ECG tracing that may be seen when specific abnormalities of cellular electrolyte concentrations occur.

1. Hypocalcemia: prolongation of the ST segment (with resulting prolongation of QT interval, Fig. 6-4).
2. Hypercalcemia: shortening of the ST segment (with resulting shortening of the QT interval, Fig. 6-4).
3. Hypokalemia (Fig. 6-5): with serum K < 2.5 mEq/L, prominent U wave, flat or diphasic T waves, and ST segment depression. Further lowering of serum K may result in prolongation of the PR interval and sinoatrial block.
4. Hyperkalemia: a progressive increase in serum K levels produces the following ECG changes (see Fig. 6-5): tall, tented T waves, best seen in the precordial leads; pro-

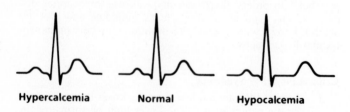

Hypercalcemia   **Normal**   **Hypocalcemia**

Figure 6-4 ECG findings of hypercalcemia and hypocalcemia. (Reproduced with permission from Park MK, Guntheroth WG: *How to Read Pediatric ECGs,* ed 3. St. Louis, Mosby Year Book, 1992, p 107.)

SERUM K

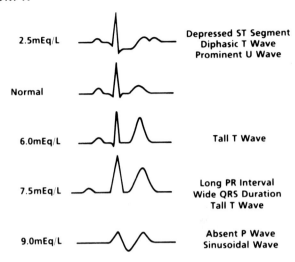

Figure 6-5 ECG findings of hypokalemia and hyperkalemia. (Reproduced with permission from Park MK, Guntheroth WG: *How to Read Pediatric ECGs,* ed 3. St. Louis, Mosby Year Book, 1992, p 108.)

longation of the QRS duration; prolongation of the PR interval; disappearance of the P waves; wide, bizarre biphasic QRS complex (sine wave), and eventual asystole.

BIBLIOGRAPHY

Guntheroth WG: *Pediatric Electrocardiography.* Philadelphia, WB Saunders, 1965.

Park MK: *The Pediatric Cardiology Handbook.* St. Louis, Mosby Year Book, 1991.

Park MK: *Pediatric Cardiology for Practitioners,* ed 2. Chicago, Yearbook Medical, 1988.

Park MK, Guntheroth WG: *How to Read Pediatric ECGs,* ed 3. St. Louis, Mosby Year Book, 1992.

CHAPTER 7

Induction, Emergence, and Extubation

Mary Ann Gurkowski
Deborah K. Rasch

The choice of anesthetic sequence for pediatric patients may vary widely depending on the child's perception of the operation, the parent's level of anxiety, the specific resources available to the anesthesiologist, and both the preexisting medical condition of the patient and the reason for which the child presents to the operating room. In some cases, the parents may be allowed to enter the operating room or induction room with the child. If the parents and child are well prepared, little or no premedication may be necessary, and induction may proceed with the parents escorted from the room after the child has lost consciousness. If premedication is not possible or the parent's anxiety is too great, then care must be taken to minimize the time between separation from the parents and anesthetic induction. Both the parents and child will remember a stormy separation period, and crying increases the risk of laryngospasm during inhalational induction, and the chance of unwanted excitement during emergence. Therefore, for elective cases, the decision of how to proceed with induction depends on the anesthesiologist's rapport with the child and the anticipated degree of patient cooperation. The basic induction techniques include (1) inhalational anesthetics, (2) intravenous medications, (3) rectal barbiturates, and (4) intramuscular ketamine. These methods of routine induction will be described with a short discussion of a few exceptional circumstances that may be encountered in healthy children. Specific recommendations for complex surgical or medical conditions will be discussed elsewhere in this handbook.

INDUCTION METHODS

Volatile Anesthetics

Inhalational Induction

Inhalational induction after premedication with oral midazolam (0.5 mg/kg) is a very common method of inducing anesthesia in the United States. Most children will accept midazolam orally when mixed in sodium citrate or concentrated Kool-Aid (1 mL/kg) fairly readily. This provides good sedation and gastric acid prophylaxis when citrate is used. If the child is cooperative, an inhalational induction can proceed and will provide a very easy and pleasant way for the child to be anesthetized. Many times after premedication, the child may be either very "drunk" or asleep. If the child is actually asleep, the patient should not be disturbed for transfer to the operating table or aroused by a noisy operating room environment. A pulse oximeter probe may be attached without awakening the patient in some cases and will supply information regarding heart rate and saturation during the early phases of induction. A high flow mixture of N_2O/O_2 at a ratio of 7 L:3 L should be administered by allowing the gases to blow over the child's face. Contact with the tubing or a mask may arouse the child; so care must be taken not to touch the face. After 1 to 2 min, halothane 0.25% is introduced and gradually increased by increments of 0.5% with every three to four breaths taken by the child to a maximum of 3 to 3.5%. If the child arouses during the early induction phases, gentle restraint, reassurance, and cuddling of the child will usually prevent undue excitement.

After the child has entered Stage II (altered consciousness and divergent pupils), they may require more forceful restraint, but they will usually have no recall of this situation. At this point in time, monitors can be placed and preparations made for obtaining intravenous (IV) access. The patient must no longer be in Stage II for insertion of the IV catheter because they may develop laryngospasm caused by manipulation during light anesthesia. After the patient is in a surgical plane of anesthesia, the N_2O concentration is often decreased to 50% if intubation is not anticipated. In cases in which endotracheal intubation is planned, the N_2O is discontinued, and the child ventilated with 100% oxygen for several breaths before laryngoscopy is attempted. This maneuver will allow a longer apneic period without hypoxemia, which can be important if the intubation is difficult. After the child has lost consciousness, ventilation may be assisted every three to four breaths, taking care to keep ventilating pressures below 20 cmH_2O when possible, because this will result in less distention of the stomach. If muscle relaxation is planned, ventilation should be controlled to ensure proper oxygenation before laryngoscopy. An oral airway, if necessary, should be inserted gently with a tongue blade, preferably when the patient is more deeply anesthetized, to prevent the oral airway itself from precipitating laryngospasm. Generally, the oral airway can be safely inserted when the eyes are no longer divergent and pupillary size has decreased, indicating that the patient is no longer in Stage II of anesthesia. Unfortunately, the greatest risk for obstruction occurs during the second stage of anesthesia, during which time placement of an oral airway has the highest risk to stimulate airway irritability. In this situation, careful dislocation of the mandible anteriorly by gentle forward pressure using two fingers at the angle of the jaw bilaterally (jaw thrust) is very effective to open the airway and improve ventilation. Lidocaine jelly applied to the end of the oral airway may also improve patient acceptance. Proper sizing of the oral airway is also important. Figure 7-1 illustrates the correct method of choosing an appropriately sized oral airway. Airways that are too large will promote inflation of the stomach or epiglottic compression, and those that are too small will displace the tongue posteriorly and worsen the obstruction.

If the decision has been made to provide anesthesia by mask, glycopyrrolate may be helpful in controlling secretions, which may otherwise cause laryngospasm. When IV access is not available, intramuscular (IM) atropine (0.02 mg/kg) and succinylcholine (3 to 4 mg/kg) may be useful in obtaining relaxation; however, onset requires 3 to 5 min to achieve relaxation for intubation by the intramuscular route. Because laryngospasm is a risk in the child undergoing an inhalational induction, it is wise not to allow the surgeons to begin painful or stimulating procedures (examining broken limbs or removing wound dressings) until the airway is safely established or the child is in a surgical plane of anesthesia.

Another situation that is also conducive to an inhalational induction is the awake or mildly sedated cooperative child who is willing to travel into the operating room (OR) with the anesthesiologist. In this instance, the child is either allowed to sit in the anesthesiologist's lap or on the table. Whether or not monitors are placed on the patient before inhalational induction is begun depends on the age of the patient and the level of cooperation. A quiet environment with constant reassurance is essential. Many children may fear the use of a mask; therefore, a "blow by" technique or allowing the child to place the end of the circuit in his/her mouth is often helpful (Fig. 7-2). Story telling, use of toys, or placing scented oils in the mask or circuit to improve tolerance of the inhalational agents are all useful tricks to help keep the child's attention without frightening him/her. Delays in proceeding with induction after the child is in the op-

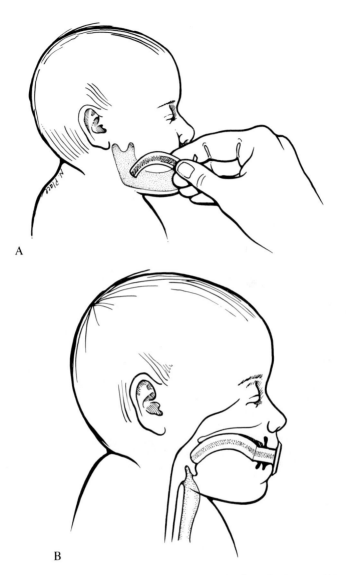

A

B

Figure 7-1 Correct method for sizing of oral airway. (A) When the flanges are located at the lip, the posterior portion of the airway should lie at the angle of the jaw. (B) When in the proper position, the tongue will be moved anteriorly to improve ventilation.

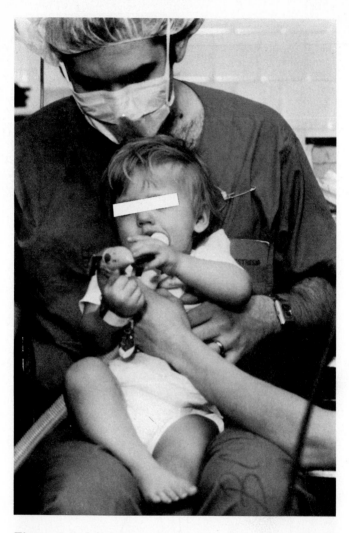

Figure 7-2 Inhalation induction in a child. Some children fear the mask. An alternate method is to remove the mask and allow the child to breathe directly through the anesthetic circuit or to cup the hand around the end of the elbow connector.

erating room should be avoided because they may result in the child losing composure. This means that surgeons need to be readily available, and the OR personnel must have equipment and instruments ready. Most of all, the anesthesia machine and monitors must be carefully checked before the patient is brought into the room.

Inhalational Anesthetic Agents

With regard to the agents used for induction, halothane is the most popular. It is well tolerated by the child, is not irritating to the airway, and causes the least respiratory depression of all currently available gases. Isoflurane has theoretic advantages over halothane. It is less soluble in blood; therefore, alveolar concentrations will rapidly approach the inspired concentration, which should result in a more rapid induction. However, because of the irritating nature of isoflurane, children often cough, hold their breath, and suffer laryngospasm during induction, which actually causes the induction to be prolonged. In addition, the laryngospasm does not appear as responsive to positive end-expiratory pressure as it does under halothane anesthesia. Enflurane is tolerated fairly well, but because of its slow induction, the excitement phase is more pronounced. Also, if the patient is hyperventilated, tonic–clonic seizure activity may result. This agent possesses the most respiratory depressant activity compared with all other currently available gases. Therefore, it is difficult to maintain adequate levels of anesthesia in spontaneously ventilating children without an elevation of pCO_2 in the 50 to 60 mmHg range or greater!

With regard to the cardiovascular system, halothane and enflurane produce a dose-related decrease in cardiac output, whereas isoflurane produces no significant decreases in cardiac output in healthy patients up to two times the minimum alveolar concentration (MAC). Barash and colleagues evaluated the cardiovascular effects of halothane anesthesia in children using an echocardiographic means to evaluate cardiac function. They found that myocardial depression in these children parallels the decrease in blood pressure and was related to both rate and contractility changes. Administration of atropine reversed the rate-dependent changes but did not improve the ejection fraction. Further studies by Neal and associates evaluating isoflurane and halothane anesthesia in children confirmed halothane's myocardial depressant effects but showed that, at end-tidal concentrations of 1.3 MAC and greater, there was a progressive decrease in blood pressure with both agents, although the heart rate remained constant. They concluded that the changes in blood pressure were caused by depression of left ventricular function by halothane and by decreases in systemic vascular resistance by isoflurane. Enflurane has also been shown to produce a dose-related decrease in systemic resistances, whereas halothane has little effect.

Epinephrine Interactions

Another area that deserves mention is the use of epinephrine-containing local anesthetic solutions in the presence of inhalational anesthetics. Halothane is known to sensitize the myocardium to circulating catecholamines, and ventricular extrasystoles may be seen with light anesthesia alone. Johnston and colleagues reported the results of varying epinephrine doses in patients under isoflurane, halothane, and enflurane anesthesia. All patients were adults with American Society of Anesthesiologists class I or II, and ventilation was controlled to prevent hypoxemia or hypercarbia. The 50 percent effective dose (ED_{50}) of epinephrine was defined as the presence of three or more premature ventricular complexes at any time after epinephrine was injected. These results are shown in Fig. 7-3. Using 0.5% lidocaine with epinephrine in adults, they concluded that the

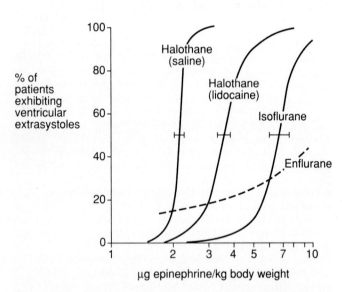

Figure 7-3 The interaction between epinephrine and the inhalational agents. The bars indicate the standard deviation from the 50 percent effective dose. (Reproduced with permission from Johnston RR, Eger EI, Wilson C: A comparative interaction of epinephrine with enflurane, isoflurane, and halothane in man. *Anesth Analg* 1976; 55:711.)

ED_{50} for halothane was 3.7 μg/kg; for isoflurane, 6.7 μg/kg; and for enflurane, 10.9 μg/kg. Since this time, a number of studies have shown that higher doses of epinephrine in children (up to 10 μg/kg) can be used without development of arrhythmias. In one of these studies, 10 mg/mL lidocaine was used as a medium for injecting epinephrine. Certainly, lidocaine can exert an antiarrhythmic effect and protect the myocardium from the interaction between halothane and epinephrine. The other concern is that toxic doses of lidocaine will be injected if 10 μg/kg of epinephrine 1:100,000 is used in these concentrations. Therefore, at our institution, we frequently allow the use of 3 to 4 μg/kg of epinephrine 1:200,000 mixed with 0.5 to 1% lidocaine under halothane anesthesia. If arrhythmias develop, the agent is switched to either isoflurane or enflurane, and the arrhythmia is treated with IV lidocaine 1 mg/kg. If rhythm disturbances persist, then other causes, including hypoxemia, hypercarbia, or acidosis, should be ruled out.

Intravenous Anesthetics

Intravenous Induction, Technique

An intravenous induction may be used for elective cases, but its most common use involves the child suspected of having a full stomach. This method allows a rapid induction of anesthesia and airway protection from aspiration of gastric contents by early insertion of the endotracheal tube. To perform an IV induction, an intravenous line must be inserted with the child awake. This can be facilitated in the holding area with the child's parents present for support, or if both child and parents are very anxious, it may be preferable to place the line in the operating room. Midazolam 0.5 mg/kg orally to a maximum of 20 mg is very helpful to allay anxiety in the child before the needle stick. After access is achieved, a rapid sequence induction under cricoid pressure and intubation of the trachea can be safely performed. Alternatively, in the child who is not an emergency case but who emotionally decompensates in the OR and will not accept the mask for induction, the butterfly technique may allow a face mask to be applied for the administration of an inhalational agent. Some anesthetists prefer the butterfly needle (Fig. 7-4) rather than the insertion of a catheter because it is often quicker and easier to insert and stabilize in the frightened, uncooperative child. After the child is anesthetized, an indwelling intravenous catheter must be inserted. If the child is cooperative for IV placement, the use of 1% lidocaine for local anesthesia of the skin and subcutaneous tissue may lessen the pain when a 22-gauge catheter or larger is inserted, particularly if the placement does not go smoothly. Other alternatives include the use of topical creams, such as

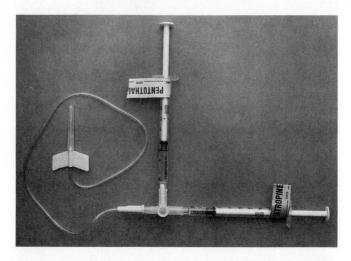

Figure 7-4 Butterfly needle for rapid induction of anesthesia. This method is useful for emergency procedures or in a child who becomes very frightened and uncooperative after arrival in the operating room.

eutectic mixture of local anesthetics (EMLA cream by Astra), before IV insertion. The disadvantage of EMLA cream is that it requires placement 1 h before insertion and should be covered with an occlusive bandage during that time. After the catheter is secured, selection of the induction agents depends on the child's medical and surgical history and the type of operation to be performed. Several drugs can be successfully used for induction, including sodium thiopental, ketamine, propofol, etomidate, and narcotics (Table 7-1).

Barbiturate Anesthetics
Barbiturate anesthetics, primarily sodium thiopental and methohexital, belong to the first group of IV induction agents used in pediatric anesthesia. Of these agents, sodium thiopental is most commonly used and has been shown to be very safe and effective in all pediatric-aged patients. The dose required to achieve an adequate plane of anesthesia for tracheal intubation or to accept bag and mask ventilation with halothane after induction varies depending on premedication and age. Infants younger than 1 month of age require 4 to 5 mg/kg in the unpremedicated state, whereas infants 1 to 6 months of age require much higher doses (6 to 8 mg/kg) under similar circumstances. Jonmarker and associates showed a progressive decrease in induction dose requirement for children aged 6 months to 4 years,

Table 7-1 Comparison of Commonly Used Induction Agents

AGENT	DOSE	ONSET	DURATION	COMMENTS
Propofol	2.5 to 3.5 mg/kg	20 to 30 s	3 to 5 min	Pain on injection, random movements during induction, hypotension possible,† low risk for nausea
Thiopental	4 to 6 mg/kg	20 to 30 s	3 to 5 min*	Hiccoughs common, nausea and vomiting postoperatively in up to 15 percent, hypotension possible,† delayed awakening in neonate
Ketamine	1 to 2 mg/kg	30 to 45 s	10 to 20 min	Increases airway secretions, maintains systemic vascular resistance, elevates intracranial pressure, moderate postoperative nausea
Midazolam	0.6 mg/kg	20 to 30 s	Variable	Unreliable as sole agent to induce anesthesia
Etomidate	0.3 mg/kg	20 to 30 s	3 to 5 min	Myoclonic activity, cardiovascular stability, decreases intracranial pressure

*Except in neonates where elimination may be prolonged.
†Use with care in patients with cardiovascular disease or hypovolemia.

115

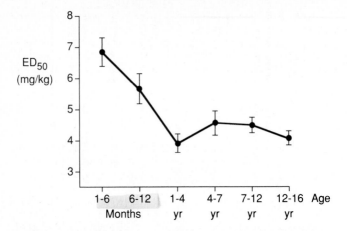

Figure 7-5 Thiopental induction dose requirements relative to age. (Reproduced with permission from Jonmarker C, Westrin P, Larssen S, et al: Thiopental requirements for induction of anesthesia in children. *Anesthesiology* 1987; 67:106.)

at which time, dose requirements seem to stabilize in the 4-mg/kg range (Fig. 7-5). The incidence of cardiovascular side effects, primarily hypotension defined as a 15 to 20 percent decrease in blood pressure from preinduction levels, varies among studies, but appears to be reversed, at least in part, by the simultaneous administration of atropine in healthy neonates and infants. Therefore, thiopental must be used with caution in debilitated infants and those with intravascular volume depletion. In regard to the recovery of consciousness after induction, thiopental's sedative effects may last several minutes to hours. This may result in delayed awakening and contribute to respiratory depression in neonates and young infants postoperatively. This may be the result of the immature hepatic metabolic pathways that lead to a slow final elimination of the drug. Therefore, for short cases in young infants, thiopental may not be the ideal induction agent.

Propofol
Propofol is another induction agent that has been studied and used more recently in pediatric patients. Just as with sodium thiopental, premedication and age have a profound effect on propofol requirements. In a study by Patel and colleagues in children aged 1 to 12 years, the induction dose required in unpremedicated children was 3 mg/kg compared with 2.5 mg/kg in

the group premedicated with trimeprazine 3 mg/kg and atropine 0.03 mg/kg orally 2 h preoperatively. The side effects encountered included moderate to severe pain on injection, random movements, and transient tremors or rigidity. Random movements could be abolished with additional doses of propofol or introduction of halothane anesthesia, and there was no correlation between the dose used and the presence of random movements up to 4.0 mg/kg. Westrin then studied infants 1 to 6 months of age and found them to require a higher dose than older children for tolerance of a mask. Infants required 3.0 mg/kg compared with 2.5 mg/kg for unpremedicated older children.

The reasons for differences in the dosing requirements between this study and other studies in older children was possibly the end point used for satisfactory induction. Apparently some patients continue to have a positive lid reflex after propofol induction, although other measures of a satisfactory induction are present (i.e., tolerance of the face mask without undue movement or agitation). Recovery times in all ages from propofol used at induction are very rapid, as in adults, and it appears to have a lower incidence of nausea and vomiting postoperatively compared with thiopental/halothane/N_2O anesthesia or inhalational anesthesia alone. There was also a decreased need for analgesic medication in the first several hours postoperatively in children when a propofol infusion was used to provide general anesthesia for short ear, nose, and throat procedures compared with thiopental/halothane/N_2O.

There are conflicting reports in the literature regarding the effects of propofol on the cardiovascular system. Westrin found no significant changes in the mean arterial pressure in children and infants receiving propofol for induction when atropine was given preoperatively. Hannallah and associates, on the other hand, demonstrated that 48 percent of children given propofol for induction followed by halothane developed a significant decrease in blood pressure($\geq$ 20 percent of preinduction levels) approximately 4 min after the bolus injection. A lower incidence of hypotension has been reported when N_2O is administered 5 min before adding a potent inhalational agent. The reason for this is unclear, although N_2O is known to have mild sympathomimetic activity. Therefore, as with sodium thiopental, care should be exercised when using propofol in children with cardiovascular disease or hypovolemia.

One of the more limiting problems with propofol in pediatric anesthesia is the pain produced on injection. Use of an antecubital vein instead of small hand veins for injection, pretreatment with lidocaine, and dilution with other intravenous fluids have been reported to help somewhat. However, a significant percentage of children will still become distressed during induction as a result of the irritating nature of the drug.

Midazolam

Midazolam has also been evaluated as an induction agent in children premedicated with narcotic plus atropine. However, even in doses up to 0.6 mg/kg, which produced a significant fall in blood pressure, the children were not reliably anesthetized. Compared with sodium thiopental, the children induced with midazolam were significantly less alert in the recovery room 30 min after termination of the procedure. Therefore, midazolam alone is generally believed to be an unsatisfactory induction agent in children. It can provide a smooth gentle induction in doses of 0.1 to 0.2 mg/kg when combined with fentanyl 10 μg/kg for longer procedures without inducing cardiovascular instability.

Ketamine and Etomidate

Ketamine and etomidate are both useful agents for inducing anesthesia rapidly and reliably in pediatric patients who are at risk for hypotension but who require rapid sequence induction and intubation. Ketamine given either IV or IM is safe for use in infants and children with cyanotic congenital heart disease (see Chap. 26) and in patients with pericardial effusion because there appears to be an augmentation of right heart function and pulmonary dilation with maintenance of systemic vascular resistance. The induction dose of ketamine is 1 to 2 mg/kg intravenously, and it should be accompanied by 0.01 mg/kg of atropine or 0.005 mg/kg of glycopyrrolate to prevent the increased salivation that may lead to laryngospasm. Therefore, because of hypersensitive airway reflexes induced by ketamine, it is not an appropriate choice for induction in a pediatric patient who may have a difficult airway. With regard to cardiovascular effects, ketamine actually has a direct dilating effect on vascular smooth muscle. This is usually overcome by sympathetic stimulation, resulting in little or no change in systemic vascular resistance. In critically ill children in whom catecholamine stores may be depleted, ketamine can be a cardiovascular depressant. Other situations in which ketamine is not an appropriate choice for anesthetic induction are in children with intracranial disease, a history of seizures, or increased intraocular pressure. It produces increased intracranial pressure, increased cerebral blood flow, and elevated cerebrospinal fluid pressures and has been reported to induce seizures in epileptic patients. Ketamine has been used safely in children undergoing tonometry, but it is usually not chosen as the induction agent for children with an open globe injury because increases in intraocular pressure are documented. All other IV induction agents are safe for use in patients undergoing ophthalmologic surgery. However, ketamine is a preferred agent for induction in children with asthma or in those at risk for bronchospasm, because ketamine has a bronchodilating effect on bronchial smooth muscle.

Etomidate 0.3 mg/kg is a very effective induction agent in pediatric neurosurgical patients and in those with hypovolemia or cardiovascular disease. As with benzodiazepines, barbiturates, and propofol, etomidate produces a decrease in cerebral oxygen requirements and intracranial pressure in a dose-related fashion. Its hemodynamic stability is desirable in these patients because cerebral perfusion pressure is more easily maintained. Compared with other rapidly acting anesthetic induction agents (e.g., barbiturates, ketamine, and propofol), etomidate produced the least hemodynamic variability, even in patients with known hypovolemia or sepsis. The only drawback to etomidate is the myoclonic spasms that sometimes occur with anesthetic induction before the onset of muscle relaxation. These movements do not represent seizure activity, are not detrimental to the patient, and do not interfere with ventilation or oxygenation. When rapid endotracheal intubation is intended, succinylcholine is the preferred muscle relaxant for use with etomidate because more forceful myoclonus, which has been reported to occur, can elevate intragastric pressure. This increases the risk of reflux and possibly aspiration pneumonia.

Intramuscular or Rectal Induction

Intramuscular Ketamine

Intramuscular ketamine can be given at any time during the transition from parents to the induction of anesthesia in the operating room if the child becomes irritable, combative, or begins to cry. In this situation, an inhalational induction might best be abandoned because it is much more pleasant for the child, parents, and anesthesiologist to consider an alternate mode of induction. Ketamine 3 to 5 mg/kg mixed with atropine 0.01 to 0.02 mg/kg is an alternative. Given IM in the deltoid muscle or vastus lateralis, the child will become calm within 2 to 3 min. The method of injection employs a 23-gauge needle on a 1-mL or 3-mL syringe, depending on the size of the child. The thumb is placed over the plunger, and the syringe is held like a dart. The child is then pricked with the needle, and the full amount injected without aspiration. By the time the child realizes he/she has been pricked, the sedative effects of the ketamine are beginning. This sequence results in minimal trauma to the child and a more pleasant separation from the parents. After sedation is achieved, the induction can be completed by the intravenous route after access is obtained or by using an inhalational agent. Atropine (0.02 mg/kg) is given in conjunction with ketamine to prevent the increase in secretions that may occur from the sympathomimetic actions of the drug. Because these secretions may lead to laryngospasm and airway obstruction, ketamine should not be administered unless oxygen, suction, and airway equipment are readily available.

Rectal Ketamine or Methohexital

Rectal ketamine or methohexital are other alternatives for induction of the uncooperative or frightened child. This route is used to sedate the child so that he/she can be quietly separated from the parents and transported into the operating room. The induction is then completed by either insertion of an intravenous catheter and administration of IV drugs or, more commonly, by using an inhalational agent. A rectally administered drug does not provide adequate anesthesia for intubation, and the child may still respond to IV placement. The most common drug given rectally is methoxital (1% or 10% solution), but ketamine (5 to 10 mg/kg) has also been used. The dose of methohexital varies, but we have had the most success using a 1% solution (15 mg/kg) for short cases and the 10% solution (25 to 30 mg/kg) for longer cases. The 1% solution, even though it has a lower concentration of drug, appears to have a more rapid onset (3 to 8 min) versus the 10% solution (10 to 15 min). This rapid onset is probably related to the fact that the larger volume delivers more drug to the colonic wall for absorption compared with the smaller volume of more concentrated drug that may be injected into stool. When the drugs are given rectally, methohexital has a faster and more predictable onset of sedation than ketamine. Rectally administered drugs provide a relatively quick and painless means for the child to fall asleep with the parents in attendance. Some older children do complain of rectal fullness, but this disappears as sedation begins. Other disadvantages include failure to sedate because of the poor bioavailability of the drug (i.e., injection into stool), defecation, and delayed recovery from anesthesia in short cases. This latter point is controversial, and in many situations, the small increase in time delay to enter the OR while waiting for the agent to work or in delaying discharge from the recovery room or outpatient facility because the child is still sedated are acceptable side effects if the agent allows for a gentle controlled induction. Remember, however, even a rectally administered induction agent can cause apnea. Do not leave a child, even with the parents present, after the drug has been administered. All inductions should be done in an area that has ready access to suction, oxygen, a positive pressure ventilation system, and airway equipment.

EMERGENCE AND EXTUBATION

Near the end of the surgery, preparations must be made for weaning the child from the general anesthesia and, often, controlled ventilation to an awake state with adequate spontaneous ventilation. The inhalational agents should be discontinued in a timely fashion, realizing that it will take several minutes to clear the agent from the child's system. Muscle relaxants must be adequately reversed. In children, a strong train-of-four should be present, but in an infant, a train-of-four stimulus may be difficult to interpret because neonates may demonstrate fade to a train-of-four stimulus before exposure to any muscle relaxant caused by immaturity of the neuromuscular junction.

Before extubation, the child should be allowed to breathe 100% oxygen at high flow rates. This process results in a well-oxygenated patient at extubation, such that if airway obstruction or laryngospasm occur during extubation, more time is allowed for correction of the problem before hypoxemia occurs. If the child has been hyperventilated, the $PaCO_2$ needs to increase to within the normal range (36 to 45 mmHg) before spontaneous ventilation will return. If the child has a full stomach, then he/she must be extubated when fully awake. It is advisable in all children, but especially in those with a full stomach, to pass an oral gastric tube or place a nasogastric tube and suction before extubation.

During emergence from anesthesia, infants and children often become restless, making it very important to keep one hand securely on the endotracheal tube to avoid accidental extubation. It is also important to ask an assistant to guard the intravenous line in an actively moving child because emergence and extubation are two common times when IV access may be lost.

Patterns of Emergence

Eye signs can be followed to determine the anesthetic depth. When deeply anesthetized, the eyes will be midline and the pupils approximately 3 mm unless narcotized. As the child begins to emerge from anesthesia, he/she will enter what is commonly called Stage II. In Stage II, the eyes will become dysconjugate (no specific direction), and the pupils may dilate. The pupillary dilation is the result of an increase in sympathetic output but may be blunted if narcotics were used intraoperatively. It is important to remember that, during Stage II, pediatric patients are more prone to laryngospasm, breath holding, and are still not able to protect their airway if vomiting were to occur. Do not extubate a child at this stage. As the sequence of emergence continues, children may pass in and out of Stage II several times. Clinically, this phenomenon is more frequent with iso-flurane than with enflurane or halothane, as is airway irritability evidenced by cough and laryngospasm. Semipurposeful movements, frowning, and conjugate eye signs generally indicate that the child is awake enough to extubate with little risk of laryngospasm and, in most cases, awake enough to maintain a patent airway.

Muscle relaxant reversal in an adult or older child is best determined by a strong hand grip and head lift for 5 s. An infant will not follow such commands, but if they can spontaneously lift their legs to create a 90° angle of flexion at the hips, then muscle strength adequate for ventilation has returned. A nerve stimulator should always be used first to determine if the reversal can be given and, then after the reversal is given, to determine the effectiveness of the reversal agents. The best location to test for muscle relaxant reversal is at the ulnar nerve at the wrist while observing the contraction of the thumb. The facial muscles represent a group whose resistance to muscle relaxation closely resembles the diaphragm. Therefore, overdosage of muscle relaxants is possible if the train-of-four stimulus is being monitored along the facial nerve. Another precaution in infants when using a nerve stimulator is that direct muscle stimulation may occur, which can lead to muscle relaxant overdosage. Therefore, a nerve stimulator with variable output should be used, and the output set at less than 40 mA.

Extubation Technique

Extubation can be performed after the child is spontaneously breathing (> 10 breaths/min for older children and ≥ 20 breaths/min for infants), shows signs of adequate muscle relaxant reversal, has a temperature of more than 35°C, and has emerged from Stage II (eyes are conjugate, no breath holding when the endotracheal tube is slightly moved, and swallowing or sucking on the endotracheal tube is present).

To prepare for extubation, the child should be breathing 100% oxygen. A face mask, functioning IV line, intubating dose of succinylcholine and atropine, appropriate-sized endotracheal tube, and laryngoscope blade should all be readily available for emergency reintubation. It is not always necessary to suction the endotracheal tube before extubation, but if suctioning has been performed, be sure to place the child back on 100% oxygen for a few assisted breaths before extubation. It is important to suction the oral cavity and posterior pharynx before extubation. An infant, especially those younger than 3 months of age, may need to have the nares gently suctioned with a soft suction catheter. They are obligate nose breathers and can become obstructed if the nares are blocked. Secretions can irritate the vocal cords and cause laryngospasm. The stomach should be emptied with an oral gastric tube before extubation if the patient has a full stomach or has swallowed air, blood, or irrigation fluid at some point in the procedure. Although this does not guarantee an empty stomach, it will lessen the chances of aspiration, may improve ventilation if the stomach is distended, and will lessen the incidence of postoperative nausea.

When extubating the child, give an assisted breath on inspiration and pull the endotracheal tube at the end of inspiration. This will fill the lungs with oxygen and, on exhalation, clear the airway of secretions. Some anesthesiologists will instill 2 to 3 mL of 2% lidocaine into the endotracheal tube to help prevent laryngospasm just before extubation. This should not be done in a child with a full stomach because it may blunt their protective reflexes.

If a child develops laryngospasm after extubation, application of continuous positive pressure (10 to 15 cmH$_2$O) to the airway using a face mask will often relieve the spasm. If unable to eliminate laryngospasm within seconds using this technique, then atropine (0.02 mg/kg IV) and succinylcholine (1 mg/kg IV or 4 mg/kg IM) will allow for improved ventilation and provide good relaxation for reintubation if necessary. If the child obstructs on extubation from the tongue adhering to the palate or the posterior pharynx, a jaw thrust, which will pull the tongue forward and open the airway, is often very effective. A nasal trumpet may be used but may cause undesirable nasal bleeding, especially in a younger child with enlarged adenoids. In addition, a nasal trumpet in a young child has a very small lumen and may obstruct easily with secretions, although reinsertion of an oral airway may be difficult because of trismus.

On certain occasions, it may be beneficial to the child to perform a deep extubation, that is, open globe surgery on the eye or tympanoplasty, because coughing and straining may endanger the results of surgery. In these cases, the child must be spontaneously breathing (100% fraction of inspired oxygen), and the inhalational anesthetic agent should be continued at anesthetic concentrations. The oropharynx and stomach should be suctioned very carefully because any secretions left behind may precipitate laryngospasm as the child emerges. Pretreatment with atropine or glycopyrrolate may lessen this problem. Lidocaine 2% at a dose of 2 to 3 mg/kg may be instilled before extubation to help prevent laryngospasm, but if the child is not still deeply anesthetized, the lidocaine may precipitate coughing and breath holding. As with awake extubation, a positive pressure breath should be given as the endotracheal tube is removed to prevent aspiration of secretions that may be pooled around the glottic opening. A tight-fitting face mask with 100% fraction of inspired oxygen should be reapplied to the face to document good air exchange by feeling the bag move and listening for breath sounds. After a good respiratory pattern is established, the inhalational agent is discontinued and the patient allowed to awaken. Laryngospasm, breath holding, and airway obstruction from the tongue or other pharyngeal structures may occur as the muscle tone increases and the depth of respiration improves. A gentle jaw thrust, as described during the induction of anesthesia, or the placement of oral or nasal airways may be necessary, particularly if the child developed airway obstruction during induction. After the child is awake and purposeful movements have returned, the child may be transported.

Finally, when transporting a child to the recovery room, the patient should be on his/her side or stomach. This position decreases the risk of airway obstruction during transport. It allows the tongue to fall forward and secretions to drain out of the mouth instead of into the posterior pharynx where they may cause airway irritability. A gentle chin lift or jaw thrust may further open the airway to promote good air exchange. Always assure yourself the child has good chest excursions before proceeding to the recovery room. It is a good idea to leave the precordial stethoscope on the chest during transport and always clinically to monitor ventilation during transport to and on arrival in the recovery room. It is always safest to transport the child to the recovery room with blow-by oxygen to minimize the risk of desaturation. If oxygen is not used for transport, its application should be the first duty performed on arrival at the recovery room.

BIBLIOGRAPHY

Ausinch B, Rayburn RL, Munson ES, et al: Ketamine and intraocular pressure in children. *Anesth Analg* 1976; 55:773–776.

Barash PG, Glanz S, Katz JD, et al: Ventricular function in children during halothane anesthesia: An echocardiographic evaluation. *Anesthesiology* 1978; 49:79–85.

Berry FA: *Anesthetic Management of Difficult and Routine Pediatric Patients.* New York, Churchill Livingstone, 1986, pp 13–55.

Borgeat A, Popovic V, Meier D, et al: Comparison of propofol and thiopental/halothane for short duration ENT surgical procedures in children. *Anesth Analg* 1990; 71:511–515.

Calvery RK, Smith NT, Jones CW, et al: Ventilatory and cardiovascular effects of enflurane anesthesia during spontaneous ventilation in man. *Anesth Analg* 1978; 57:610–614.

Fisher DM, Robinson S, Brett C: Comparison of enflurane, halothane and isoflurane for pediatric anesthesia. *Anesthesiology* 1984; 61:A427.

Hannallah RS, Baker SP, Casey W, et al: Propofol: Effective dose and induction characteristics in unpremedicated children. *Anesthesiology* 1991; 74:217–219.

Idvall J, Holasek J, Stenberg P: Rectal ketamine for induction of anaesthesia in children. *Anaesthesia* 1983; 38:60–64.

Johnston RR, Eger EI, Wilson C: A comparative infraction of epinephrine with enflurane, isoflurane, and halothane in man. *Anesth Analg* 1976; 55:709–712.

Jonmarker C, Westrin P, Larsson S, et al: Thiopental requirements for induction of anesthesia in children. *Anesthesiology* 1987; 67:104–107.

Karl HW, Swedlon DB, Lee KL, et al: Epinephrine, halothane interactions in children. *Anesthesiology* 1983; 58:142–145.

Kettler D, Sonntag H, Donath U, et al: Haemodynamic, myocardial function, oxygen requirements and oxygen supply to the human heart after administration of etomidate. *Anaesthetist* 1974; 23:116–118.

Laishley RS, O'Callahan AC, Lerman J: Effects of dose and concentration of rectal methohexitone for induction of anaesthesia in children. *Can J Anaesth* 1986; 33:427–432.

Liu LM, Gaudrealt P, Friedman PA, et al: Methohexital plasma concentrations in children following rectal administration. *Anesthesiology* 1985; 62:567–570.

Markku S, Kanto J, Iisalo E, et al: Midazolam an induction agent in children: A pharmacokinetic and clinical study. *Anesth Analg* 1987; 66:625–628.

Mirakhur RK: Induction characteristics of propofol in children: Comparison with thiopentone. *Anaesthesia* 1988; 43:593–598.

Neal MB, Peterson MD, Gloyna D, et al: Hemodynamic and cardiovascular effects of halothane and isoflurane anesthesia in children. *Anesthesiology* 1984; 61:A437–A448.

Patel DK, Keeling PA, Newman GB, et al: Induction dose of propofol in children. *Anaesthesia* 1988; 43:949–952.

Ryan JF, Coté CJ, Todres ID, et al: *A Practice of Anesthesia for Infants and Children.* New York, Grune and Stratton, 1986, pp 77–104.

Salonen M, Kanto J, Iisalo E: Induction of general anesthesia in children with midazolam: Is there an induction dose. *Int J Clin Pharmacol Ther Toxicol* 1987; 25:613–615.

Tweed WA, Minuck M, Mymin D: Circulatory responses to ketamine anesthesia. *Anesthesiology* 1972; 37:613–615.

Veda W, Hirakawa M, Mae O: Appraisal of epinephrine administration to patients under halothane anesthesia for closure of cleft palate. *Anesthesiology* 1983; 58:574–576.

Westrin P: The induction dose of propofol in infants 1-6 months of age and children 10-16 years of age. *Anesthesiology* 1991; 74:455–458.

Westrin P, Jonmarker C, Werner O: Thiopental requirements for induction of anesthesia in the neonate and in infants 1-6 months of age. *Anesthesiology* 1989; 71:344–346.

CHAPTER 8

The Pediatric Patient in the Postanesthesia Care Unit

Dawn E. Webster

After completion of a successful general or regional anesthetic, the pediatric patient continues to require close supervision. The following is a discussion of some of the common problems encountered in children during the early postoperative period. Recommendations for management are also provided. Airway obstruction, vomiting, laryngospasm, and agitation are all common problems that may have disastrous results if they are not recognized and managed early.

POSTOPERATIVE PLANNING

Postoperative care begins preoperatively during the patient evaluation. The patient's condition, medical history, and scheduled procedure are all factors in determining whether a child may be a satisfactory candidate for outpatient surgery, whether postoperative hospital admission or apnea monitoring is required, or whether admission to the intensive care unit might be desirable. In the latter two instances, the availability of appropriate monitors or of an intensive care unit bed should be confirmed to prevent delays. In addition, children who may require prolonged ventilation may be identified at this time. These plans may be modified during the intraoperative period as changes in the surgical procedure, complications, or the patient's condition dictate.

TRANSPORT

Transport to the Postanesthesia Care Unit (PACU) is a critical time. Airway obstruction, hypoventilation, hypoxia, and a host of other problems may occur at this time. In extubated patients, transport should occur only after the patency of the airway and the adequacy of respiration have been confirmed. The lateral position is favored for transport to encourage pooling of secretions in the side of the mouth rather than in the posterior pharynx where they may produce laryngospasm or be aspirated into the child's lungs. Studies have shown a high incidence (21 to 28 percent) of unrecognized low oxygen saturation in pediatric patients transported to the PACU while breathing room air; it is now common practice to transport pediatric patients with supplemental oxygen. Patients who are to remain intubated should remain sedated and carefully restrained during transport. If ventilation is accomplished using a modified Mapleson D system attached to an oxygen tank, a self-inflating bag should be readily available if, for any reason, the oxygen source is lost. All equipment and drugs that may be needed for rapid reintubation should also be within easy reach of the anesthesiologist during transport.

Monitoring during transport depends on the judgment of the anesthesiologist. A healthy, sleeping, or sedated child may be monitored with a precordial stethoscope and careful attention to clinical parameters, such as chest wall movement and skin color. Critically ill children may require as many monitors for transport as they did for intraoperative care, possibly including pulse oximetry, electrocardiography (ECG), and blood pressure monitoring. Infants and children should be transported with guard rails up and careful attention lest they decide to escape from the crib or bed!

Intravenous (IV) access is easily lost during transport of the awake, healthy child. Carefully checking and securing the IV line before moving the child may help to prevent this complication. The lost or infiltrated IV may be a minor issue in an awake child who recovers quickly and can take fluids readily, but it may be a serious problem in the child who develops respiratory or cardiac compromise on arrival in the PACU and requires urgent intervention.

Care should be taken to maintain temperature homeostasis during transport. Heated transport units are available for newborn and premature infants, which permit easy observation of the infant while ensuring a warm environment. These units should be plugged in and kept warm during the operative procedure. Older infants and children should be covered with a warm blanket when traveling through cold hallways.

ARRIVAL

On arrival in the PACU, continue to administer oxygen. A towel wrapped around thick corrugated oxygen tubing and pointed at the child's face is tolerated better than most face masks, tents, or nasal cannulas. Reevaluate the patency of the airway and the adequacy of ventilation of the extubated child. If the child is intubated and is placed on a ventilator, the presence of bilateral

Table 8-1   Report to PACU

Type of surgery
Current medical problems
Significant MH or SH
Medications (antibiotics given and when due)
Allergies
Premedications
Anesthesia agents/techniques (i.e., was a caudal block placed
    after the procedure?)
Blood loss and fluid replacement
Problems during surgery or anesthesia
Anticipated problems

MH = medical history; SH = surgical history.

breath sounds and chest wall excursion should be confirmed
and the adequacy of the ventilator settings for that particular
child, reevaluated. End-tidal CO_2 monitoring and pulse oximetry are useful tools in these cases. Minimal monitors in the
PACU should include noninvasive blood pressure monitoring,
pulse oximetry, and ECG.

After the respiratory status is confirmed and the monitors
are placed, the patency and security of any vascular access
lines should be determined. A disconnected arterial or even IV
line may result in rapid, significant blood loss. For optimal care,
a complete report should be given to the nurse who will be caring for the patient. Recommended topics to include in the report
are listed in Table 8-1.

SPECIFIC PROBLEMS IN THE
POSTANESTHESIA CARE UNIT

Pain

Postoperative pain varies for a given procedure and patient.
There is no "right" amount of pain for a procedure, and a child
who complains of pain should always be believed. Many children are either unwilling or unable to complain of pain; so it is
important that the anesthesiologist maintain a high index of suspicion for this problem. If the amount of pain a patient is ex-
periencing seems unusual, an evaluation for the causes of pain,
other than the operative procedure, should be sought, for example, sharp instruments left under the patient, Foley catheters, traction on a chest tube or drain, a full bladder, and compartment syndrome after orthopedic procedures. Chapter 18
discusses the evaluation of pain in the infant, preverbal, and
young child more fully. Pain is a noxious stimulus and requires
treatment for that reason alone. It may also cause tachycardia,

hypertension, nausea, vomiting, and anxiety and may exacerbate emergence delirium.

The mainstay of postoperative pain relief is pharmacologic. Acetaminophen (10 to 15 mg/kg) may be all that is needed in some cases. For more severe pain, IV narcotics are frequently used. Infants older than age 3 months have no more predilection to respiratory depression after narcotics than do adults, and narcotics should not be withheld during the acute postoperative period because of an exaggerated fear of this complication. Infants younger than 3 months of age may require more intensive monitoring for respiratory depression and judicious titration of narcotics, but they also should have the benefit of postoperative pain relief. Patient-controlled analgesia is very useful in the adolescent population, who appreciate having some sense of control over their environment. It has also been used successfully in younger patients. Patient and family selection are very important when this modality is used. Family (and visitors) must be educated to never "push the button" for the sleeping or sedated child who seems uncomfortable. In all cases, intramuscular injections should be avoided in the pediatric patient when an oral or IV route for analgesic administration is available. Table 8-2 includes some commonly used postoperative analgesics and doses. Whenever opioids are used, monitoring for respiratory depression and drugs and airway equipment for intervention must be readily available.

Ideally, postoperative pain can be abolished or attenuated intraoperatively by the use of appropriate local, topical, or regional anesthetics. For example, the pain of circumcision is markedly reduced by the use of either the penile block or topical administration of lidocaine jelly. The pain of herniorrhaphy may be reduced by caudal block or infiltration of the wound with 0.25% bupivacaine. Regional techniques may be employed in many cases. Blocks that have been used with success include caudal, femoral, ilioinguinal, iliohypogastric, penile, and intercostal nerve blocks; interpleural catheters; brachial plexus blocks; and epidural anesthesia. These are discussed in more detail in Chap. 10. Generally, regional techniques are performed on heavily sedated or anesthetized children because the positioning, immobility, and needle sticks involved may be frightening and uncomfortable to the young child. The use of opioids or infusions of local anesthetics into the epidural or intrathecal space can extend postoperative pain relief long into the recovery period; this should be done only when the patient is to remain an inpatient and may be monitored for apnea.

In addition to pain at the operative site, sore throat pain and headache are common postoperative complaints. The incidence of sore throat has been reported as high as 91 percent. Although traditionally associated with intubation, it is present in up to 28

Table 8-2 Starting Doses for Postoperative Analgesia

DRUG	DOSE
Acetaminophen	10 to 15 mg/kg PO q 4 h or PR q 4 h
Codeine	0.5 to 1 mg/kg PO q 4 h
Fentanyl	0.5 to 2 μg/kg IV q 1 to 2 h
Morphine	0.05 to 0.1 mg/kg IV q 2 h or 0.2 to 0.4 mg/kg PO q 4 h
Meperidine	0.8 to 1 mg/kg IV q 2 h or 0.8 to 1.3 mg/kg IM/SC q 3 to 4 h
An example of:	
Starting PCA pump settings	0.025 mg/kg morphine sulfate, 15-min lockout time, 4-h maximum of 0.4 mg/kg (may be used with continuous infusion to provide pain relief during sleep)
Starting morphine sulfate infusion	15 μg/kg/h after a 20 to 30-μg/kg bolus to achieve adequate drug levels for pain relief
Ketorolac tromethamine	1 mg/kg load, then 0.5 mg/kg every 6 h IV
Naloxone drip	3 to 10 μg/kg/h

PO = oral; q = every; PR = rectal; IV = intravenous; IM = intramuscular; SC = subcutaneous; PCA = patient-controlled analgesia.

percent of patients who were not intubated. The presence or absence of an oral airway does not appear to be implicated in the development of sore throat, but vigorous suctioning may contribute because sore throat was more common when blood was found on suction apparatus. The incidence of headache is about 12 percent. Both may be treated with nonnarcotic analgesics such as acetaminophen 10 to 15 mg/kg.

Myalgias may occur in the pediatric postoperative patient also. These are usually related to the intraoperative use of succinylcholine and may be minimized by pretreatment with curare or atracurium.

Agitation

Agitation on emergence occurs in as many as 15 percent of pediatric patients. The exact cause of this phenomenon is unknown, although it may be exacerbated by the presence of pain. Although pain relief and the presence of a parent may readily treat the majority of these cases, we must be sure to exclude serious causes of agitation, including respiratory or cardiovas-

Table 8-3   Causes of Agitation in the PACU

Hypoxemia
Hypercarbia
Hypotension (poor cerebral perfusion)
Hypoglycemia
Hyponatremia
Increased intracranial pressure
Excitatory drugs (ketamine or scopolamine)
Pain
Emergence delirium from inhalation anesthetics

cular insufficiency and glucose or electrolyte abnormalities. Table 8-3 lists possible causes of agitation in the PACU.

Nausea and Vomiting

Postoperative nausea and vomiting remains a big problem in pediatric anesthesia. The incidence has been reported to be from 10 to 48 percent and up to 80 percent in patients recovering from strabismus surgery. An increased risk has been noted in the latter (up to 80 percent) and in patients undergoing orchiopexy, herniorrhaphy, tonsilloadenoidectomy, middle ear surgery, and prolonged procedures (greater than 2 h). In addition, inexperienced airway management during induction leading to inflation of the stomach, premature oral fluids, and early postoperative ambulation are also contributory factors.

Prevention of postoperative nausea and vomiting begins in the operating room, where the stomach should be emptied with an orogastric tube and adequate hydration ensured before transport to the PACU. In certain cases, the perioperative use of antiemetic prophylaxis with droperidol, metoclopramide, or ondansitron is warranted, as in strabismus patients.

Treatment of nausea and vomiting in the PACU begins by avoiding the premature introduction of oral fluids. Hunger appears to be a better sign than thirst that the child is ready for fluids. If a child becomes nauseated on changing position, the adequacy of volume replacement should be evaluated, and an IV fluid challenge attempted. If nausea persists, promethazine 0.25 to 0.5 mg/kg or metoclopramide 0.1 mg/kg (max: 5 mg) may be administered. If vomiting persists, volume and electrolyte disturbances may occur and may require treatment with IV fluids.

Delayed Awakening

Prolonged drowsiness after an anesthetic is usually the result of a residual narcotic or inhalational anesthetic effect. Knowledge

Table 8-4   Delayed Awakening in the PACU

Hypoxemia
Hypercarbia
Hypovolemia (poor cerebral perfusion)
Hypoglycemia
Residual anesthetic
Residual neuromuscular blockade
Increased intracranial pressure
Water or electrolyte imbalance
Postictal state
Malignant hyperthermia

of the patient's medical history and intraoperative course and a physical examination of the patient may lead the anesthesiologist to suspect a more serious underlying disorder. In these instances, a blood glucose, electrolyte, and arterial blood gas analysis and a careful examination to exclude other disorders is called for. Possible causes of delayed awakening are found in Table 8-4.

Respiratory Insufficiency

At all times during the recovery phase, transport, arrival in the PACU, and PACU stay, the adequacy of ventilation must be ensured. Respiratory insufficiency may present as anxiety, agitation, unresponsiveness, tachycardia, bradycardia, hypertension, cardiac arrhythmias, or arrest. The patency of the airway and the adequacy of ventilation must be evaluated continuously during the recovery phase by the use of capable nursing personnel who are familiar with the pediatric patient and comfortable with the pediatric airway and by monitoring with pulse oximetry. When called to the PACU to evaluate a child exhibiting any of these aforementioned problems, the anesthesiologist must have a high index of suspicion concerning the adequacy of ventilation. Table 8-5 contains a summary of frequent causes of respiratory insufficiency in the postoperative period.

Inadequate ventilation occurs because of central respiratory depression, muscle weakness, or upper airway obstruction. The most commonly encountered problem is upper airway obstruction caused by displacement of the tongue posteriorly against the palate or enlarged adenoids and tonsils. The patient may demonstrate absent or diminished breath sounds with evidence of respiratory effort. The obstruction may be relieved by positioning the patient on the side, thrusting the jaw forward, and/or gently placing an airway. Oral airways are not well tolerated in conscious patients but may be useful in the child who has been extubated "deep." Nasal airways may precipitate adenoidal bleeding and should never be forced into position. A cut endotracheal tube measuring from the tragus of the ear to the ipsilateral naris can serve as a nasal airway.

Laryngospasm may occur at any time during transport to or stay in the PACU and can quickly become a life-threatening event. The child may present with rapidly decreasing oxygen saturation and absent breath sounds despite respiratory effort. It is treated as it would be during the induction of anesthesia, that is, with displacement of the mandible forward (jaw thrust) and positive pressure ventilation with 100% oxygen. Succinylcholine is the muscle relaxant of choice for the treatment of laryngospasm. An intubating dose is 2 mg/kg; however, it is possible to relax the laryngeal musculature and allow positive pressure ventilation with smaller doses (0.5 mg/kg). Atropine may be used to prevent or reverse a succinylcholine-induced bradycardia. Bradycardia that does not immediately respond to improved oxygenation may respond to atropine but will sometimes require epinephrine. (In neonates, epinephrine is the drug of choice.) The decision to intubate is variable and will depend on the individual child and the circumstances leading to the laryngospasm. Laryngospasm can be caused by the presence of secretions or blood in the airway, by stimulation from oral or nasal airways, or by an improperly timed extubation. If the cause of the laryngospasm will still be present after the muscle relaxant wears off (i.e., continued bleeding or secretions), intubation may be preferable.

Patients with obstructive sleep apnea pose a special problem in the PACU because they are prone to obstruction when sedated from an anesthetic. If they have had a tonsilloadenoidectomy to correct their sleep apnea, the tissues may still be edematous, and the musculature lax. Therefore, they are still at risk for obstruction and apnea. These patients should receive no narcotics during the operative period and should have narcotics titrated very carefully during the postoperative period. They may require frequent maneuvers to relieve airway obstruction and require careful attention.

Postintubation stridor usually occurs within 2 h of extubation. It is most common in children aged 1 to 4 years and is associated with a tightly fitting endotracheal tube, traumatic intubation, movement of the head during surgery, neck surgery, and prolonged intubation. Children with Down's syndrome are also at increased risk. Prevention of postintubation stridor begins in the operating room by ensuring that there is a leak between 15 and 25 cmH$_2$O pressure around the endotracheal tube. A tightly fitting endotracheal tube needs to be exchanged for the proper size. Minimize trauma to the airway during intubation and head movement during the case, if at all possible. Dexamethasone (0.2 to 0.4 mg/kg) before extubation may be

Table 8-5 Common Causes of Respiratory Insufficiency in the PACU

TYPE	CAUSE	TREATMENT	COMMENTS
Upper airway obstruction	Secretions	Administer O_2, suction	
	Residual anesthetic resulting in inability to maintain airway	Administer O_2, reposition head, oral airway reintubation in some cases	
	Edema of tongue and soft tissues	Administer O_2, oral airway if not contraindicated by surgical procedure, may require reintubation	Most common in cleft palate repair, pharyngeal reconstructive surgery, tonsillectomy
	Laryngospasm	Administer O_2, positive pressure ventilation, may need muscle relaxant and reintubation, suction secretions	May be caused by secretions aggravated by Stage II anesthesia

| Subglottic obstruction or pulmonary complications | Postextubation subglottic edema | Cool mist, racemic epinephrine 0.05 mL/kg dose of 2.25% solution diluted to 3 mL with normal saline and administered by nebulizer. Do not administer more frequently than every 2 h. Rebound airway edema may occur. Dexamethasone (for severe cases): loading dose, 0.5 mg/kg; maintenance dose, 1 mg/kg/day given in divided doses every 6 h | Contributing factors: tube size, movement of head, duration of case, age of patient, traumatic intubation |
| | Bronchospasm | Administer O_2, inhalational bronchodilator treatment, aminophylline, terbutaline, isoprotenol drip (extreme cases), steroids (extreme cases), doses (see Chap. 3) | |

(Continued)

Table 8-5 *(Continued)*

TYPE	CAUSE	TREATMENT	COMMENTS
Decreased respiratory effort or efficiency	Residual neuromuscular block	Administer O_2, reverse block, reintubate, and ventilate until block wears off. If necessary; aminoglycosides and polymyxins may potentiate an incompletely reversed neuromuscular block	
	Residual narcotics	Administer O_2, intravenous naloxone 5 to 10 μg/kg, reintubate and ventilate until residual narcotic effect is gone, if necessary	
	Pain on inspiration	Pain relief	
	Restrictive bandages	Revise dressings appropriately	
	Abdominal distention	Decompress stomach with nasogastric or orogastric tube	

136

useful in children who are at risk for developing airway edema. In addition, these children should receive humidified oxygen-enriched mist in the recovery room. Treatment of postextubation stridor with 2.25% racemic epinephrine 0.05 mL/kg to a maximum of 0.5 mL, administered by hand-held nebulizer, may improve the symptoms. The use of racemic epinephrine in post-extubation stridor is associated with a rebound effect during which the symptoms may return. For this reason, these patients should be observed carefully for 4 to 6 h after treatment. If they require a second dose of racemic epinephrine, they require continued observation, which usually results in hospital admission and overnight observation.

Premature and ex-premature infants are at increased risk for postoperative apnea and require 24-h apnea monitoring after an anesthetic. Controversy exists as to the exact cutoff age at which apnea monitoring is no longer indicated. At our institution, we admit any ex-premature infant younger than 60 weeks postconceptual age and any other infant with a history of apnea for observation and apnea monitoring. Although the use of caffeine (10 mg/kg) has been demonstrated to control apnea in ex-premature infants between 37 and 44 weeks postconceptual age who have not received narcotics, this does not replace the need for careful postoperative monitoring. Infants anesthetized with a regional technique also fall under the same monitoring guidelines.

Other causes of respiratory insufficiency or respiratory distress in the PACU include atelectasis, aspiration, pulmonary edema, pneumothorax, and preexisting pulmonary disease. A current or recent upper respiratory infection also increases the risk of respiratory complications encountered in the postoperative period.

Cardiovascular Instability

The most frequent cardiovascular problem encountered in the pediatric postoperative patient is hypotension. Arrhythmias, hypertension, and oliguria may also occur and will also be discussed.

Bradycardia in the pediatric patient may be caused by hypoxia, a vagal response to stimulation (suctioning), or drugs such as narcotics. Rarely, bradycardia may be cardiac in origin or may be the result of elevated intracranial pressure. Any child with bradycardia should be evaluated immediately for possible hypoxemia. Pulse oximetry readings and physical examination will usually allow a quick evaluation for hypoxemia. The presence of or a history of vagal stimuli and the medication record should then be sought. Treatment of bradycardia depends on the cause. If the child is hypoxic, improved oxygenation should result in a rapid increase in the heart rate. If it does not or if bradycardia is related to narcotic or cardiac disease or does not cease when vagal stimulation is stopped, atropine 0.02 mg/kg may be used. Bradycardia resistant to atropine should be treated with epinephrine 0.1 mL/kg of a 1:10,000 solution if the child is unstable.

Sinus tachycardia may be caused by pain, hypovolemia, or inadequate ventilation. The treatment depends on the cause. If ventilation is assessed as adequate, attention should be directed to the child's volume status. This is best evaluated by assessing end-organ perfusion, that is, urine output, skin temperature, capillary refill time, and central nervous system perfusion. Blood pressure evaluation may also be helpful, although older infants and children can maintain a normal blood pressure in the face of volume depletion by peripheral vasoconstriction. Inadequate replacement of intraoperative or ongoing fluid losses may be corrected by fluid boluses of colloid or nonglucose-containing isoosmotic crystalloid solutions at 5 to 20 mL/kg, depending on the degree of volume resuscitation that is needed. Generally, if the child is not hypotensive, 5 mL/kg boluses may be repeated until the volume status is optimal. If the child is hypotensive, a 25 mL/kg bolus will be well tolerated by most children. Pain relief has already been discussed.

Arrhythmias other than sinus arrhythmia, sinus tachycardia, and bradycardia are infrequent in children and warrant immediate investigation.

The most common reason for hypotension is hypovolemia from inadequate intraoperative volume replacement. If the hypotension does not resolve with volume resuscitation or does not make sense from the evaluation of the patient's fluid intake and output, the patient should be evaluated for ongoing blood loss.

Hypertension is less frequent than hypotension and may be spurious if the blood pressure cuff in use is the improper size. The cuff should cover two-thirds the length of the patient's upper arm. Hypervolemia, pain, and a distended bladder are common causes of postoperative hypertension, but hypercarbia from inadequate ventilation should also be considered. If none of these factors is present, underlying renal or cardiac disease (i.e., coarctation of the aorta) may be suspected. A summary of causes of hypo- and hypertension in the PACU is covered in Table 8-6.

Oliguria is usually a result of hypovolemia. A urine output of 1 mL/kg/h usually indicates that the volume status is adequate. If a Foley catheter is present, it should be checked and irrigated and the bladder palpated before oliguria is assumed. The child with no Foley in place may not urinate because of a loss of the voiding reflex and may have a full bladder. Diuretics

Table 8-6   Causes of Hypotension and Hypertension in the PACU

Hypotension
  Hypovolemia
  Drugs
  Myocardial depression
  Increased temperature (vasodilation)
  Interference with venous return:
    Tension pneumothorax
    Pericardial tamponade
    Compression of intravenous catheter

Hypertension
  Too small blood pressure cuff
  Hypervolemia
  Pain
  Distended bladder
  Hypercarbia
  Drugs (ketamine)
  Underlying disease (renal, endocrine, or coarctation)

should not be given to treat oliguria unless the patient shows clear signs of volume overload (pulmonary edema or enlarged heart on chest x-ray).

Temperature Abnormalities

Hyperthermia in the PACU may be caused by overwarming, bacterial sepsis, dehydration, pneumonia or other underlying infection, a pyrogenic reaction to the infusion of blood products, and malignant hyperthermia. The elevated temperature may be treated with acetaminophen, cooling blankets, use of a fan, and if necessary, ice packs. If the elevated temperature does not respond quickly to these measures or if signs of hypermetabolism (tachycardia or tachypnea) or the patient's history or examination indicates, further workup may require an arterial blood gas analysis, chest x-ray, blood cultures, and possibly a complete blood count. Malignant hyperthermia is discussed thoroughly in Chapter 16. It can occur in the PACU, and a high index of suspicion is necessary for rapid detection and treatment.

Hypothermia is usually a result of inadequate intraoperative warming. It may result in acidosis and cardiac depression, apnea (in small infants), prolonged action of muscle relaxants, delayed awakening, and shivering. It is best prevented, but if it occurs, it should be treated with warming lights. Warming lights must be kept far enough from the skin to prevent burns. Extubated patients should be watched for any evidence of apnea or muscle weakness. Intubated patients should remain intubated until they are normothermic.

Glucose Abnormalities

Blood glucose levels usually remain stable or slightly increased during surgery in older infants and children. Small infants and newborns may require glucose measurement intra- and post-operatively. A low blood glucose level may be treated with an infusion of 5 to 7 mg/kg/min of dextrose. There is no absolute value accepted by the American Academy of Pediatrics for "hypoglycemia." Frequently used guidelines include 36 mg/dL for full-term infants and 20 mg/dL in premature babies.

If glucose-containing solutions are administered intra- or postoperatively to the older infant or child, hyperglycemia may result. This may cause an osmotic diuresis resulting in hypovolemia. Hyperglycemia also aggravates neuronal injury in the setting of global cerebral insult. This may be deleterious if an untoward event occurs resulting in hypoxia.

DISCHARGE GUIDELINES

Before discharge from the PACU, the child must be fully awake and have no evidence of untreated surgical or anesthetic complications. The Aldrete scoring system used in adults (Table 8-7) is not easily applied to infants and small children. An alternative scoring system called Steward's postanesthetic score (Table 8-8) may be used. A full score and stable vital signs are recommended before discharge. Careful consideration is involved in the disposition of the patient to an appropriate place. The child who requires an apnea monitor or pulse oximeter needs to be placed in a location that is close to the nurses' station or in an intermediate care setting. Most neonatal and pediatric intensive care patients return to their previous beds. Provisions should be made early (i.e., before the patient is anesthetized) for an intensive care unit bed for the child who requires extensive nursing care in the postoperative period. A child who has had a spinal, epidural, or caudal anesthetic should show evidence of a receding block in addition to other parameters for discharge. Provisions for postoperative pain management (patient-controlled analgesia pump, centrally administered opioids, opioid infusions, or other) should be ensured before discharge.

Patients discharged to the outpatient unit and then to home require special consideration because they will receive no further monitoring on leaving the outpatient unit. It is essential that these children be carefully evaluated. At our institution, day-surgery patients recover in the same unit as inpatients.

Table 8-7   Aldrete Postanesthesia Recovery Score

CRITERION	SCORE
Activity	
Able to move four extremities voluntarily or on command	2
Able to move two extremities voluntarily or on command	1
Able to move no extremities voluntarily or on command	0
Respiration	
Able to breathe deeply and cough freely	2
Dyspnea or limited breathing	1
Apneic	0
Circulation	
BP ± 20 percent of preanesthetic level	2
BP ± 20 to 50 percent of preanesthetic level	1
BP ± 50 percent of preanesthetic level	0
Consciousness	
Fully awake	2
Arousable on calling	1
Not responding	0
Color	
Pink	2
Pale, dusky, blotchy, jaundiced, other	1
Cyanotic	0

Reproduced with permission from Aldrete JA, Kroulik D: A post-anesthetic recovery system for the post-operative recovery room. *Can Anaesth Soc J* 1975; 22:111.

They are then discharged to the day-surgery unit for further, less intensive observation and preparation for home. Before discharged home from the outpatient unit, day-surgery patients must be observed long enough to ensure that they do not develop late respiratory complications (3 to 4 h) from intubation. They should have no evidence of respiratory compromise (stridor, wheezing, dyspnea, cyanosis, retractions or nasal flaring, or croupy cough). They should exhibit an intact gag and swallow reflex, minimal nausea and vomiting, and the ability to retain oral fluids. They should have no evidence of dehydration. They should have minimal to no dizziness. The activity level (e.g., ambulation or crawling) and consciousness level must be consistent with normal activities for that individual child.

All day-surgery patients must have an escort home. The adult who is to take them home and care for them should be

Table 8-8 Steward's Postanesthesia Scoring System

CRITERION	SCORE
Consciousness	
Awake	2
Responding to stimuli	1
Not responding	0
Airway	
Coughing on command or crying	2
Maintaining good airway	1
Airway requires maintenance	0
Movement	
Moving limbs purposefully	2
Nonpurposeful movements	1
Not moving	0

Reproduced with permission from Steward G: Steward's postanesthesia scoring system. *Can Anaesth Soc J* 1975; 22:111.

responsible and capable of understanding and following postoperative instructions. Caretakers should understand that their child may not attain a usual level of activity for 1 to 2 days after surgery and that sore throat, nausea and vomiting, and headaches are fairly common. They should be instructed in the management of their child's pain using medications prescribed by the surgeon, and they should be instructed about indications for bringing the child back to the emergency room or surgery center (vomiting and inability to take oral fluids, respiratory distress, bleeding, development of a high fever or rigidity, or change in level of consciousness). If a regional block has been used (i.e., an axillary block for postoperative analgesia for upper extremity surgery), the parent must be taught to protect the child from hurting themselves because the child will have no or a limited pain reflex. The caretaker should also receive instructions on wound care and follow-up surgical or medical care. Instructions should be both verbal and written, and a phone number to call for questions should be included.

CONCLUSION

The postoperative period can be as stressful for the pediatric patient as the preoperative period because of pain, strange surroundings, and separation from parents. The practice of allowing one parent into the PACU as soon as the child is awake and stable is to be encouraged. Careful attention to the child's respiratory and cardiovascular status and to pain management is critical to a safe and comfortable stay in the PACU.

BIBLIOGRAPHY

Abramowitz MD, Oh TH, Epstein BH: The antiemetic effect of dro-peridol following strabismus surgery in children. *Anesthesiology* 1983; 59:579–583.

Amar D, Brodman E, Winikoff S, et al: An alternative oxygen deliv-ery system for infants and children in the post anesthesia care unit. *Can J Anaesth* 1991; 38:149–153.

Berde CB, Lehn BM, Yee DJ, et al: Patient-controlled analgesia in children and adolescents: A randomized, prospective comparison with intramuscular administration of morphine for postoperative analgesia. *J Pediatr* 1991; 118:460–466.

Berde CB, Todres ID: Recovery from anesthesia and the postopera-tive recovery room, in Ryan J, Todres D, Coté C, Goudsouzian N (eds): *A Practice of Anesthesia for Infants and Children*. New York, Grune & Stratton, 1986, pp 261–270.

Berry F: Anesthesia complications occurring primarily in the very young, in Benumof J, Saidman L (eds): *Anesthesia and Perioper-ative Complications*. Chicago, Mosby Year Book, 1992, pp 548–571.

Chripko D, Bevan JC, Archer DP, et al: Decreases in arterial oxygen saturation in paediatric outpatients during transfer to the postan-aesthetic recovery room. *Can J Anaesth* 1989; 36:128–132.

Epstein B, Hannallah R: Gregory G (ed): *Outpatient anesthesia,* in *Pediatric Anesthesia,* ed. 2. New York, Churchill Livingstone, 1989, 727–766.

Hannallah RS: *Ambulatory Surgery for Pediatric Patients: ASA Re-fresher Course Lectures.* Philadelphia, JP Lippincott, 1991, 172.

Hartwell PN: Recovery room care. *Int Anesthesiol Clin* 1983; 21:107–114.

Hertzaka RE, Gauntlett IS, Fisher DM: Fentanyl-induced ventila-tory depression: Effects of age. *Anesthesiology* 1989; 70:213–218.

Jung D, Mroszczak E, Bynum L, et al: Pharmacokinetics of ketorolac tromethamine in humans after intravenous, intramuscular, and oral administration. *Eur J Clin Pharmacol* 1988; 35:423–425.

Koka BV, Jeon LS, Andre JM, et al: Post intubation croup in chil-dren. *Anesth Analg* 1977; 56:501–505.

Laycock GJ, McNicol LR: Hypoxaemia during recovery from anaes-thesia: An audit of children after general anaesthesia for routine elective surgery. *Anaesthesia* 1988; 43:985–987.

Liu LMP, Coté CJ, Goudsouzian NG, et al: Life threatening apnea in infants recovering from anesthesia. *Anesthesiology* 1983; 59:506–510.

McConachie IW, Day A, Morris P: Recovery from anaesthesia in children. *Anaesthesia* 1989; 44:986–990.

Mikawa K, Maekawa N, Goto R, et al: Effects of exogenous intra-venous glucose on plasma glucose and lipid homeostasis in anes-thetized children. *Anesthesiology* 1991; 74:1017–1022.

Olkkola KT, Maunuksela EL: The pharmacokinetics of postopera-tive intravenous ketorolac tromethamine in children. *Br J Clin Pharmacol* 1991; 31:182–184.

Patel RI, Norden J, Hannallah RS: Oxygen administration prevents hypoxemia during post-anesthetic transport in children. *Anesthe-siology* 1988; 69:616–618.

Patel RI, Rice LJ: Special considerations in recovery of children from anesthesia. *Int Anesthesiol Clin* 1991; 29:55–68.

Patel RI, Hannallah RS: Anesthetic complications following pediatric ambulatory surgery: A 3-yr study. *Anesthesiology* 1988; 69: 1009–1012.

Shannon M, Berde CB: Pharmacologic management of pain in children and adolescents. *Pediatr Clin North Am* 1989; 36:855–872,

Soliman IE, Patel RI, Ehrenpreis MB, et al: Recovery scores do not correlate with postoperative hypoxemia in children. *Anesth Analg* 1988; 67:53–56.

Wachta MF, Jones MB, Lagueruela RG, et al: Comparison of ketorolac and morphine as adjuvants during pediatric surgery. *Anesthesiology* 1992; 76:368–372.

Watcha MF, Simeon RM, White PF, et al: Effect of propofol on the incidence of postoperative vomiting after strabismus surgery in pediatric outpatients. *Anesthesiology* 1991; 75:204–209.

Wright TE, Orr RJ, Haberkern CM, et al: Complications during spinal anesthesia in infants: High spinal blockade. *Anesthesiology* 1990; 73:1290–1292.

CHAPTER 9

Fluid Balance in Pediatric Anesthesia

Deborah K. Rasch
Bonny Carter

Fluid balance is one of the primary concerns facing the anesthesiologist when caring for children in the operating room. Certain basic facts are valid in the management of children despite the many differences and continuing changes in the maturing child. Regardless of age, circulating blood volume must be maintained at a normal level to prevent activation of the body's homeostatic mechanisms. These homeostatic mechanisms impair peripheral tissue oxygenation to provide blood flow to essential organs. Just as in adults, pediatric patients respond to regional hypoxia, surgery, and trauma by a translocation of fluid from the intravascular compartment to a third-space compartment, both in the injured tissues and, in severe cases, to a generalized accumulation that is not retrievable by the body's homeostatic forces to offset the intravascular losses. Those losses must also be calculated and replaced adequately. When the affected cell membranes regain their integrity, this fluid then shifts back into the vascular compartment and relative fluid overload occurs, which must also be managed. Therefore, the differences in body fluid composition at varying ages will be discussed and a rational approach to fluid therapy will be outlined.

GENERAL CONSIDERATIONS

Cardiovascular System

The cardiovascular system is an important consideration for judging perioperative fluid requirements, although it is not the limiting factor in fluid and electrolyte therapy of the infant and child, with the rare exception of those patients with structural heart disease. There are specific differences between adult and infant cardiovascular dynamics that have a bearing on fluid management. Infant myocardium has fewer contractile elements, and the cellular arrangement is poorly organized, with the myofibrils having a more random orientation than in the adult heart. Furthermore, the cardiac sympathetic innervation is not fully developed at birth. In in vitro experiments, these differences correspond to reduced compliance and reduced contractile force compared with the mature myocardium.

The hemodynamic effects produced by this immaturity of the infant myocardium are still not clearly defined. It is thought that the fetal heart performs at or near its peak capacity, even during normal conditions, and has a very limited ability to change stroke volume. Therefore, fetal and neonatal cardiac output should be almost entirely dependent on heart rate. However, this premise has been recently questioned in fetal and neonatal lamb studies and in human fetal and neonatal studies.

If it is true that the heart rate is the primary determinant of cardiac output, then maintaining or increasing demands on the heart can only be met by increasing the heart rate and not by adjustments in stroke volume. The heart rate is also the most sensitive guide to fluid replacement because blood pressure is maintained in children until more than 10 percent of body water is lost, but the heart rate progressively increases with this increasing fluid loss. The final comment regarding the cardiovascular system in children is the fact that anatomic right to left shunts may exist at the atrial or pulmonary arterial levels, which make the child at risk for air embolism directly into the arterial circulation. Therefore, care must be taken to remove all bubbles from intravenous (IV) tubing before fluids are infused. This includes the air frequently found in the injection ports of intravenous fluid administration sets.

Renal Maturation

Renal maturation is the limiting factor in fluid and electrolyte balance during the first few weeks of life. The glomerular filtration rate (GFR) at birth is 15 to 30 percent of normal adult values. Adult values are reached by approximately 1 year. By day 5 of life, however, a relatively rapid maturation occurs, and by 1 month of age, the term infant's kidneys have reached 80 to 90 percent of adult capacity. Specific deficiencies during the first weeks of life include obligatory salt loss and inability to concentrate the urine maximally. Because of this low GFR and decreased concentrating ability, newborns tolerate water deprivation or salt loads poorly.

Obligatory Salt Loss

Infants given free water only without a maintenance of 3 to 4 mEq/kg/day of NaCl will become hyponatremic, even in the absence of the stress of surgery. Urinary sodium excretion continues despite a decreasing serum Na^+ concentration. The cause of this salt wasting is unknown, because antidiuretic hormone, cortisol, and aldosterone levels are normal.

Reduced Concentrating Ability

The other problem with the immature renal system involves inadequate concentrating ability. The adult kidney has a concentrating capacity of 1000 to 1400 mosm/kg, whereas neonates can produce urine with a concentration of only 700 mosm/kg during the first week of life. The neonatal kidney responds appropriately to both exogenous and endogenous vasopressin. Limitations to the concentrating capacity of the kidney are multifactorial. An important factor is increased renal prostaglandin E_2 synthesis, which can interfere with vasopressin-mediated water permeability of the collecting duct and reduce the medullary gradient by impairing the movement of urea out of the tubular fluid into the medullary interstitium, inhibiting NaCl transport along the ascending thick limb and increasing juxtamedullary blood flow to produce washout of the gradient.

Glucosuria, observed often at birth and during postnatal life in normoglycemic infants less than 30 weeks gestational age, decreases with postnatal age as the extracellular fluid compartment decreases, but the glomerulotubular balance for glucose occurs from birth even in preterm infants. Neonates appear to have a lower threshold for glucose, such that only mildly increased serum glucose levels may result in glycosuria and an osmotic diuresis.

The combination of obligatory salt loss and inability to concentrate puts the infant with immature renal function at even greater risk for dehydration. In preterm infants, renal function matures somewhat slower, although by 1 month postdelivery, even a 30- to 32-week preemie can attain nearly adult functional levels. Fluid loss (and hence replacement requirement) is related to insensible fluid loss, urine output, and metabolic rate. Insensible fluid losses are relatively high during infancy, a major factor being the high level of minute ventilation. Fluid losses are increased by the use of radiant heat and phototherapy. Because of the infant's proportionally increased water turnover and limited ability to concentrate urine and conserve water, dehydration develops rapidly when intake is restricted or losses occur. Therefore, rather than being more susceptible to overhydration, infants are at greater risk for dehydration when kept without oral intake (NPO) for elective procedures or when they have been vomiting or not eating well in the preoperative period.

Table 9-1   Body Water as a Percent of Total Body Weight

AGE	PERCENT TBW (%)	PERCENT ECF (%)
Premature infant	90	50 to 60
Term infant	75 to 80	40
2 mo to 1 yr	75	40
1 yr to adolescence	70	30
Adult	60	20

TBW = total body water; ECF = extracellular fluid as a percent of total body water.

Body Fluid Distribution

Another consideration when managing pediatric fluid require-ments is the fact that total body water and, thus, the extracel-lular fluid compartment represent a larger portion of body weight compared with the adult (Table 9-1). In addition, esti-mated blood volume and hematocrit differ with age (Table 9-2). Therefore, calculations must be adjusted depending on the age and weight of the patient when transfusion is necessary. That is, a newborn with a hematocrit of 33 percent would be con-sidered severely anemic, and transfusion may be appropriate before transport to the operating room. On the other hand, a 3-month-old otherwise healthy infant with a hematocrit of 29 percent would be considered normal and would not be a can-didate for transfusion until the hematocrit dropped into the 22 to 25 percent range, provided the hemodynamics were stable.

These physiologic differences in body fluid distribution pre-dispose the infant to an even greater risk for dehydration when abnormal losses occur or when maintenance fluids are withheld such as during the NPO interval before anesthesia and surgery. With these considerations in mind, we can now discuss a ra-tional approach to fluid management, including preoperative

Table 9-2   Blood Volume and Hematocrit at Varying Ages

AGE	ESTIMATED BLOOD VOLUME (mL/kg)	HEMATOCRIT (%)
Premature infant	90	40 to 50
Term infant	80	50 to 60
3 mo	80	30 to 35
6 mo to 1 yr	80	35 to 40
1 yr to adolescence	70 to 75	35 to 40
Adult	55 to 65	40 to 45

and intraoperative deficits and maintenance fluids. The most important premise to remember is that fluids obey a dose–response relationship, and administration should be subject to change on a minute-to-minute basis.

MAINTENANCE FLUIDS

Rate of Administration

There are several ways to calculate daily requirements for fluids and, thus, an hourly rate for IV fluid administration. One of the easiest methods is the rule of 4-2-1 (Table 9-3). This method allows rapid assessment of fluid requirements with the use of only one variable, that is, weight.

Another way to calculate fluid maintenance is by the use of surface area. A normogram is necessary for estimating the surface area from known height and weight variables and, therefore, may require a little more time for computation. The maintenance fluid requirement is estimated at 1500 mL/m²/day. This method may be preferable for patients with intracranial hypertension from a mass effect or head injury and those with renal insufficiency because it results in a more conservative estimate of fluid administration rates. Table 9-4 gives a listing of estimated surface areas according to age and weight.

Composition

Maintenance electrolyte requirements must also be taken into account when formulating perioperative fluids (Table 9-5). Fortunately, we do not have to calculate these separately because dextrose 5% in 0.2% saline with 20 mEq KCl added to each liter satisfies this requirement when given at maintenance rates according to the previous formulas. For rates of infusion faster than twice maintenance, as might be necessary for rehydration

Table 9-3   Maintenance Fluids: 4–2–1 Rule

WEIGHT	INTRAVENOUS FLUID RATE
10 kg	4 mL/kg/h
11–20 kg	40 + 2 mL/kg/h for every 1 kg weight over 10 kg
> 20 kg	60 + 1 mL/kg/h for every 1 kg weight over 20 kg

Adapted from Firestone L, Leibowitz P: *Clinical Anesthesia Procedures of the Massachusetts General Hospital.* Boston, Little Brown, 1988, p. 398.

Table 9-4   Age, Weight, and Surface Area Approximations

AGE	WEIGHT (kg)	SURFACE AREA
Birth	3.0	0.2
6 mo	7.5	0.35
1 yr	10.0	0.5
5 yr	20.0	0.75
8 yr	30.0	1.00
Adult	70.0	1.73

of an infant with pyloric stenosis, the glucose content should be reduced or a sugar-free solution piggybacked into the intravenous lines to prevent hyperglycemia and glucosuria, which would defeat the purpose of giving extra IV fluids.

There is some controversy regarding the administration of glucose intraoperatively because hyperglycemia may be detrimental in low perfusion states. Adult studies suggest that the neurologic outcome after cardiopulmonary arrest is improved in those patients who had normal or only slightly elevated serum glucose levels. Certainly, serum glucose concentrations greater than 150 mg/dL are often associated with glycosuria and an osmotic diuresis. The ideal glucose concentration is not known, but probably levels between 80 to 200 mg/dL would provide adequate serum levels of glucose without inducing diuresis. Other problems associated with hyperglycemia include reduced phagocytic function and delayed gastric emptying. The latter of these may add significant risk to the induction of or emergence from general anesthesia.

The argument for the use of glucose stems from the fact that the newborn infant's metabolic rate, oxygen consumption, and cardiac index are almost double that of the adult and they have reduced hepatic glycogen stores, which predisposes them to hypoglycemia. Early studies would suggest that the incidence of hypoglycemia in infants and children younger than age 5 years who are not receiving glucose infusions was as high as

Table 9-5   Daily Electrolyte Requirements
for Infants

ELECTROLYTE	CONCENTRATION
Na^+	2 to 3 mEq/kg/day
Cl^-	3 to 5 mEq/kg/day
K^+	2 to 4 mEq/kg/day
Glucose	100 to 200 mg/kg/h

15.2 percent. In the same study, the incidence was 28 percent in those below a body weight of 15 kg. More recently, these statistics have been challenged, suggesting that, in otherwise healthy infants, only the very young infant (younger than 2 months of age) is at risk for hypoglycemia. Perhaps the best way to judge the need for glucose is to follow serum values in longer cases or where prematurity, young age, chronic debilitating conditions, hyperalimentation, or liver disease put the patient at increased risk.

PREOPERATIVE DEFICIT

Assessment

Pediatric fluid management should begin at the time of the preoperative visit to assess the patient's state of hydration. In routine elective cases, this is easy to calculate by knowing the maintenance fluid rates and the number of hours NPO. In hospitalized patients, the assessment of hydration status may be somewhat more complicated, and both acute and chronic deficits must be evaluated. Acute deficits may exist in the form of, for example, hemorrhage, burns, profuse osmotic diuresis from contrast material for CT scan or cardiac catheterization, or peritonitis. Chronic deficits, such as nasogastric tube losses, vomiting, diarrhea, perspiration (cystic fibrosis), or cerebrospinal fluid losses from repeated lumbar puncture or ventriculostomy, produce less recognizable changes in cardiovascular status than acute losses and are, therefore, harder to quantify. The bedside physical examination and a review of intake and output sheets are invaluable for making decisions regarding appropriate fluid management. Table 9-6 describes physical findings that

Table 9-6   Physical Signs of Dehydration

AGE OF CHILD (yr)	PERCENT DEHYDRATION	PHYSICAL FINDINGS
< 10 (> 10)	5% (3%)	No specific findings, child appears wan and drawn to parents
< 10 (> 10)	10% (6%)	Sunken eyes, no tears, dry mucous membranes, tachypnea, tachycardia, may have poor tissue turgor
< 10 (> 10)	15% (9%)	Vascular collapse with hypotension and altered sensorium

can help quantify the degree of intravascular volume depletion in a child. Bedside nursing notes can be extremely informative, especially in those patients hospitalized more than 24 h. Pay careful attention to weight and intake/output records. Normal weight gain in pediatric patients is 30 to 50 g per day when eating a full diet. One gram of weight lost or gained is essentially equal to 1 mL of fluid. With regard to intake and output, we can expect a difference of 400 to 500 mL/m²/day because of insensible loss through evaporation. Excess loss may denote dehydration, or excess gains may represent fluid overload, depending on the initial body fluid status of the patient.

Urine output in the normal child without cardiovascular or renal disease should be at least 1 mL/kg/h when adequate hydration is present. For abnormal losses, such as vomiting and diarrhea, losses should be replaced with the following solutions at a rate of 1 mL replaced for each milliliter lost.

1. Fecal losses: colon, 24 to 90 mEq/L Na⁺; small bowel, 120 to 130 mEq/L Na⁺.
2. Nasogastric losses: 50 to 70 mEq/L Na⁺.
3. Isotonic fluid loss: Na content is the same as plasma. Occurs in peritonitis, trauma, and burns. 120 to 150 mEq/L Na⁺.
4. Fever: 10 to 14 percent over maintenance fluid requirements should be given for every degree rise in temperature above 38.5°C.

In pediatric patients, the heart rate is the vital sign that is the most sensitive to changes in intravascular volume. In older children, the tilt test may be helpful, that is, blood pressure readings taken in supine and sitting positions. Decreases in blood pressure from supine to sitting of 15 percent or heart rate increases of 10 to 15 percent are considered significant for intravascular dehydration. In these cases, 10 to 20 mL/kg of isotonic fluids should be given and the test repeated before anesthetic induction is undertaken. Physical characteristics, capillary refill (normal less than 1.5 s), skin turgor, and clinical examination of the fontanel and orbits are also important clues of fluid status. In cases of fluid deficit or overload, the fontanel and orbits are one of the first areas to show water loss or gain by tissues. This occurs because the interstitial fluid compartment acts as a "volume buffer." Within 4 to 6 h of plasma loss, fluids shift from the interstitial fluid compartment to plasma in an attempt to restore circulating volume, thus altering skin turgor, which in severe cases, will result in persistent skin tenting over the abdomen.

Invasive Monitoring

When is invasive hemodynamic monitoring necessary in the pediatric patient? At our institution, we use invasive monitoring when any of the following is true: (1) when a blood loss of 15 to 20 percent of the estimated blood volume or more is expected, (2) in neurosurgical procedures in which adequate circulating volume needs to be maintained yet cerebral edema minimized by both reducing fluids to below maintenance requirements and by using diuretics, and (3) in patients with a compromised cardiovascular system, that is, sepsis, congenital heart disease, or cardiomyopathy. These are not the only indications for arterial and central venous pressure monitoring nor is invasive monitoring always needed under these circumstances, but we have certainly found these monitors useful to guide fluid replacement in such patients.

Rate of Administration and Choice of Fluid

Acute fluid losses may be replaced rapidly, often in less than 1 h, to restore the circulating volume. The major goal of fluid therapy is the return of a more normal heart rate and better capillary refill before transport to the operating room when possible. In acute hemorrhage, necrotizing enterocolitis, and sepsis, isotonic fluids are best for this purpose (Normosol, Ringer's, 0.9% physiologic saline, plasma protein fraction, 5% albumin, or blood products). For chronic losses and less emergent procedures (i.e., pyloric stenosis), fluids and electrolytes should be replaced over 24 to 48 h and the surgical procedure postponed. For healthy patients undergoing elective procedures, the deficit is merely the hourly maintenance times the hours the patient was NPO. This amount of replacement is usually given by the following guidelines.

1st h: one-half fluid deficit and maintenance + ongoing losses.

2nd h: one-quarter fluid deficit and maintenance + ongoing losses.

3rd h: one-quarter fluid deficit and maintenance + ongoing losses.

If the procedure duration is shorter than 3 h, this rehydration should continue in the recovery room either in the form of IV fluids or by allowing the child to take liquids orally. Whenever possible, no patient should be taken to the operating room until dehydration has been substantially corrected, and adequate

Table 9-7 NPO Interval in Pediatrics

	AGES			
	NEWBORN TO 1 YR	1 TO 14 YR	14 TO 19 YR	ADULT
UTHSC guidelines	Regular formula feeds until 5 h preoperatively, clear liquids until 2 h preoperatively	Solids until midnight, clear liquids until 3 h preoperatively	Nothing after midnight	Nothing after midnight
New guidelines based on recent studies	Regular formula feeds with last feeding being clear liquids 3 h preoperatively	2 mL/kg of clear liquids up to 2 h preoperatively	Unlimited clear liquids until 3 h preoperatively	240 mL of clear liquids 2 h preoperatively

UTHSC = University of Texas Health Science Center.

154

volumes of urine with a specific gravity of less than 1.020 are present. Anesthetics decrease the compensatory mechanisms to hypovolemia, such that correction of deficits preoperatively reduces the adverse effects of intraoperative blood and fluid losses.

NPO Recommendations

High metabolic rate, a large body surface-to-weight ratio, and a relatively high percentage of body weight represented by the extracellular fluid compartment make infants and children more susceptible to dehydration. They therefore require an alteration in the NPO time period before surgery. In general, they also have a more rapid gastrointestinal transit time, which allows the shorter NPO interval without increasing the risk of aspiration. The recommendations followed by our institution are listed in Table 9-7. By shortening the NPO period or offering a clear liquid breakfast, compliance may be improved, especially with older children who are capable of "helping themselves" to food or drink without the nursing staff or the parents being aware. Indeed, recent evidence would suggest that prolonged fasting not only fails to protect against aspiration, but also the ingestion of clear fluids actually reduces the resting gastric volume because gastric peristalsis is stimulated by a bolus of clear liquids.

INTRAOPERATIVE FLUID MANAGEMENT

The goals of intraoperative fluid therapy are to maintain the cardiovascular homeostasis by supporting the circulating volume and providing adequate tissue oxygenation to maintain adequate renal function, usually defined as urine output greater than 1 mL/kg/h, and to maintain normal body fluid kinetics. This involves regulation of intravascular and interstitial fluid compartment relationships, electrolyte balance, osmolarity, and hematocrit.

To achieve these goals, five sources of fluid loss/requirement must be taken into account. These are:

1. Maintenance fluids.
2. NPO deficit.
3. Translocation of fluids from surgical trauma.
4. Respiratory losses.
5. Blood loss.

The first two of these have been discussed previously. Translocation fluid loss includes insensible losses from exposed tissue and third-space accumulations of fluids in injured tissues that are not readily accessible to the intravascular compartment.

The amount depends on the extent and location of the surgical procedure and, in some cases, the patient's disease (e.g., peritonitis; Table 9-8). It is most extensive during the first 2 to 3 h after injury or operation and must be replaced with isotonic fluids or blood. For superficial procedures (Table 9-8) that produce very little trauma to the tissues, an additional 1 to 2 mL/kg/h intraoperatively is necessary, in addition to maintenance requirements, to offset translocation fluid loss. Examples of this type of procedure include tonsillectomy, club foot repair, and minor plastic surgical procedures. Moderate tissue trauma occurs with elective intraabdominal and intrathoracic procedures and requires an additional 3 to 5 mL/kg/h of isotonic fluids. Severe tissue injury occurs with multiple trauma, burns, or peritonitis. These situations require an additional 6 to 8 mL/kg/h of fluid replacement. The choice of isotonic fluid depends on the individual anesthesiologist's preference and whether large volumes of fluids are anticipated. Colloid is preferred for massive trauma and in septic patients because of reduced lung morbidity in the postoperative period. Normal saline should not be used when large volumes of resuscitation fluids are needed because the pH is very low (pH, 5.5) and the chloride content is high (150 mEq/L), which can lead to a profound hyperchloremic metabolic acidosis.

Respiratory losses are not often considered when caring for adults, but in small infants, these may represent 20 to 25 percent of the maintenance fluid rate. Depending on the fresh gas flow, minute ventilation, and ambient temperature, the use of a nonrebreathing anesthesia system connected to the endotracheal tube will incur additional losses of 1 to 2 mL/kg/h on average. The circle system will incur losses of approximately one half this amount when using low flows. Other reasons for humidification of inspired gases include better mucociliary function and heat conservation.

Table 9-8   Translocation Fluid (Third-Space) Requirements

TYPE OF PROCEDURE	ADD TO MAINTENANCE (mL/kg/h)
Superficial procedures (i.e., orthopedic or cleft repair)	1 to 2
Moderate trauma (elective intraabdominal or intrathoracic procedures)	3 to 5
Severe trauma (multiple injuries or peritonitis)	6 to 8

The fifth consideration in fluid management is intraoperative blood loss. For all pediatric cases, a graduated suction trap should be inserted and the sponges weighed to obtain a more accurate estimate of blood loss (1 g weight = 1 mL blood loss). Before each patient comes into the operating room, there are several calculations that should be completed. Estimated blood volume (EBV) is calculated according to the guidelines listed in Table 9-2.

Knowing the blood volume, the allowable blood loss before transfusion becomes necessary can be calculated. The ideal hematocrit to begin transfusion is variable. With the concerns over transfer of acquired immunodeficiency syndrome, hepatitis, and cytomegalovirus infection in transfused blood products, many anesthetists are accepting lower levels of hematocrit, provided that cardiovascular stability and normal acid–base status are present. Other factors involved in this decision are oxygen requirements, normal hematocrit for age, presence of cyanotic congenital heart disease, and anticipation of further losses in the postoperative period. After a minimum permissible hematocrit is selected, estimated allowable blood loss (EABL) can be calculated by the following equation.

$$\text{EABL} = \frac{\text{Hct now} - \text{Hct allowed}}{\text{Hct average*}} \times \text{EBV}$$
*equals the average of Hct now and Hct allowed;
HCT = hematocrit.

Before achieving this amount of loss, the blood loss is replaced as in adults at a rate of 3:1 (i.e., three volumes of replacement solution for each volume of blood lost) using a crystalloid fluid (Normosol or lactated Ringer's). When colloid is used, such as 5% albumin or plasma protein fraction, the ratio of colloid solution to blood loss is 2:1. Also, we must remember that these calculations represent estimates and transfusion therapy is best guided by hematocrits measured intraoperatively. To decide how much blood should be transfused, we again must choose a level to which we wish to raise the patient's hematocrit. After this is decided, the formulas in Table 9-9 can be used to calculate the volume of packed red blood cells that is needed to raise the patient's hematocrit to the desired level.

Case Scenario

Now that we have discussed an approach to fluid management in the pediatric patient, we will discuss a case scenario to illustrate some of these points.

A 1000-g premature infant with necrotizing enterocolitis is scheduled for an exploratory laparotomy. The infant is intu-

Table 9-9   Calculations of Blood Replacement

AGE	FORMULA
Infant to 1 yr	1.2 mL PRBC × weight (kg) × desired change in Hct = transfusion volume
1 yr to adolescence	1 mL PRBC × weight (kg) × desired change in Hct = transfusion volume
Adolescent to adult	0.8 mL PRBC × weight (kg) × desired change in Hct = transfusion volume

PRBC = packed red blood cells; Hct = hematocrit.

bated and on a ventilator. He is very edematous, yet his urine output is only 0.5 mL/kg/h. Capillary refill times in the fingers and toes are 5 s (normal, less than 1.5 s). His heart rate is 190 beats/min, and his blood pressure is 48/26 mmHg (normal, 45 to 60/20 to 40 mmHg). What is this baby's fluid status?

The infant is total body fluid overloaded, as evidenced by edema, but his intravascular compartment is depleted, as evidenced by his fast heart rate, slow capillary refill, and low urine output. Appropriate fluid intervention before transport to the operating room or skin incision would be administration of 10 to 20 mL/kg of isotonic fluid (5% albumin, Normosol, or lactated Ringer's) or perhaps blood products if the baby had physical or laboratory signs of coagulopathy. End points for isotonic fluid administration would be a decrease in the heart rate and improved perfusion. It is not uncommon for septic patients with an intraabdominal catastrophe to require fluid boluses of 40 to 60 mL/kg to restore their circulating volume. This fluid may be given over a 10- to 15-min period, carefully observing the cardiovascular response.

After transport to the operating room, what should be a reasonable estimate of this infant's hourly fluid requirements, not including blood loss? This could be calculated by giving maintenance fluids plus translocation third-space losses. Maintenance fluids would be calculated as 1.0 kg × 4 mL/h or 4.0 mL/h. Translocation losses would be approximately 7 mL/kg/h or 1.0 × 7, which is 7.0 mL/h. Therefore, not including blood or peritoneal fluid loss, the baby needs a basal rate of 11.0 mL/h. If the blood loss were 15 mL in the first 15 min of the procedure and volume expansion fluids were used instead of packed red blood cells, a ratio of 3:1 for crystalloid or 2:1 for colloid should be followed. Thus, an additional 30 to 45 mL of albumin, Normosol, or Ringer's lactate would be necessary to maintain the circulating blood volume. In reality, these infants often require tremendous amounts of fluids to maintain hemodynamic stability.

If this infant's hematocrit at the end of the procedure is 33 percent and we wish to transfuse to a level of 40 percent, using Table 9-9 as a reference, the estimated amount of packed red blood cells necessary would be (1.2 mL of cells) × 1 kg × (7 points of change) = approximately 8.4 mL of cells transfused. As with other formulas, this calculation is an estimate. The best method for assessing the adequacy of transfusion is a posttransfusion hematocrit.

In summary, we have discussed a rational approach to perioperative fluid management in the pediatric patient. The calculations presented in this chapter are reasonable estimates of fluid requirements for the individual patient. However, an important premise to remember is that fluids obey a dose–response relationship and the type of fluid administered and the rate of delivery should be subject to change on a minute-to-minute basis according to the cardiovascular response of the patient.

BIBLIOGRAPHY

Anderson PAW, Glick KL, Killam AP, et al: The effect of heart rate on in utero left ventricular output in the fetal sheep. *J Physiol (Lond)* 1986; 372:557–573.

Arant BS Jr: The newborn kidney, in Rudolph A (ed): *Pediatrics*, ed 19. Norwalk, CT, Appleton and Lange, 1991, p 1233.

Aun CST, Panesar NS: Paediatric glucose homeostasis during anaesthesia. *Br J Anaesth* 1990; 64:413–418.

Baylen BG, Ogata H, Oguchi K, et al: Left ventricular performance and contractility before and after volume infusion: A comparative study of preterm and full-term newborn lambs. *Circulation* 1985; 73:1042–1049.

Bennett EJ, Daughety M, Jenkens MT: Some controversial aspects of fluids for the anesthetized neonate. *Anesth Analg* 1970; 49:478–486.

Clyman RI, Mauray F, Heyman MA, et al: Cardiovascular effects of patent ductus arteriosus in preterm lambs with respiratory distress. *J Pediatr* 1987; 111:579–587.

Coté CJ: NPO after midnight for children: A reappraisal. *Anesthesiology* 1990; 72:589–592.

Crawford M, Lerman J, Christensen S, et al: Effects of duration of fasting on gastric fluid pH and volume in healthy children. *Anesth Analg* 1990; 71:400–403.

DeBruin WJ, Greenwald BM, Notterman D: Fluid resuscitation in pediatrics. *Critical Care Clin* 1992; 8:423–438.

Firestone L, Lebowitz P: *Clinical Anesthesia Procedures of the Massachusetts General Hospital.* Boston, Little Brown, 1988, p. 387, 398.

Fisher J, Towbin J: Maturation of the heart. *Clin Perinatol* 1988; 15:421–445.

Friedman WF: The intrinsic physiologic properties of the developing heart. *Prog Cardiovasc Dis* 1972; 15:87–111.

Friedman WF, Pool PE, Jacobowitz D, et al: Sympathetic innervation of the developing rabbit heart: Biochemical and histochemical comparisons of fetal, neonatal, and adult myocardium. *Circ Res* 1968; 23:2532.

Kempe CH, Silver HK, O'Brien D: *Current Pediatric Diagnosis and Treatment,* ed 9. Norwalk, CT, Appleton and Lange, 1987, p 453.

Kirkpatrick SE, Pitlick PT, Naliboff J, et al: Frank-Starling relationship as an important determination of fetal cardiac output. *Am J Physiol* 1976; 231:495–500.

Lindner W, Seidel M, Versmold HT, et al: Stroke volume and left ventricular output in preterm infants with patent ductus arteriosus. *Pediatr Res* 1990; 27:278–281.

Lingman G, Marsal K: Circulatory effects of fetal cardiac arrhythmias. *Pediatr Cardiol* 1986; 7:67–74.

Rudolph A: The circulatory system, in Rudolph A (ed): *Rudolph's Pediatrics,* ed 19. Norwalk, CT, Appleton & Lange, 1991, p 1310.

Rudolph AM: Cardiac output in the fetal lamb: The effects of spontaneous and induced changes of heart rate on right and left ventricular output. *Am J Obstet Gynecol* 1976; 124:183–192.

Rudolph AM: Fetal circulation and cardiovascular adjustments after birth, in Rudolph AM, Hoffman J (eds): *Pediatrics.* Norwalk, CT, Appleton and Lange, 1987, pp 1219–1222.

Schreiner MS, Triebwasser A, Keon TP: Ingestion of liquids with preoperative fasting in pediatric outpatients. *Anesthesiology* 1990; 72:593–597.

Shevde K, Trivedi N: Effects of clear liquids on gastric volume and pH in healthy volunteers. *Anesth Analg* 1991; 72:528–531.

Splinter WM, Schaefer JD: Ingestion of clear fluids is safe for adolescents up to 3 h before anaesthesia. *Br J Anaesth* 1991; 66:48–52.

Splinter WM, Stewart JA, Muir JG: Large volumes of apple juice preoperatively do not affect gastric pH and volume in children. *Can J Anaesth* 1990; 37:36–39.

Steward DJ: *Manual of Pediatric Anesthesia,* ed 3. New York, Churchill Livingstone, 1990, pp 33–34.

Strafford M, Jeon A, Pascucci R: Pre and post-induction blood glucose concentrations in healthy fasting children. *Anesthesiology* 1985; 63:A350.

Thomas DKM: Hypoglycemia in children before operation: Its incidence and prevention. *Br J Anaesth* 1974; 46:66–68.

Tonge HM, Wladimiroff JW, Noordam MJ, et al: Fetal cardiac arrhythmias and their effect on volume blood flow in descending aorta of human fetus. *J Clin Ultrasound* 1986; 14:607–612.

Van der Walt JH, Carter JA: The effect of different preoperative feeding regimens on plasma glucose and gastric volume and pH in infancy. *Anesth Intensive Care* 1986; 14:352–359.

Winberg P, Lundell BPW: Left ventricular stroke volume and output in healthy term infants. *Am J Perinatol* 1990; 7:223–226.

CHAPTER 10

Pediatric Regional Anesthesia

Deborah K. Rasch

The use of regional anesthesia for pediatric patients has become more prevalent in recent years owing, at least in part, to an increased number of premature nursery graduates with acute and chronic lung disease presenting for operation. These infants are at greater risk for development of postoperative apnea and respiratory compromise compared with age-matched healthy infants born at term. When considering regional anesthesia for older children, the operative site, patient age, presence of other medical conditions, degree of anticipated cooperation, and parental preference are all important variables that must be weighed in the balance before making a final decision. This chapter deals with patient preparation, the regional anesthetic techniques that are most useful in general practice, and a brief discussion of postoperative analgesia.

ADVANTAGES OF REGIONAL ANESTHESIA

Many preschool or school-age children with accidental burns or congenital defects will require multiple anesthetics. When the operative site is conducive to a regional nerve block, either for operative anesthesia or postoperative analgesia, the reduction of postoperative pain in these patients might be expected to encourage more rapid return of appetite and promote a better attitude regarding the hospitalization than in those patients in whom postoperative analgesia was not afforded. In our experience, even preschoolers are capable of requesting repeat injection of epidural or caudal catheters when they are beginning to sense the return of pain. In the operating room, regional nerve block can provide profound muscle relaxation below the level of the blockade, obviating the need for other muscle relaxants and reducing the depth of general anesthesia required. Variability in vital signs because of changes in surgical stimulus is diminished. Spinal or caudal anesthesia also eliminates the bradycardiac response to manipulation of the mesentery or spermatic cord during operations of the genitourinary tract or lower abdomen. Other advantages include immobility of the extremity after tendon or nerve repair in young children unable to cooperate with postoperative instructions not to use the involved extremity.

DISADVANTAGES OF
REGIONAL ANESTHESIA

As with any technique, there are also disadvantages to regional anesthesia in children. Performance of various types of regional block requires skills and training that may not be possessed by all anesthesiologists and is a bit more time consuming than a general anesthetic alone. In addition, when regional anesthesia is provided in conjunction with a general anesthetic, two persons experienced in managing pediatric patients under anesthesia are often required so that one person may concentrate on administering a safe general anesthetic while the other is performing the regional block. When local anesthetics are administered, some degree of muscle weakness in the lower extremities may be present. This is usually not a problem for the physician but must be explained to the cognizant child who may be frightened by the sensation of weakness.

Contraindications to regional blockade in children are much the same as in adults. These include the presence of a significant spinal defect, infection in the skin or subcutaneous tissues in the area where the block is to be performed, clotting abnormalities, or patients with ongoing neurologic defects, such as demyelinating diseases of the central nervous system. The latter is more of a medicolegal contraindication because there are no scientific data to support the fact that a regional anesthetic would worsen such conditions.

PREPARATION OF THE CHILD FOR
A REGIONAL ANESTHETIC

Whether a child will accept a regional technique as the primary anesthetic depends on several variables, including age, parental support, maturity, and previous operating room experience. However, it is not realistic to expect most children to be still for the insertion of a regional block without either first inducing general anesthesia or administering significant sedation (Table 10-1). In infants up to approximately 6 months of age, intramuscular ketamine 4 to 5 mg/kg plus 0.01 mg/kg of atropine mixed in the same syringe works nicely to induce the calm needed for performance of the block. Also, an intravenous catheter can be placed more easily for hydration of patients in whom spinal or epidural anesthesia is anticipated. However, if

Table 10-1   Sedation for Regional Blockade*

Ketamine 4 to 5 mg/kg and atropine 0.01 mg/kg IM for infants
up to 6 mo of age
Methohexital 15 to 20 mg/kg rectally
Fentanyl 1 to 2 μg/kg and midazolam 0.05 to 0.1 mg/kg IV in
older children
Midazolam 0.2 mg/kg intranasally or 0.5 mg/kg orally
Diphenhydramine 1 to 2 mg/kg IV or chloral hydrate 20 to 30
mg/kg PO for premature nursery graduates

IM = intramuscular; IV = intravenous; PO = oral.
*In most instances, general anesthesia is preferred in outpatients.

the major objective for using a regional anesthetic is the prevention of apnea in the preterm or ex-premature infant, then ketamine is not recommended because several authors have reported apnea after ketamine to have a frequency similar to that
of general inhalational anesthesia. Small doses of chloral hydrate 20 to 30 mg/kg orally or diphenhydramine 1 to 2 mg/kg
intravenously provide sedation with a very low risk for apnea
or hypoventilation.

For outpatient procedures, induction of general anesthesia is
preferred for insertion of the block because ketamine and other
sedatives may cause delayed awakening in children that could
necessitate hospitalization postoperatively. Another option is
the administration of 15 to 20 mg/kg rectally of methohexital for
sedation, oral midazolam 0.5 mg/kg, or intranasal administration of midazolam 0.2 mg/kg. Often, an intravenous line can
then be inserted without further anesthesia and the block performed.

In older children, an intravenous catheter can be inserted
preoperatively for sedation with a variety of agents. In our experience, a combination of midazolam given in incremental
doses of 0.025 mg/kg up to 0.1 mg/kg combined with fentanyl 1
to 2 μg/kg often affords excellent sedation for insertion of the
block.

Sedation during the procedure when general anesthesia is
not utilized can be achieved with a variety of agents. In small infants, a pacifier is often all that is necessary. In older infants and
children, supplemental ketamine or midazolam may be required.

REGIONAL ANESTHETIC
TECHNIQUES

Spinal Anesthesia

Subarachnoid block (SAB) can be used for any surgical procedure below the diaphragm during which blood loss will be min-

imal. The most common local anesthetics used are 5% lidocaine or 1% tetracaine mixed with dextrose 10% in water. The precise dose of the drug employed for SAB in pediatric patients, much like in adults, is influenced by the depth and spread of anesthesia desired for a particular procedure. Refer to Table 10-2 for some of the recommendations designed to achieve a T6 to T8 level block.

We have experienced more predictable results using 0.4 to 0.6 mg/kg of tetracaine mixed in equal parts of dextrose 10% in water for infants. Some authors also add epinephrine to the solution to increase the duration of the block. Abajian and colleagues recommend addition of 0.02 mL of epinephrine (1:1000) to the anesthetic solution and report no complications. Without epinephrine, tetracaine anesthesia lasts approximately 45 min. The duration of anesthesia may be prolonged by as much as 25 percent when epinephrine is added.

Before administering spinal anesthesia in children, volume loading of the patient is done to counteract the sympathectomy produced by SAB. However, some authors believe this is not necessary in infants because their sympathetic nervous system is poorly developed and they have a very low baseline systemic vascular resistance.

In our experience, in children who do not have a preoperative deficit (i.e., intravenous fluids have been given up to the time of operation or the no oral intake period is 4 h or less), no volume loading is required. For other infants and children, 8 to 10 mL/kg of an isotonic saline solution is administered. Just as in adults, if the patient is hemodynamically unstable or large volume shifts are anticipated with surgery, general anesthesia might be a better choice.

The technique of lumbar puncture (LP) for placement of the SAB differs somewhat in infants compared with adults because the conus medullaris of the newborn ends at L2 rather than T12 to L1. Therefore, LP should be performed no higher than the L3 to L4 interspace, preferentially at L4 to L5. Also, many of these infants are premature nursery graduates with residual lung disease; therefore, care should be taken not to flex the neck. We recommend the use of either a pulse oximeter or a transcutaneous O_2 monitor during performance of the block because Gleason and associates have found that neck flexion produces as much as a 28 mmHg decrease in transcutaneous oxygen pressure in normal infants undergoing LP.

After the infant is prepared with antiseptic solution and placed in the lateral decubitus position, the block is performed using a midline approach with either a 25- or 22-gauge 1-in. spinal needle. Piercing the skin with an 18-gauge hypodermic needle before inserting the spinal needle will reduce the risk of accidentally transversing the spinal canal because the spinal

Table 10-2 Recommended Doses for Subarachnoid Block in Children

AUTHOR	ANESTHETIC SOLUTION	DOSES (mg/kg)	AMOUNT D10W
Gouveia	Lidocaine 5%	1 to 2	Equal parts
Berkowitz et al.	Tetracaine 1%	0.2	Equal parts
Blaise and Roy	Tetracaine 1%	0.4	0.04 mL/kg
Melman et al. (infants up to 10 kg)	Lidocaine 5%	1.5 to 2.5	—
Welborn et al.	Tetracaine 1%	0.4 to 0.6	Equal parts

D10W = dextrose 10% in water.

needle is inserted through the tough epidermis in a newborn. Once below the skin, the needle must be advanced very slowly. In infants younger than age 12 months, the subarachnoid space is usually entered between 1 and 1.5 cm from the skin surface. If clear cerebrospinal fluid (CSF) is obtained, then a 1.0-mL tuberculin syringe is attached to the needle and an attempt made to aspirate the CSF. If CSF is easily obtained, then the local anesthetic solution may be injected at the rate of approximately 0.5 mL/s for upper abdominal procedures and somewhat slower for mid to lower abdominal procedures. In infants fasted for greater than 6 h, it is not uncommon to experience a dry tap. Occasionally, aspiration with a tuberculin syringe will allow confirmation of proper needle placement. Another minor problem is the bloody tap. If the CSF is only pink tinged and clears after aspiration of approximately 0.5 to 1 mL of CSF, then the injection of local anesthetic can proceed. If more blood is present or it does not clear, another interspace may be tried or general anesthesia employed. Do not inject local anesthetic under these circumstances because intravascular injection may result.

Caudal or Lumbar Epidural Anesthesia

Caudal anesthesia is best utilized in cases where genitourinary or lower abdominal procedures, such as inguinal herniorrhaphy or circumcision, are performed. It is a simple procedure to accomplish in small infants compared with a lumbar epidural, which is difficult to perform in children younger than age 18 months to 2 years, primarily because of patient size. Also, because access to the caudal epidural space is easy and passage of a catheter into the lumbar or thoracic epidural space by the caudal approach is possible in young infants and children, lumbar epidural anesthesia and analgesia is usually reserved for those infants weighing 10 kg or more. For both caudal and lumbar epidural anesthesia, the most common agents employed are bupivacaine (0.125%, 0.25%, or 0.5%) or lidocaine (0.5% and 1%). Various formulas have been suggested for calculating the dose of the agent. For infants less than 15 kg, the following equation is used.

$$\text{Volume needed} = 0.1 \text{ mL local anesthetic solution (LAS)} \\ \times \text{ weight (kg)} \\ \times \text{ number of spinal segments blocked}$$

For example, a 3-kg infant presents for herniorrhaphy. A T10 level is required, therefore:

Volume needed = 0.1 mL LAS × 3 kg
      × [5 (sacral) + 5 (lumbar) + 2 (thoracic)
      = 12 segments] or 3.6 mL of LAS

Another similar equation that has been recommended for children older than age 2 years is:

0.1 mL × age (yr) × spinal segments blocked
= volume needed

Depending on the agent used, we must then calculate the maximum safe dose of the particular anesthetic (3 mg/kg of bupivacaine or 6 to 7 mg/kg of lidocaine) to ensure that a toxic dose of the agent will not be given. When using 0.25% bupivicaine or 0.5% lidocaine to achieve a T8 level block, we have good success using 1 mL/kg of LAS. The addition of epinephrine 1:200,000 helps warn against intravascular injection of local anesthetic but does not appear to affect the duration of the nerve block.

The caudal epidural space can be approached either with the patient in the prone position or in the lateral decubitus position. We favor the lateral decubitus position because there is less chance of endangering the airway. After the child has been prepped and draped, the sacral hiatus can be palpated by placing a thumb or finger between the sacral cornua (Fig. 10-1). In infants, the hiatus will be at or approximately 1 to 2 mm above a line drawn through the cornua, whereas in older children, the hiatus will actually be about the same distance below that point. A 22- to 23-gauge regional block needle or butterfly needle is then inserted through the sacral hiatus at an angle of 30° to 45° from the skin surface (Fig. 10-2). Penetration of the sacrococcygeal ligament will be felt as a slight "pop" approximately 2 to 4 mm from the skin surface in neonates and 1 to 1.5 cm in the adolescent. By contrast with adults and older children, the needle is not advanced any further into the caudal canal of the neonate because the dural sac may end as low as S4 in this age group. Therefore, accidental dural puncture and spinal anesthesia can occur if the needle is advanced more than a few millimeters beyond the sacral hiatus. At this point, aspiration is performed to ensure that the tip of the needle is neither in a blood vessel or in the subarachnoid space. The local anesthetic solution is then injected slowly in four equally divided portions of the total calculated dose. If subcutaneous infiltration is noted, just advance the needle 1 to 2 mm more and try again. Potential complications of caudal anesthesia include inadvertent injection either in the dural sac or intravascularly, periosteal injection of the LAS, or penetration of the anterior table of the sacrum and

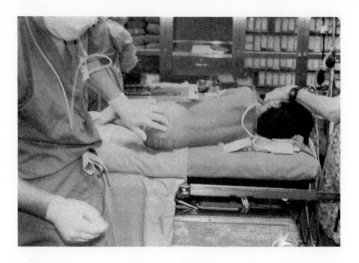

Figure 10-1 Sacral hiatus for caudal anesthesia can be palpated as a "window" between the sacral cornua.

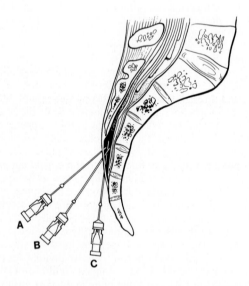

Figure 10-2 Needle position for caudal anesthesia at various ages. (A) The needle is inserted at 30° to 45° angle to the skin in neonates until the sacrococcygeal ligament is penetrated. (B and C) For older children the needle must be "walked" into the caudal canal.

perforation of pelvic viscera. If either urine or fecal material is aspirated from the needle, the caudal block should be aborted, and the child should receive intravenous antibiotics for 48 h. However, in our performance of more than 3500 caudal anesthetics, we have encountered none of these complications.

If a caudal epidural is desired for a longer case that may require a repeat injection, a 22-gauge intravenous catheter can be inserted into the caudal space using the technique previously described. The flexible catheter is then threaded over the needle into the caudal space and attached to sterile low-volume intravenous extension tubing (Fig. 10-3). The catheter is taped in place, and the tubing is positioned to provide an easily accessible port for injection. Aspiration and injection precautions have already been described and are similar to those used in the single-shot caudal.

Lumbar epidural anesthesia is achieved using the same loss of resistance techniques as in adults. An 18-gauge Touhey needle with a 20-gauge epidural catheter is preferred for performance of the block in children 3 years of age or older. For children between the ages of 2 to 3 years, a 20-gauge 1-in. Touhey needle is selected to perform the block (Fig. 10-4). The selected interspace is identified by palpation of the spinous processes, and the epidural needle is inserted in the midline approximately 1 to 1.5 cm, at which time the ligamentum flavum will be en-

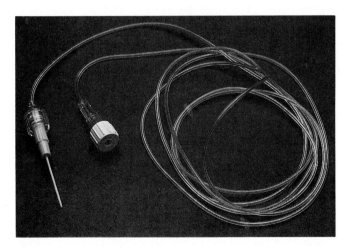

Figure 10-3   Catheter over needle technique for short-term use to provide caudal epidural analgesia in neonates. The catheter is connected to low-volume extension tubing to provide a reinjection port.

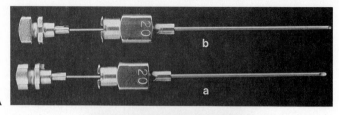

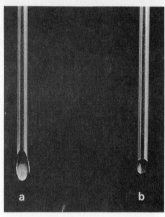

Figure 10-4 (A) A 20-gauge Touhey needle (a) for lumbar or thoracic epidural anesthesia in the pediatric patient and a 20-gauge Crawford needle (b) for continuous caudal epidural anesthesia. (B) A close-up view of the needle tips. Note that the Crawford needle has a blunter end, which allows for a more distinct pop as the needle pierces the sacrococcygeal ligament. The straight design also allows a smooth introduction of the epidural catheter into the caudal canal. A Touhey needle, because of the gentle curve at the end, is often not satisfactory for caudal catheter insertion because, as the catheter exits the needle, it may be directed toward the ligament rather than into the caudal canal.

gaged by the tip of the needle. Just as in adults, the midline approach is chosen in pediatric patients because (1) the epidural space is widest in that area, (2) there is less risk for vascular disruption because the greatest density of blood vessels is located laterally in the epidural space, and (3) the ligamentum flavum is thickest in the midline so loss of resistance is much more distinct.

After the ligamentum flavum is identified by a slight increase in resistance to passage of the needle (approximately 1 to 1.5 cm from the skin surface), the stylet is removed, and a 3-mL

Luer-Lock syringe filled with 1 to 2 mL of saline or 1 mL of air is attached to the hub of the needle. Constant gentle pressure is exerted against the plunger of the syringe, and the needle is advanced slowly until the ligamentum flavum is pierced. At this time, the plunger on the syringe will easily be depressed, identifying the epidural space. For single-injection anesthesia, the calculated dose of LAS may be given in incremental parts (usually one quarter of the total volume as a test dose). If a catheter technique is to be used, insertion of the catheter may proceed at this point, and the remainder of the LAS may be injected after the catheter is secured using a transparent dressing and tape.

In children younger than age 2 years or less than approximately 10 kg, we have used the caudal approach for insertion of lumbar and thoracic epidural catheters. This technique is accomplished using either an 18-gauge flexible catheter over a blunt needle (Burron continuous brachial plexus kit, Fig. 10-5) or a 20-gauge Crawford needle (Preferred Medical Prod, Fig. 10-6). When using the former, the sacrococcygeal ligament is punctured, the entire apparatus is inserted 1 to 2 mm farther, and the catheter is threaded off the needle into the caudal epidural space. If the Crawford needle is used, after the caudal space is identified by loss of resistance, the needle is advanced 1 to 2 mm and stabilized while the stylet is removed. One to 2

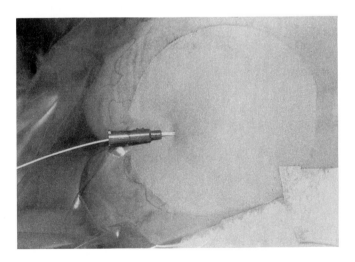

Figure 10-5 Continuous caudal epidural anesthesia. The caudal canal is entered with a soft catheter-over-needle technique. Then a 20-gauge epidural catheter can be inserted to the desired length.

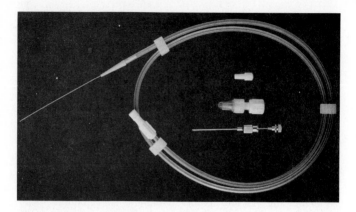

Figure 10-6 A 20-gauge Crawford needle with a 24-gauge epidural catheter for continuous epidural anesthesia by the caudal approach.

mL of sterile saline is injected through the introducer catheter or Crawford needle for distention of the caudal epidural space after aspiration is performed to check for either CSF or blood. Then the epidural catheter (20 or 24-gauge) can be inserted to a premeasured length, depending on the operative site, into the lumbar or thoracic epidural space. The plastic introducer catheter or Crawford needle is then removed and the epidural taped in place. Aspiration is again performed to document proper placement of the catheter before a local anesthetic with epinephrine 1:200,000 is injected. The volume of local anesthetic to be administered is calculated according to the following equation for both caudally inserted catheters and direct lumbar epidurals.

$$\text{Volume needed} = 0.05 \text{ mL} \times \text{weight (kg)} \\ \times \text{number of spinal segments blocked}$$

Postoperatively, prolonged analgesia is easily provided using preservative-free morphine sulfate 0.05 mg/kg/dose. The duration of action is 12 to 36 h, and the incidence of delayed apnea is rare, even in neonates. Fentanyl (1 μg/kg/h) by continuous infusion may offer some advantages because analgesia is continuous and does not require repeated injections and, therefore, does not allow for lapses in pain control. However, neonates require a much lower dose, and even at low doses, an accumulation may occur, leading to apnea. We reserve the use of fentanyl to children 2 years of age or older. Local anesthetics (bupivacaine) are safest as a single injection in outpatients and afford 6 to 8 h of postoperative pain relief. Infants and children receiving narcotics epidurally should be monitored in an intermediate care or intensive care unit setting to observe for postoperative apnea. We require pulse oximetry and apnea monitors on these patients.

Axillary Block of the Brachial Plexus

This technique is useful for operations of the upper extremity at or below the elbow. As in the adult, complications from this technique are rare, most commonly production of a small axillary hematoma. In most cases, this occurrence is benign, provided the patient has normal clotting function. Preparation to treat accidental intravascular injection of the LAS should be made, as in all cases where regional anesthesia is employed. The most common LAS used is 0.25% bupivacaine or 1% lidocaine. As with epidural and spinal anesthesia, various formulas have been suggested to determine the local anesthetic doses for infants and children. We usually use 1.5 to 2 mg/kg of 0.25% bupivacaine or 3 mg/kg of 0.5% bupivacaine if a motor block is desired. Alternatively 6 mg/kg of 1% lidocaine may be used. Good results may be obtained when using a single agent. When combinations of LAS are chosen, the volume of solution injected is 0.3 to 0.4 mL/kg. Axillary block is most easily performed with the patient in the supine position and the arm abducted 90°. Because pediatric patients are often either heavily sedated or under general anesthesia at the time of the block, a nerve stimulator is very useful to locate the brachial plexus. To use this technique, a nerve stimulator that allows variation in output is necessary. The axillary pulse is palpated, and a point is selected as high in the axilla as is practical for injection. The output is initially set at approximately 1 mA, and a 22-gauge short bevel needle is inserted at a 45° angle to the skin along an axis tangential to the artery and advanced very slowly. When the needle penetrates the sheath surrounding the neurovascular bundle, often a pop is felt. The sheath in children is very superficial (approximately, 2 to 3 mm below the skin in a neonate); so in small infants, care must be taken not to enter the artery when making the skin wheal.

The needle is then directed immediately lateral to the axillary pulse, watching for a twitch along the distribution of median, ulnar, or radial nerves. After a twitch is encountered, the output of the nerve stimulator is decreased to 0.5 mA or less. If a twitch is still present, the needle point lies within the neurovascular sheath. Usually, as the LAS is injected, the twitch will either temporarily disappear or decrease in amplitude. When the injection is halted, the twitch will return to near-initial intensity as the solution diffuses into the sheath. The LAS should be injected slowly, and aspiration should be done for each one-quarter of the solution injected. Routine search for a second twitch along a different nerve distribution before injecting the LAS is not helpful and may result in misplacement of the needle into the axillary vessels as they are compressed by the local anesthetic in the sheath. Equally effective is the transarterial approach, but there is increased risk of rapid uptake of the anesthetic.

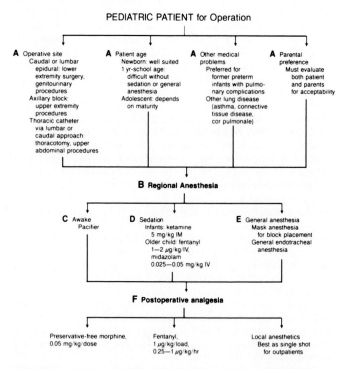

Figure 10-7 Management of a pediatric patient for regional anesthesia. (Reproduced with permission from Rasch DK: Pediatric regional anesthesia, in Bready L, Smith RB (eds): *Decision Making in Anesthesiology*, ed 2. St. Louis, MO, Mosby-Year Book, 1992, p 247.)

CONCLUSION

Regional anesthesia in pediatric patients is useful for postoperative analgesia and intraoperative anesthesia. Figure 10-7 is a summary of the approach to regional anesthesia in a child. Regardless of the technique chosen for each individual case, our goal should be to provide a painless operation and minimize discomfort in the postoperative period.

BIBLIOGRAPHY

Abajian JC, Mellis PWP, Browne AE, et al: Spinal anesthesia for surgery in the high risk infant. *Anesth Analg* 1984; 63:359–362.

Berkowitz S, Green BA: Spinal anesthesia in children: Report based on 350 patients under 13 years of age. *Anesthesiology* 1951; 12:376.

Blaise G, Roy L: Spinal anesthesia in children [letter]. *Anesth Analg* 1984; 63:359–362.

Broadman LM: *Pediatric Regional Anesthesia: ASA Refresher Course*. vol 14, chap 4. Philadelphia, JP Lippincott, pp 43–60.

Crelin ES: *Anatomy of the Newborn*. London, Henry Kimpton, 1969.

Eather KF: Axillary brachial plexus block. *Anesthesiology* 1985; 19:683–685.

Eriksson E: Axillary brachial plexus anesthesia in children with citanest. *Acta Anesthesiol Scand* 1965; 16:291.

Gleason CA, Martin PJ, Anderson JV, et al: Optimal position for a spinal tap in preterm infants. *Pediatrics* 1983; 71:31–35.

Gouveia MA: Raqui anestesia para pacientes pediatricos–experiencia personal en 50 casos. *Rev Bras Anest* 1970; 20:501–504.

Gunter JB, Watcha MF, Forester JE, et al: Caudal epidural anesthesia in conscious premature and high risk infants. *J Pediatr Surg* 1991; 21:9–14.

Jensen BH: Caudal block for postoperative pain relief in children after genital operations: A comparison of bupivacaine and morphine. *Acta Anesthesiol Scan* 1981; 25:373–375.

Melman E, Pennelas A, Maruffo E: Regional anesthesia in children. *Anesth Analg* 1975; 54:387–392.

Niesel HC, Rodriguez P, Ilsman I: Regional anesthesia der oberen extremitat der kindern [English abstract]. *Anaesthesist* 1974; 23:178.

Schulte-Steinberg O, Rahlfs VW: Spread of extradural analgesia following caudal injection in children. *Br J Anaesth* 1977; 49:1027–1033.

Selander D, Dhuner K-G, Lundborg G: Peripheral nerve injury due to injection needles used for regional anesthesia. *Acta Anesthesiol Scand* 1977; 21:182–188.

Steward DJ: Preterm infants are more prone to develop complication after minor surgery than are term infants. *Anesthesiology* 1982; 56:304–306.

Takasaki M, Dohi S, Kawabata Y, et al: Dosage of lidocaine for caudal anesthesia in infants and children. *Anesthesiology* 1977; 47:527–529.

Webster AC, McKishnie JD, Kenyon CF, et al: Spinal anesthesia for inguinal hernia repair in high risk neonates. *Can J Anaesth* 1991; 38:281–286.

Welborn LG, Rice LJ, Hannallah RS, et al: Postoperative apnea in former preterm infants: Prospective comparison of spinal and general anesthesia. *Anesthesiology* 1990; 72:838–842.

Yaster M, Maxwell LG: Pediatric regional anesthesia. *Anesthesiology* 1989; 70:324–338.

CHAPTER 11

The Pediatric Outpatient

Kelly Gordon Knape

Up to 75 percent of pediatric surgical cases can be managed successfully on an outpatient basis. This area of care has developed, not only because of pressure from third-party payers, but also because it offers the following distinct advantages: (1) children should have less prolonged psychological upset compared with that which is associated with separation from parents caused by hospital stays lasting 2 days or more; (2) there is a minimized risk of acquiring a nosocomial infection; (3) the child's feeding schedule is less disrupted; and (4) there are lower associated costs and also increased hospital bed availability. The first three are the most important.

PREOPERATIVE SCREENING

Critical to the safe management of these children is proper patient selection. The criteria should include American Society of Anesthesiologists (ASA) status, the reliability of the parent or guardian, the kind of operative procedure planned, and whether there is a history of prematurity.

ASA Status

These children should be classified as ASA I or II. ASA III patients are considered only if their chronic problem that "limits activity" is well controlled and should be evaluated by the anesthesiologist well in advance of the day of surgery. An example of an ASA III patient who would benefit from a well-planned outpatient procedure is a child with mental and/or motor handicaps and a well-controlled seizure disorder who needs operative dental care.

Reliable Parent or Guardian

This responsible adult must provide the child's complete medical history. They must also ensure that all preoperative instructions are carried out thoroughly, especially the nothing by mouth (NPO) orders. These adults also are critical to the overall outcome because they must intelligently provide postoperative care after careful instructions are given.

Short, Atraumatic Surgery

The surgical procedure must be brief and associated with minimal physiologic insult, especially blood loss. Examples include myringotomy and tympanoplasty, herniorrhaphy, circumcision, and dental rehabilitation. Outpatient adenotonsillectomy is recommended only in children 3 years of age and older. Tom and colleagues demonstrated a high incidence of serious complications in children younger than this age. Specifically, they found that about 50 percent of these patients suffered airway complications, 8.5 percent required intravenous therapy (fluids and medications) for vomiting, and 8 percent required postoperative care in an intensive care unit. Anesthetic technique was not a factor. If tonsillectomy is performed as an outpatient procedure, the patient should live nearby and have a reliable caregiver capable of providing ready transportation to the hospital if postoperative bleeding occurs.

History of Prematurity

Children with a history of prematurity must be carefully considered and evaluated. The guidelines vary among institutions and include admitting former premature infants ("premies") postoperatively for at least the night after surgery who are younger than 3 months postnatal age. Better determinants for postoperative admission include: (1) all ex-premies younger than 45 to 60 weeks postconceptual age (PCA) and (2) any symptomatic infant regardless of age. The average PCA used by most centers is 55 weeks. These patients are at an increased risk of postoperative apnea and should also be monitored for bradycardia and desaturation. They must be monitored at least overnight and longer if there is a history of apneic spells, intubation, and/or ventilatory support (especially for bronchopulmonary dysplasia) in their postnatal course. Caffeine citrate (10 mg/kg) has been used to reduce perioperative apnea. Those children already receiving theophylline should have it restarted as soon as they can tolerate oral liquids.

Infants born at term, who are otherwise healthy, should not be scheduled for procedures until after the age of at least 1 month (44 weeks PCA). Postoperative apnea is still possible, and so, they too should be monitored for at least 4 h before considering discharge.

SCREENING ON THE DAY
OF SURGERY

Preoperative preparation on the day of surgery should include not only a good history and physical, but also assurance that the parent has followed the preoperative instructions completely. The preoperative evaluation is similar to that performed in inpatients (see Chap. 4). We allow the parent to be present and even hold the small child as long as possible, and the following points should be emphasized in the history while the physical examination is performed.

NPO Status

The goal is to minimize the risk of a full stomach, dehydration, and hypoglycemia (rare). Milk, orange juice, and other solids are withheld from all children. Clear liquids are allowed more liberally (see Chap. 4 for NPO guidelines). This has been shown to not only not leave gastric pH or volume unaltered, but also keep the child happier. Children can be very clever in finding food; therefore, parents should be forewarned and the child questioned carefully (but gently). Hard candy and chewing gum are also considered clear liquids and are treated as such.

The Runny Nose?

Parents should be questioned about whether the child has had a recent upper respiratory infection or any other acute change in their health (see Chap. 4 for further discussion of this subject).

Congenital Heart Disease

Any previously undiagnosed murmur is most likely to be an innocent one, but a trained ear auscultatory examination, preferably by a pediatric cardiologist, should confirm the diagnosis. Antibiotic prophylaxis according to American Heart Association guidelines may be required because oral and upper respiratory tract procedures are common in the pediatric outpatient. Careful attention to the avoidance of bubbles in the intravenous lines must be maintained because of the possible risk of systemic embolization through intracardiac communications.

Other Medical Problems

Be alert for problems that may occur even during a routine anesthetic in patients with supposedly well-controlled disease.

Sickle Cell

Tourniquets, acidosis, hypothermia, hypoxia, and hypotension promote sickling. Patients with significant end-organ disease or a crisis within the last 12 months who are noncompliant with therapy, live a long distance from care, and/or would have probable inadequate follow-up are best handled as inpatients.

Asthma

These children should be questioned closely about recent wheezing and the presence of foul-smelling green sputum (and, if it has increased significantly in the past 24 h, in those with concomitant cystic fibrosis). Asthmatic patients are also at an increased risk of arrhythmias with halothane, especially if the theophylline level is high.

Down's Syndrome

There is a high incidence of atlantoaxial subluxation, subglottic stenosis, apnea, and congenital heart disease in this patient population.

To prevent delays, most of the evaluation should be done before the day of surgery, including the laboratory work. Most centers require a hematocrit because anemia is not uncommon in infants. Urinalysis is not usually required unless there is some genitourinary complaint.

Psychological preparation is crucial to the success of the perioperative care. Always allow for questions from both the parent or guardian and the child (especially older ones). With some understanding of the procedures and a familiarity with the surroundings and personnel, the child and the parent are less anxious, which promotes a smooth induction and perioperative course.

OPERATIVE PHASE

Premedication

When a sympathetic, compassionate presentation is insufficient or when a child is especially anxious and time allows, premedication may be considered, especially for those older than 8 to 10 months of age. Midazolam may be used in doses of 0.2 mg/kg intranasally, 0.5 to 1.0 mg/kg PO (maximum, 15 mg), or 1 mg/kg rectally. Pentobarbital has also been used in doses of 4 to 6 mg/kg PO. The child should not be left unattended after the premedication is given.

After the patient changes into hospital garb and all paperwork and preoperative assessments are thoroughly complete the patient and parent (to avoid premature separation) come to the designated operating room (OR) holding area together. A pleasant mode of transportation, such as a little red wagon, is frequently employed with favorable results. Children should be allowed to bring their favorite toy along into the OR.

Induction

The goal of outpatient anesthesia is safety and rapid return to the awake ready-for-home state. With this in mind, induction techniques are planned based on the medical status, age, and demeanor of the child. Rectal induction is the only method performed outside the OR, and the parent is always present. Techniques performed in the OR are occasionally attended by parents when the child has severe separation anxiety. It is useful to have a Plan A and a Plan B because children will often change their minds or suddenly become uncooperative when they actually arrive in the OR, especially if the parent or guardian is not with them. Many induction techniques are suitable for outpatients.

Rectal Methohexital

Methohexital allows for smooth induction while not significantly affecting recovery time. A 1.0% solution at a dose of 15 mg/kg given rectally provides the most rapid onset (mean, 6.3 min) with the least chance of expulsion or defecation. This method is best for children aged 1 to 3 years.

Inhalation Induction

A very popular technique using nitrous oxide (N_2O) and a volatile agent is generally simple but requires a cooperative patient. It is usually better tolerated if the child is allowed to sit on the OR table or cradled in the anesthetist's arms and lap, with the mask lightly scented with the child's favorite flavor. Halothane is preferred for induction; however, isoflurane may offer a slightly faster return-to-normal-at-home status. Therefore, after inhalation induction with halothane, some practitioners prefer to switch to isoflurane for maintenance.

Intravenous Induction

Using a quick pinch with a butterfly needle while the child is distracted, thiopental is administered at a dose of 5 to 6 mg/kg. These patients are sleepier than those who undergo inhalational induction only during the first 15 min of recovery. Methohexital has faster elimination but may produce pain or hiccoughs associated with injection. Propofol may be used with rapid recovery and minimal nausea, but injection may be painful unless large antecubital veins are used.

Intramuscular Induction

Because of its painful nature, this technique is reserved for those with behavioral problems. Ketamine in low doses (2 to 3 mg/kg) produces only slightly longer recovery times than inhalation induction and has a lower incidence of emergence phenomena or dreams than do larger doses. Methohexital (5% solution, 6 to 8 mg/kg) may induce sleep in less than 5 min with no lasting soreness or local reaction. For intubation, succinylcholine in a dose of 4 mg/kg intramuscularly may be used if IV access is not available. Glycopyrrolate should be administered with ketamine to help reduce secretions.

Intubation

Outpatients should be intubated according to the same set of criteria that inpatients would be. If postextubation stridor occurs, aerosolized racemic epinephrine (0.1 mL/kg to a maximum dose of 0.5 mL in 2.5 mL of normal saline) usually is sufficient for treatment. Admission is recommended if the stridor required treatment with racemic epinephrine because of the chance of rebound. Steroids for prophylaxis or treatment of postextubation stridor are controversial but are probably of no benefit. Patients requiring intubation may have some laryngeal incompetence; therefore, oral intake is generally delayed until 1 h after extubation.

Monitoring

Monitoring standards for outpatients are no different than those for inpatients. Insurance carriers focus on the need for minimal monitoring to include at least two monitors. The most preferred include precordial stethoscope, noninvasive blood pressure, electrocardiography, pulse oximetry, and temperature.

Perioperative Intravenous Fluids

The length of the patient's NPO period, the length of the procedure, and the risk of postoperative vomiting will determine whether an IV catheter and maintenance fluids are started. Short procedures, like PE tube placement, are often done without an IV line, but procedures lasting at least 30 to 60 min would be best performed with IV access. The IV solution can still be started after or during an inhalation induction. In many cases, inhalational induction will facilitate placement of an IV catheter because of venodilation.

Maintenance

Generally, inhalational agents are preferred. The addition of short-acting muscle relaxants will reduce the amount of inhalational agent used. Mivacurium is approved for use in children older than the age of 2 years, but it requires larger doses (induction, 0.2 mg/kg; 95 percent effective dose, 0.1 mg/kg) and is shorter acting than in adults. Short-acting narcotics (fentanyl, 1.0 to 2.0 μg/kg) may also reduce the amount of agent and provide residual analgesia postoperatively without significantly increasing the risk of delayed recovery or nausea/vomiting. Intraoperative regional techniques, which are growing in popularity, also reduce the dose of volatile agents, thus speeding recovery and minimizing nausea, and provide postoperative analgesia.

POSTOPERATIVE CARE

Postanesthesia care unit care should be no different than that for inpatients. However, as soon as the child has normal ventilation with reflexes intact and with the absence of bleeding, a parent should be called to the patient's bedside in the postanesthesia care unit, where they will provide considerable comfort, reassurance, and familiarity to the awakening child. As awareness improves, they are often moved to an isolation room for privacy and more quiet surroundings, if there is no separate outpatient recovery area.

Analgesia

With infants younger than 6 months of age, a combination of rocking, cuddling, and nursing a bottle may be sufficient for comfort after some procedures. Most children, however, require analgesia. For the relief of the mild pain from peripheral procedures, acetaminophen orally or rectally (10 mg/kg) may be sufficient. For persistent and more intense pain, acetaminophen with codeine (1 mL per year of age or 120 mg and 12 mg per 5 mL, respectively) can be used. Codeine causes less nausea and respiratory depression than morphine. Intramuscular codeine (1.0 to 1.5 mg/kg) or meperidine (0.5 mg/kg) can be used for those without an IV line.

Regional techniques provide long-lasting analgesia without nausea or additive sedation. Caudal epidural blockade is used for circumcision, herniorrhaphy, orchidopexy, or similar procedures below the umbilicus. Infiltrative penile block of the dorsal nerve is often used for circumcision. Bupivacaine (0.25% at a dose of 0.5 to 0.7 mL/kg; maximum, 2 to 3 mg/kg) is the preferred agent because of its long duration (at least 4 to 6 h) and minimal motor blockade. Combining 1.0% lidocaine (1.0 mg/kg) with 0.25% bupivacaine (0.25 mg/kg) for penile block may reduce the potential for toxicity without affecting the quality or duration. Postural hypotension is unlikely, but patients should have a normal upright blood pressure and be able to ambulate without dizziness (if ambulatory). Most patients receiving a regional anesthetic can be discharged home within 2 h of admission to the postanesthesia care unit.

Infiltration of the tonsillar fossa after tonsillectomy with a local anesthetic and epinephrine to reduce pain and bleeding is controversial. Jebles and colleagues showed that infiltration with 0.25% bupivacaine and 1:200,000 epinephrine significantly reduced pain for at least 10 days postoperatively.

Vomiting

Nausea and vomiting are the most common complications seen after outpatient surgery and anesthesia. Although the overall incidence of emesis in children is 10 to 20 percent, it is as high as 76 percent in patients who have had eye (strabismus) surgery. Procedures with an incidence greater than 50 percent include herniorrhaphy, tonsillectomy/adenoidectomy, and orchidopexy. These children may benefit from droperidol 50 to 70 μg/kg IV intraoperatively for prophylaxis and/or 5 μg/kg for treatment of persistent postoperative vomiting. Metoclopramide has also been used for prophylaxis and treatment (0.1 mg/kg). Ondansetron has also been used effectively in children (0.15 mg/kg). An IV line should remain in place until the child is tolerating oral liquids because this will minimize the risk of dehydration.

Discharge Criteria

Before discharging the child home, all of the following must be met:

1. Appropriate and stable vital signs.
2. Ability to swallow fluids and cough or demonstrate a gag.
3. Activity/ambulation consistent with development.
4. Absence of respiratory difficulty.
5. Awareness/consciousness appropriate to development.
6. Ability to retain oral fluids without vomiting.
7. Absent or manageable nausea and dizziness.
8. Absence of complications including persistent pain, bleeding, or unexpected swelling.

All children, as with any outpatient, must have a responsible escort to take them home. The family should be given written instructions and demonstrate understanding; they also are given a phone number to call if there are problems or questions. A phone number for the family must also be on record. All outpatient facilities must have follow-up procedures to ensure that all outpatients have an uncomplicated postoperative course.

Complications

Generally, postoperative problems are easily managed, still allowing discharge home. The most frequently reported occurrences at home include loss of appetite (38 percent), upset stomach (21 percent), and sore throat (14 percent). When admission to the hospital after an outpatient procedure is necessary, it is infrequent (less than 1 to 2 percent) and is generally caused by vomiting (50 percent), pain (10 percent), and bleeding (8 percent). Other reasons include not only croup and fever, but also the family's apprehension about postoperative care at home. Up to 9 percent of parents surveyed would choose admission if they had to repeat the experience.

SUMMARY

With the increasing demand for outpatient procedures, it has been demonstrated that the majority of children can be successfully treated in this manner if patients are carefully selected and evaluated, appropriate anesthetic management is followed, and the postoperative condition is closely scrutinized.

BIBLIOGRAPHY

Broadman LM, Ceruzzi W, Patane PS, et al: Metoclopramide reduces the incidence of vomiting following strabismus surgery in children. *Anesthesiology* 1990; 72:245–248.

Cohen MM, Cameron CB: Should you cancel the operation when a child has an upper respiratory infection? *Anesth Analg* 1991; 72:282–288.

Dunbar BS: *Anesthetic Considerations for the Pediatric Outpatient: American Society of Anesthesiologists (ASA) 1987 Annual Refresher Course Lectures.* 126:1–5.

Gibbons PA: *Anesthetic Considerations for the Pediatric Outpatient: American Society of Anesthesiologists (ASA) 1986 Annual Refresher Course Lectures.* 274:1–6.

Hannallah RS: *Anesthesia for Pediatric Outpatients: American Society of Anesthesiology (ASA) 1992 Annual Refresher Course Lectures.* 133:1–7.

Hannallah RS, Epstein BS: Management of the pediatric patient, in Wetchler BV (ed): *Anesthesia for Ambulatory Surgery,* ed 2. Philadelphia, JB Lippincott, 1991, pp 131–195.

Jebles J, Reilly J, Gutierrez J, et al: The effect of pre-incisional infiltration of tonsils with bupivacaine on the pain following tonsillectomy under general anesthesia. *Pain* 1991; 47:305.

Kapur PA: *Ambulatory Anesthesia: International Anesthesia Research Society (IARS) 1992 Review Course Lecture.* pp 114–119.

Schreiner MS, Triebwasser A, Keon TP: Ingestion of liquids compared with preoperative fasting in pediatric outpatients. *Anesthesiology* 1990; 72:593–597.

Sfez M, Mapihan YL, Mazoit X, et al: Local anesthetic serum concentrations after penile nerve block in children. *Anesth Analg* 1990; 71:423–426.

Steward DJ: *Manual of Pediatric Anesthesia,* ed 2. pp 83–86.

Tellez DW, Galvis AG, Storgion SA, et al: Dexamethasone in the prevention of postextubation stridor in children. *J Pediatr* 1991; 118:289–294.

Tom LWC, DeDio RM, Cohen DE. Is outpatient tonsillectomy appropriate for young children? *Laryngoscope* 1992; 102:277–280.

Part II

Special Problems in Pediatric Anesthesia

CHAPTER 12

The Pediatric Trauma Patient

Dawn E. Webster

Trauma is the leading cause of death in the pediatric population. The care of the critically injured child requires rapid assessment and treatment to preserve life and limit morbidity. The medical care received during the first critical posttrauma hour strongly affects the outcome; therefore, a well-organized approach to the pediatric trauma patient is essential. Although the pediatric general surgeon usually directs the resuscitation of the pediatric trauma patient, the anesthesiologist may be consulted for airway management and cardiovascular resuscitation of these patients in the emergency room and in the operating room.

This chapter will describe the basic principles in resuscitation of the pediatric trauma patient and discuss injuries of particular interest to the anesthesiologist.

ANATOMY AND THE PEDIATRIC TRAUMA PATIENT

Several anatomic differences exist between the child and the adult. These differences have an impact on how injury affects children and how management may differ between the pediatric and adult trauma patient. Compared with the adult, the child's head is larger in mass and comprises a larger relative proportion of body surface area. Because the head is a source of heat loss, the relatively larger size renders the child more susceptible to hypothermia after environmental exposure and after resuscitation attempts in a cool environment. Bony sutures remain open for 12 to 18 months, allowing palpation of anterior and posterior fontanelles to aid in assessment of intracranial pressure and volume status. In addition, the open fontanelle affords a degree of protection against the development of increased intracranial pressure in the head-injured infant, although this protection is not unlimited. The child's brain has a higher percentage of white matter, which may be responsible for the greater resilience children demonstrate after head injury.

189

Perhaps because of the head's relatively greater size and the fact that the child's neck is less muscular and offers less support, head injury is extremely common in the pediatric trauma victim and is an important factor in morbidity and mortality. Maxillofacial injury is much less common in children than in adults because the brunt of the energy applied to the face is absorbed by the relatively larger frontal bone and cranium.

The pediatric neck is shorter, fatter, less muscular, and more cartilaginous than that of the adult. Evaluation of the neck veins and trachea may be difficult, and landmarks for central venous access may be obscure. The larynx is located more anteriorly and cephalad than that of the adult, making intubation more difficult and rendering blind nasal intubation less successful. The child's occiput is prominent until the age of 10 years, making the "sniff position" used to enhance visualization of the airway for intubation automatic in some children; others require a pad under the shoulders to avoid hyperflexion of the neck. The narrowest part of the pediatric airway, the cricoid cartilage (rather than the vocal cords as in the adult) is lined with loose columnar epithelium, which is easily damaged and scars as a response to pressure necrosis or infection. Therefore, the proper size of endotracheal tube must be chosen to prevent airway complications postintubation. The narrowness of the airway at the level of the cricoid cartilage also renders needle cricothyrotomy and emergency tracheostomy more difficult and hazardous than is a similar procedure in the adult. The larynx is positioned high in the neck; therefore, some protection against trauma is provided by the mandible. Rather than actual fracture of the larynx, injury to the neck tends to cause soft tissue damage. This is because the tracheal rings are cartilaginous in children, and the airway is supported by an abundance of loose connective tissue.

The thorax of the child is more pliable, less bony, and more cartilaginous than that of the adult, with less overlying muscle and fat to protect the ribs and underlying chest structures. Therefore, blunt trauma is more easily transmitted to the underlying structures, and significant injury may be present with little external evidence of damage. The sternum and ribs are cartilaginous. If they are fractured, the force required would have been massive, and damage to underlying structures is likely. The mediastinum of the child is not firmly fixed and is subject to wide excursions in the presence of pneumothorax.

Tension pneumothorax in children, therefore, develops more rapidly and has more devastating consequences than in adults. Until a child is 12 years old, the diaphragm is inserted horizontally and is more distensible than in the adult. This respiratory compromise from distention of gastric contents, diaphragmatic irritation, and diaphragmatic injury is more likely because the horizontal insertion of both ribs and diaphragm is less efficient than in the adult configuration.

The child's abdomen has less overlying muscle and fat to protect internal organs. In addition, the ribs insert horizontally, providing less protection to the liver and spleen and placing them in a more anterior and caudad position, more exposed to injury. Therefore, seemingly insignificant forces can cause serious abdominal injury. Measurement of abdominal girth provides valuable information in the ongoing assessment of abdominal trauma and possible internal hemorrhage. Even small changes in abdominal girth can reflect significant internal blood loss.

ABCs: THE INITIAL APPROACH TO THE PEDIATRIC TRAUMA PATIENT

The first priority in the severely traumatized patient is (1) to diagnose and treat life-threatening injuries, (2) then to diagnose injuries requiring emergent operative intervention, and (3) finally, to manage nonlife-threatening injuries. To this end, the initial use of the "Primary Survey" is recommended by the American College of Emergency Physicians, American Academy of Pediatrics, and the American College of Surgeons. This may be remembered easily by use of the mnemonic ABCDE.

A: Airway and cervical spine (c-spine) stabilization.

B: Breathing and ventilation.

C: Circulation and hemorrhage control.

D: Disability (neurologic screening examination).

E: Exposure and environment.

The Primary Survey addresses life-threatening issues first and requires that resuscitative measures be carried out simultaneously with evaluation. Because the anesthesiologist rarely evaluates A without planning to ensure the adequacy of B, the two will be discussed together after a few words about c-spine injury.

C-Spine Stabilization

Pediatric patients comprise 5 to 10 percent of cervical spine injuries. All patients who may have had c-spine injury must have neck stabilization and protection, particularly during airway manipulation. Two thirds of pediatric patients who have c-spine injuries do not show radiographic evidence. An awake patient who complains of neck pain, dysesthesias, or weakness should be evaluated carefully for occult injury. C-spine stabilization and study is suggested in:

1. All patients with head injury.
2. All patients with significant supraclavicular injury.
3. Any patient knocked down by a motor vehicle.
4. Any patient unrestrained in a motor vehicle.
5. Any unconscious patient who has sustained significant trauma.

Appropriate study includes CT scan (the so-called gold standard) or three plain radiographic views: cross table lateral, anteroposterior, and open mouth. If c-spine injury has not been ruled out, stabilization of the neck with sandbags and tape or tongs is recommended. Special care must be taken during airway manipulation, when flexion and extension of the neck is common. During airway manipulation, in-line stabilization (Fig. 12-1) by an assistant may help prevent c-spine damage. Care must be taken that the head is not pulled during stabilization

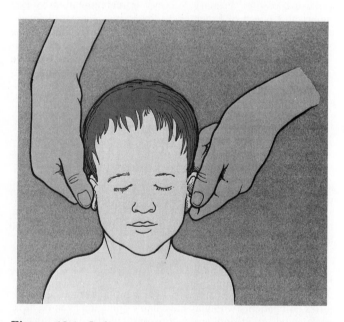

Figure 12-1 In-line stabilization may help prevent spinal cord damage during laryngoscopy and intubation. It is accomplished by grasping the child's ears and holding the head and neck in a neutral position, without pulling the head.

because this stretches the cord and may worsen an injury. Stabilization of the c-spine by cervical collar is of little value during airway manipulation. Studies in adults have shown that a soft collar allows as much as 75 percent of normal neck movement. Rigid collars reduce flexion and extension to about 30 percent of normal and laterally, to 50 percent. Although a jaw thrust is typically taught as the method for opening the airway in the c-spine-injured patient, both the jaw thrust and chin lift caused significant widening of the disk space in one cadaver study. Oral and nasopharyngeal airways caused minimal movement and may be the preferred technique when they can be used. The technique for securing the airway in the child with a known or suspected c-spine injury depends on the urgency of the situation, the skills of the practitioner, and the child's associated injuries and airway anatomy. Direct laryngoscopy is the fastest, surest way to achieve intubation in these children. In-line stabilization is recommended by the American Heart Association. Although studies have not proved its benefit, there appears to be a low risk associated with this method. Failed intubation is the biggest hazard with this technique. Many factors can occur that make intubation difficult. Inability to extend the neck fully with poor visualization, blood in the pharynx, facial and pharyngeal edema, and even hematoma and edema formation around the larynx can impair visualization of the airway and intubation. Other methods that can be used also have their drawbacks. Cricothyroidotomy has a high failure and complication rate in adults (and even more so, in children). Transtracheal ventilation also has a high complication rate and is difficult to perform if the head cannot be extended. Awake tracheal intubation, either the blind nasal technique or a fiberoptic technique, is frequently used in adults. Awake procedures require a cooperative patient; in children, this may require the use of significant sedation. Struggling, coughing, and bucking during intubation attempts will also threaten an injured neck. An awake nasal intubation requires multiple attempts (up to 90 percent of patients in one adult series). This will be poorly tolerated by most children and may precipitate adenoidal bleeding, making further intubation attempts difficult. In summary, no one technique for airway management has been proved to be superior in the c-spine-injured child. The urgency of intervention, the equipment at hand, and the skill of the practitioner must all be considered in managing these patients. In-line stabilization and direct laryngoscopy is the surest, fastest method to secure the airway. Other techniques that are useful in adults, such as cricothyrotomy, transtracheal ventilation, retrograde tracheal intubation, and awake techniques, may be unsatisfactory for most children. If a muscle relaxant is required, succinylcholine can be used during the first 48 h of injury.

Airway and Breathing

Upper airway obstruction in the injured child is usually caused by the tongue falling back against the child's soft palate. Other causes include secretions, vomitus, blood, or aspiration of loose bone fragments, teeth, or other debris. Suction may be the first step to clearing the airway. Other maneuvers to clear the airway may include repositioning of the airway using chin lift or, if c-spine injury is suspected, a jaw thrust maneuver. Oral or nasal airways, intubation, or in certain extreme circumstances, surgical or needle cricothyrotomy may be required to provide an airway.

An oral airway is poorly tolerated in an awake patient, but in an unconscious patient, it may be used to pull the tongue forward. The most common mistake in the use of the oral airway in pediatric patients is in placement. The tongue should be pulled down and forward with a tongue blade or laryngoscope before the airway is placed. Otherwise, the airway may push the tongue further back and worsen the obstruction. The proper size is chosen by placing the airway against the child's cheek. When the flanged end is at the upper incisors, the other end should reach the angle of the mandible (see Fig. 7-1). A small airway may push the tongue back; a large airway may push the epiglottis over the vocal cords. Each will cause further obstruction.

Nasal airways are used infrequently because they may cause significant adenoidal bleeding when placed in the young child. They may be more useful in teen-agers. In infants, a cut endotracheal tube may be used in place of a nasal airway because it can be adjusted to the proper size for each infant and the lumen is larger in proportion to the total diameter of the airway.

Ideally, intubation should be preceded by ventilation and oxygenation of the patient with bag valve mask devices using a 100 percent fraction of inspired oxygen. However, if the airway is obstructed and cannot be relieved enough to allow adequate ventilation, either spontaneous or assisted, preoxygenation may not be possible.

If intubation is necessary to obtain an airway, the choice of correctly sized equipment is essential to avoid iatrogenic airway trauma. A quick estimate of tube size is possible by choosing a tube the same diameter as the nares or one that matches the diameter of the little finger. The formula 16 + age (in years)/4 also provides a useful estimate. Straight blades usually allow the best displacement of soft tissue and visualization of the cords in small children and infants and can be used to lift the epiglottis. At age 4 or 5 years, either a Miller 2 or MacIntosh 2 may be used.

The adequacy of ventilation can be assessed by observation

of the child's respiratory rate and depth and by the presence or absence of indicators of distress, that is, retractions, use of accessory muscles, nasal flaring, wheezing, and stridor. Arterial blood gases may be helpful but must be used in conjunction with the examination. Blood gases may be normal in a child who is close to respiratory arrest secondary to fatigue but is still managing to compensate. If breathing must be assisted, bag valve mask ventilation is the best initial way to do this. After the airway is clear, the adequacy of assisted ventilation should be evaluated by chest excursion and auscultation of breath sounds. Difficulty with mask ventilation unrelated to upper airway obstruction may be encountered in:

1. The struggling child.
2. The patient with direct laryngeal injury.
3. Massive aspiration.
4. Pneumothorax with increased airway pressure.
5. Massive pulmonary artery obstruction.
6. Gastric dilatation.
7. Laryngospasm.

Intubation may be required for many reasons as follows:

1. Inadequate ventilation by bag and mask.
2. Need for prolonged control of the airway.
3. Prevention of aspiration.
4. Need for positive pressure ventilation or controlled hyperventilation.
5. Presence of a flail chest.
6. Shock unresponsive to volume.

All children who have sustained trauma are considered to have a full stomach and may possibly have an ileus. They are at increased risk for aspiration if their airway reflexes are diminished for any reason (e.g., induction of anesthesia, head injury, or sedation). When ventilating or attempting to intubate these patients, the use of the Sellick maneuver (Fig. 12-2) to prevent air from entering the stomach and passive aspiration is recommended. Placement of a gastric tube to decompress the stomach may be done after intubation to facilitate ventilation and minimize aspiration on extubation. If a distended stomach is inhibiting ventilatory efforts during bag–mask ventilation or positive pressure ventilation is causing the child to swallow a great deal of air, placement of an oral gastric tube may be necessary before intubation. An awake, struggling child may not tolerate awake gastric decompression, and placement of the tube in these patients may precipitate vomiting.

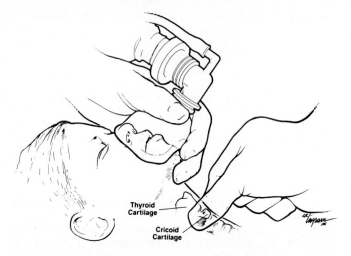

Figure 12-2 Sellick maneuver. Firm pressure is held over the cricoid cartilage by the thumb and forefinger. The cricoid is the only cartilaginous ring of the trachea that forms a complete ring. Firm pressure on the cricoid cartilage will effectively occlude the esophagus and prevent passive regurgitation of gastric contents before tracheal intubation is accomplished. (Reproduced with permission from the *New York State Journal of Medicine,* copyright by the Medical Society of the State of New York. Rasch DK, Pollard TG: Near-drowning in children: Management and outcome. *NY State J Med* 1988; 88:427–433.)

Circulation

Shock is a clinical state in which perfusion is inadequate to meet the metabolic needs of the end organs. Shock may still be present even though the blood pressure is normal. This is considered "compensated" shock. When the sympathetic system no longer can maintain enough peripheral vasoconstriction to maintain a normal blood pressure, shock is "decompensated." The goal of the circulatory evaluation is to detect the subtle signs and symptoms of shock and treat compensated shock before it becomes uncompensated. End-organ perfusion is the best indicator of circulatory status. Capillary refill, level of consciousness, and urine output are useful to evaluate end-organ perfusion, but in the immediate resuscitation phase, the urine output is not always known. Heart rate is also a valuable indicator, but blood pressure can be misleading. During the assessment of circulatory status, it is necessary to assess end-organ perfusion, obtain venous access, send blood for typing and

Table 12-1   Normal Heart and Respiratory Rates in Children

	INFANTS	PRE-SCHOOLERS	SCHOOL-AGE CHILDREN
Respiratory rate	20 to 30	16 to 20	12 to 15
Heart rate (upper limit)	140	120	100

crossmatching, and diagnose and control external and internal hemorrhage.

Evaluation of the circulatory status of children is frequently hampered by a lack of familiarity with the normal blood pressures and pulse values in children. Tables 12-1 and 12-2 present a simplified guide for normal heart rates in children and a useful formula for calculating normal systolic and diastolic blood pressures.

Tachycardia is the earliest response of the young child to hypovolemia. An increase in heart rate should alert the clinician to possible hypovolemia or unrecognized, ongoing blood loss. The blood pressure is a less useful means of evaluating the circulatory status. Although blood pressure varies directly with volume status in the very young infant, as the sympathetic nervous system develops, older infants and children may vasoconstrict enough to keep both blood and central venous pressure normal until 25 percent of the blood volume is lost. When a tachycardic child also displays hypotension, blood loss may be 30 to 50 percent of the blood volume, or more! Capillary refill is a good indicator of the peripheral perfusion and circulatory status. A normal capillary refill time is 2 s. To perform the capillary refill test, compress the skin or nail beds for 5 s; then release them and note the time until color returns. A delayed capillary refill indicates that perfusion is poor. In the pediatric trauma patient, this is usually because of hypovolemia. A child who is cold may have delayed capillary refill in the face of ad-

Table 12-2   Calculation of Normal Blood Pressure

80 + (2 × age in yr) = normal systolic BP for age.

70 + (2 × age in yr) = lower limit of normal systolic BP for age.

BP = blood pressure.

equate circulating volume. A child who is exhibiting tachycardia and delayed capillary refill needs urgent volume resuscitation to prevent shock. There are several rules of thumb that can be used in calculating fluid replacement.

> Blood volume = 80 mL/kg
> Replace 25 percent of this volume rapidly *or*
> Fluid bolus with 20 mL/kg

Regardless of which rule is used, repeated assessment of fluid status is necessary to guide replacement of previous or ongoing losses. Many fluid boluses may be necessary to obtain hemodynamic stability. Appropriate fluids for resuscitation include nonglucose-containing, isotonic crystalloid, colloid, or blood products. In massive hemorrhage, either type-specific or O negative red blood cells may be used. Massive transfusion is covered elsewhere in this text. Glucose-containing fluids should be avoided because they may induce a hyperosmolar diuresis and result in further volume depletion and because hyperglycemia is associated with a poor outcome in head-injured children. An exception to this would be the child who is documented to be hypoglycemic, in whom one 20 mL/kg bolus of a 5% dextrose solution may substitute for correction with 25% dextrose (1 to 2 mL/kg).

Obviously, administration of volume to the injured child requires establishment of venous access—no easy task in the hypovolemic, vasoconstricted child or chubby infant. Many techniques are available. Percutaneous peripheral venous cannulation is usually the first method attempted. After 90 s have passed in an attempt to obtain peripheral percutaneous cannulation, other methods need to be considered, for example, intraosseous cannulation, peripheral cutdown, or percutaneous central line placement. The method used should be the one that allows the most fluid to be given most rapidly with a minimum of complications, and it will vary according to the expertise of the available personnel.

Intraosseous cannulation (Fig. 12-3) is easy to accomplish and has minimal associated complications. Its use has been recommended by the American Heart Association in children younger than 6 years of age, but it can and has been used in other age groups. Cannulas have been made especially for this purpose, but any 14- or 16-gauge needle, a Jamsheedy bone marrow needle, or a large-bore spinal needle may be used. Traditionally, the site of cannulation is just below the tibial tuberosity on the medial aspect of the bone. The needle is held at a 90° angle and pushed through the bony cortex until it pops into the medullary space. Evidence that the needle is in place in-

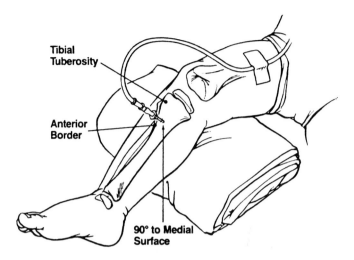

Tibial
Tuberosity

Anterior
Border

90° to Medial
Surface

Figure 12-3 Intraosseous cannulation provides a rapid, easily accomplished route for drug and fluid resuscitation.

cludes a pop or loss of resistance when the needle pushes through the cortex, the return of bone marrow into a syringe when aspirated, and infusion of fluid (sometimes requiring pressure) with a minimum of subcutaneous infiltration. All types of fluids and medications have been infused through an intraosseous line without complication. Considerable pressure may be needed to do rapid volume resuscitation because flow through the line depends on the perfusion pressure.

Complications include leakage from the site after the needle is removed and minimal subcutaneous infiltration. Osteomyelitis has been reported in a small percentage of patients in whom the line was used for a prolonged period of time. Intraosseous cannulation is not recommended in a fractured extremity.

If central venous cannulation is desired, the femoral vein has the advantage of being away from the airway, which may be requiring simultaneous manipulation. In addition, cannulation at this site is easier for most practitioners and has no risk of pneumothorax or carotid artery cannulation. If severe intraabdominal hemorrhage is suspected, however, an upper extremity or central line site above the diaphragm is preferred.

Prolonged, fruitless efforts to obtain percutaneous peripheral venous access should be avoided. Use of a 90-s limit followed by intraosseous cannulation has been shown markedly to reduce the time until attainment of vascular access.

Hemorrhage in the trauma patient may be external or internal. Do not assume that the obvious injury is the only injury. A child with one injury should be suspected of having others until proved otherwise. External hemorrhage can usually be controlled by pressure and, possibly, by elevation of the hemorrhaging extremity. Scalp and facial wounds can be a source of considerable blood loss in children and should not be treated lightly. Internal hemorrhage occurs in five body areas: chest, abdomen, retroperitoneum, pelvis, and thigh. Signs and symptoms of impending shock from blood loss may be subtle in children, for reasons previously discussed, and repeated evaluation of heart rate, capillary refill, and blood pressure are essential. In addition, the presence of pain or swelling must be observed because they are signs of occult hemorrhage.

The Pneumatic Antishock
Garment in Children

Occasionally, a pediatric patient will require placement of a pneumatic antishock garment for stabilization of circulatory status. This garment works by increasing the total peripheral vascular resistance, decreasing circulation to the area inflated, possibly tamponading further hemorrhage, and providing a 5 to 10 percent autotransfusion effect. Indications for placement in the pediatric population have not been well studied but, presently, include a systolic blood pressure less than two-thirds of normal and signs and symptoms of shock.

Trousers are placed (usually in the field but sometimes in the emergency room) by first removing the clothing and placing the garment under the child without rotating, flexing, or extending the spine. The legs are inflated one at a time, followed by the abdominal compartment, if necessary. Inflation should be done only to the point at which the vital signs are normal. Pedal pulses should be monitored before and after placement and should not be occluded. Antishock trousers can remain in place for 2 h with minimal detrimental effects.

The most frequent problem encountered with them is premature removal or rapid deflation. The garment should be released only when the vital signs are stable and, then, slowly. The abdominal compartment is released first. If blood pressure drops by 5 to 10 percent, the garment should be reinflated and further volume resuscitation done. In the patient with intraabdominal bleeding, deflation is best done in the operating room, after anesthesia has been induced, when blood products are readily available and exploration is imminent. Sudden deflation of the garment results in a decrease in cardiac output for several reasons as follows: sudden redistribution of blood flow to the pelvis and lower extremities, rebleeding from a previously tamponaded site, and possibly the release of large quantities of lactic acid from poorly perfused extremities.

Disability

Head injury is discussed in detail later in this text. However, after urgent stabilization of respiratory and cardiac function is accomplished, a simple but rapid evaluation of neurologic status is extremely helpful for further management. The Glasgow coma scale or the modified infant Glasgow coma scale may be used for this purpose, but if time or memory does not allow, information should be assessed in a simplified manner using a simple mnemonic AVPU.

A: Alert.

V: Responds to verbal stimuli.

P: Responds to painful stimuli.

U: Unresponsive.

This is more objective information than terms like semicomatose and aids in the immediate decision-making concerning the trauma victim. An objective starting point by which improvement or deterioration may be evaluated is offered by this system. Although a head-injured child is usually given minimal intravenous fluids, if the child is also in shock, volume resuscitation is necessary to maintain perfusion and normalize vital signs.

Exposure and Environment

Infants and small children become hypothermic easily. The fibrillation threshold for children is about 27 to 30° C. Exposure at the site of accident and resuscitation of an unclothed child in a drafty emergency room can contribute to a difficult resuscitation. Attempts should be made to maintain the body temperature in the 36 to 37° range by warming the room, using warming lights, and warming fluids. If the patient is intubated, humidify and warm the inspired gases. Peritoneal lavage and even cardiopulmonary bypass may be necessary to rewarm a severely hypothermic child.

The minimal laboratory results in the primary survey include blood typing and crossmatching, hematocrit, hemoglobin, leukocyte count, urinalysis, amylase level, cardiac and liver enzymes, and arterial blood gases. The latter may be normal in a compensated child who is near respiratory failure from fatigue. The hematocrit may not reflect acute blood loss in the child who has received no fluid resuscitation.

SPECIFIC INJURIES

After initial stabilization has been accomplished, a secondary survey is conducted to evaluate the body from head to toe (Table 12-3). During this critical postresuscitation time, frequent reassessment of the child's airway, breathing, and circulation are important. A quick medical history (Table 12-4) should also be obtained from the parents, if possible. Although

Table 12-3 The Secondary Survey

Head	Check pupillary size, conjunctiva, reaction of pupils, fundal appearance, and vision. Examine face for maxillofacial trauma. Check dentition. Examine scalp for laceration of soft tissue injury. Look for signs of basilar skull fracture (battle sign, raccoon eyes, hemotympanum, and cerebrospinal fluid rhinorrhea or otorrhea). Check for symmetric voluntary movement and neurologic function of facial muscles.
Neck	Palpate cervical spine. Check for subcutaneous emphysema, abnormal tracheal position, hematoma, and localized pain. Evaluate neck veins for distention.
Chest	Check for bilateral chest excursion, asymmetry of wall motion, and flail segments. Palpate chest. Auscultate lung fields and cardiovascular system.
Abdomen	Repeated measurement of girth may help diagnose unsuspected bleeding. Inspect for ease of movement with respiration, bruises, lacerations, and bowel sound. Palpate for localized findings. Observe and palpate flanks.
Pelvis	Palpate bony prominences for tenderness or instability. Check for laceration, hematoma, and active bleeding. Check urethral meatus for blood.
Rectum	Do a rectal examination, including the integrity of the wall, muscle tone, prostatic injury, and occult GI hemorrhage.
Extremity	Check for signs of fracture, dislocation, abrasion, contusion, and hematoma. Note bony instability. Do a neurologic examination.
Back	Examine only if spinal cord injury is not suspected.
Skin	Look for petechiae, burns, and contusions.
Neurologic	In-depth neurologic examination.

Table 12-4   Quick Medical History: AMPLE

A:	Allergies/anesthetic history.
M:	Medications.
P:	Past illnesses/surgeries.
L:	Last meal.
E:	Events preceding injury.

the majority of pediatric trauma patients are relatively healthy, some have significant underlying disease, and some may have unrecognized congenital abnormalities, which may complicate resuscitation attempts.

Head Injury

Head injury is present in greater than 75 percent of pediatric multiple trauma victims and is a big factor in morbidity and mortality. The outcome of the head-injured child depends largely on the primary injury. It is the responsibility of the medical team to minimize damage caused by secondary insult (hypoxia, hypercarbia, shock, and mismanagement of the c-spine) and to provide an optimum chance for the patient to recover. Fortunately, the pediatric brain is resilient, warranting aggressive treatment. Accurate assessment of the child's neurologic status is necessary to allow classification of the severity of the injury, to predict the outcome, and to monitor deterioration of the neurologic status. The Glasgow coma scale is objective and reproducible (Table 12-5). It has limited usefulness in the preverbal child. A modified infant version is available. Its use has not yet been validated. Some practitioners use the adult one but assign a full verbal score to those infants who can cry (Table 12-5). A change in status of two points on the Glasgow coma scale is important, and a change of three points is considered a neurosurgical emergency.

The child with a massive intracranial hemorrhage or a rapidly expanding hematoma with threatened herniation is a candidate for immediate surgery. These injuries are less common in children than adults. Basic therapy for the majority of head-injured patients is as follows:

1. Maintain or establish airway and circulation.
2. Protect the c-spine at all times until CT or three-view radiologic study has been accomplished.
3. Early neurosurgical consultation.
4. Minimize intracranial pressure (ICP). Cerebral perfusion pressure equals the mean arterial pressure (MAP) minus the ICP. After the MAP is stabilized, attempts to mini-

Table 12-5 Glasgow Coma Score

ACTIVITY	BEST RESPONSE	SCORE
Eye opening	Spontaneous	4
	To verbal stimuli	3
	To pain	2
	None	1
Verbal	Oriented	5
	Confused	4
	Inappropriate words	3
	Nonspecific sounds	2
	None	1
Motor	Follows commands	6
	Localizes pain	5
	Withdraws in response to pain	4
	Flexion in response to pain	3
	Extension in response to pain	2
	None	1

mize the ICP are warranted, with the goal being to maintain cerebral perfusion pressure. Methods for reduction of ICP include elevation of the head of the bed by 30 to 40° and keeping the head midline, hyperventilating to a $PaCO_2$ of 25 to 28 mmHg to increase the cerebrovasoconstriction and reduce the blood flow. Prevention of seizures will also minimize an ICP increase. The use of diuretics and steroids is controversial and best done at the recommendation of a neurosurgical consultant.

5. Control hemorrhage. Unlike adults, children with head injuries can lose a large proportion of their blood volume in the subgaleal or intracranial space, resulting in shock from head injury alone. The two areas most prone to hemorrhage are the scalp veins and the dural sinuses. Bleeding from scalp veins may be controlled by pressure, hemostats, and pressure dressings. Uncontrollable bleeding may be the result of a dural sinus tear, which requires surgical intervention.

6. Control seizures. Seizures greatly elevate the oxygen requirement of the brain. They can be treated with phenytoin 10 mg/kg given slowly.

7. Give antibiotics if the wound is penetrating.

Securing the airway of the head-injured child is a challenge. The anesthesiologist who is consulted to help with these children in the emergency room must sometimes work in less than optimal conditions. Careful assessment, planning, and flexibility are required in these circumstances. Drug choices for facilitation of intubation are made according to the availability and pharmacology of the drug in question, the patient's volume status, airway anatomy, ICP status (known or suspected), and mental status (comatose or uncooperative). Nasal intubation is contraindicated in the presence of basilar skull fracture because the cribriform plate may be penetrated and the brain stem also intubated. Awake nasal intubation is poorly tolerated and difficult to perform in children and is probably not useful in the head-injured child in whom the ICP may be further elevated by struggling and coughing. Figure 12-4 is an algorithm for airway management in the head-injured child. This algorithm may not be appropriate for every patient or every circumstance, but it does provide a general guideline for airway management.

The goal of airway intervention in the head-injured child is to secure the airway safely and rapidly with an endotracheal tube with a minimal decrease in MAP and a minimal increase in ICP. With this in mind, the muscle relaxant of choice depends largely on the situation. Nondepolarizing muscle relaxants may be preferable to succinylcholine because of the increase in ICP associated with succinylcholine. If rapid intubating conditions are required, relatively larger doses of pancuronium (0.2 mg/kg) or vecuronium (0.28 mg/kg) may be used, with a corresponding increase in duration. The use of succinylcholine offers an advantage when rapid onset and short duration are required. If difficulty with ventilation and intubation is suspected (difficult anatomy or injured airway), muscle relaxants may be omitted altogether and spontaneous ventilation maintained.

The Injured Airway

Attention to the airway and adequacy of ventilation are essential in the urgent care of the pediatric trauma patient. When the airway itself is damaged, the anesthesiologist faces a challenge. The following is a discussion of trauma of the upper airway, neck, and tracheobronchial tree.

Maxillofacial trauma is unusual in children because their relatively larger cranium tends to absorb the energy of impact. When present, associated injuries, particularly head injury, are common. The most frequent causes of maxillofacial trauma are motor vehicle accidents, fights, child abuse, and falls. Trauma of the midface may be associated with head injury and severe bleeding from the carotid artery. Nasal intubation is contraindicated in midface fracture and fractures of the bones of the sinuses because of the danger of cranial placement of the endotracheal tube. Mandibular fracture is the most frequent of maxillofacial trauma in the pediatric population. Although airway obstruction in this group is frequently a concern, at least

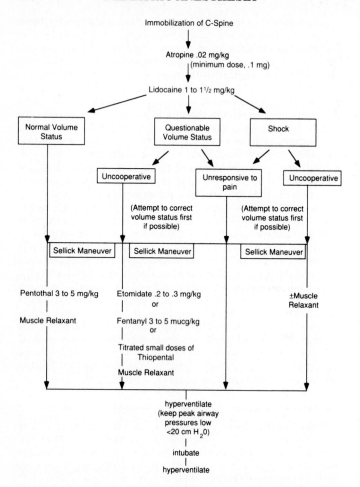

Figure 12-4 Airway management of the head-injured child.

one series showed it to be unusual. Airway compromise in these patients is more often secondary to the tongue falling backward on the soft palate and is easily relieved by placement of an oral airway or laryngoscopy and intubation. Foreign bodies, loose teeth, bone fragments, blood, secretions, and significant edema can make intubation difficult.

Neck trauma may either be blunt or penetrating. Penetrating neck trauma is rare in children, but blunt trauma may be more common than previously suspected. Blunt trauma to the neck may exhibit very little in the way of external evidence. A history consistent with strangulation, hanging, or motor vehicle accident should alert the physician to this possibility. The child's larynx is somewhat protected by the mandible because of its cephalad location in the neck. However, the small size of the airway, the narrowed laryngeal opening, and the abundance of loose connective tissue predispose the child to soft tissue injury with significant swelling. Injury from blunt impact includes arytenoid dislocation, anteroposterior collapse of the larynx, and vocal cord paralysis. Because of the flexible cartilaginous nature of the child's not yet mature tracheal rings and larynx, laryngeal fracture is not common. These injuries in an adult would probably be handled with an awake tracheostomy. This would be difficult to achieve in a pediatric patient. These children are usually endoscoped in the operating room by an ear, nose, and throat surgeon experienced in pediatric care. The induction for these children will be discussed in the following section and is similar to that of a child with epiglottitis. Pneumothorax and c-spine injury must be ruled out in these children.

Tracheobronchial injury is rare in children. Although penetrating trauma is the most common cause of tracheobronchial injury in the adult, violent blunt injury to the upper chest is the most common cause in the child. This type of injury should also be suspected with penetrating injuries of the lower neck and thorax. (Note: Gunshot wounds cause tissue damage far from the site of entry and exit. This is of particular importance in the neck and thorax.) Subcutaneous emphysema is also a frequent finding (92 percent). A child who has a pneumothorax that persists despite chest tube drainage may have a tracheobronchial injury. The most frequent sites of injury are the posterior trachea and the right or left main bronchus. Rapid deceleration injuries tend to tear the trachea at the cricoid cartilage and at the carina, where it is fixed. Crushing anteroposterior injuries against a closed glottis tend to pull the lungs apart at the carina or can burst the trachea. Hemorrhage in a tracheobronchial injury is usually from the bronchial vessels (25 percent of patients) and contributes to hemoptysis. Major vessel injuries are rare but serious. Signs of great vessel injury include a widened mediastinum and opacification of the thoracic apex. In one series, about one-third of children with tracheobronchial rupture required immediate operation. A large percentage of these patients die before they even reach the emergency room. Overall, the mortality is about 77 percent. Treatment requires rapid evaluation, treatment of tension pneumothorax, and rapid access to the airway distal to the site of rupture. If the injury lies below the end of the endotracheal tube, a tube must be placed distal to the site of injury or directly into the uninvolved bronchus by thoracostomy. In some cases, a long endotracheal tube can be passed translaryngeally and a one-sided intubation done. Double-lumen tubes are not available for pediatric patients.

Anesthetic care for children with suspected laryngeal or tracheal injury is exciting, to say the least. The goal is to maintain spontaneous ventilation until the airway can be inspected and secured, either with intubation or tracheostomy. The following is the method for induction commonly used at our institution:

1. Preoxygenation.
2. Intravenous line and monitors.
3. Atropine 0.01 mg/kg.
4. Lidocaine 1 mg/kg.
5. O_2/halothane induction; avoid nitrous oxide.
6. When surgical plane of anesthesia is attained, spray cords with lidocaine 2 mg/kg.
7. Endoscopy by surgeon; ventilate through the side port of a rigid scope.
8. Tracheostomy, intubation, or ventilation through a bronchoscope.

Occasionally, the intravenous lidocaine will be omitted and the cords sprayed with 4 mg/kg of lidocaine.

Thoracic Injury

Thoracic injury requires rapid assessment and appropriate therapy because some of these injuries are an immediate threat to life. Blunt injury comprises the majority of thoracic injury in children. All children who receive blunt chest trauma should receive supplemental O_2, even if they seem to have no respiratory distress. The signs of chest injury may be subtle, and rapid deterioration may occur. Most children with severe cardiorespiratory compromise secondary to thoracic injury have one of the following:

1. Airway obstruction.
2. Tension pneumothorax.
3. Large hemo- or hemo-/pneumothorax.
4. Flail chest.
5. Open pneumothorax.
6. Pericardial tamponade.

More rare injuries include pulmonary crush injuries, injury to the heart or great vessels, rupture of the tracheal bronchial tree, and rupture of the esophagus. Many of these problems can be detected by physical examination of the child. Table 12-6 shows the associated physical signs related to specific injuries.

The emergency airway management for complete airway obstruction unresponsive to bag valve mask ventilation or intubation is cricothyrotomy, which is considered faster and slightly less risky than an emergency pediatric tracheostomy. The procedure is difficult, in part, because it must be performed in the

Table 12-6   Signs of Thoracic Injury

SIGN	INJURY	COMMENT
Neck vein distention	Cardiac tamponade	Classic signs often missing in the hypovolemic child
Asymmetric chest wall motion	Pneumothorax, tension pneumothorax, flail chest, foreign-body aspiration	
Deviated trachea	Tension pneumothorax	
Decreased breath sounds	Pneumo-/hemothorax, foreign-body aspiration	Hemothorax dull to percussion, tension pneumothorax hyperresonant
Chest wall tenderness, subcutaneous emphysema	Rib fractures	Considerable force needed to fracture ribs; observe for injury to underlying organs
Stridor, suprasternal or intercostal retraction, wheezing	Lower airway obstruction	
Petechiae, conjunctival hemorrhage, decreased level of consciousness	Massive pulmonary crush injury	Cardiac and pulmonary contusion may be associated

narrowest part of the pediatric airway. Cricothyrotomy (Fig. 12-5) is accomplished by placing the neck in gentle extension. A 14-gauge catheter over the needle is inserted at a perpendicular angle through the cricoid cartilage. When air is aspirated, the needle bevel is in the trachea, and the catheter can be advanced off the needle into the trachea. Air should be aspirated after the catheter is placed to ensure that the posterior wall of the trachea has not been perforated. A 3.5 I.D. endotracheal tube connector may be connected to the hub of the catheter and

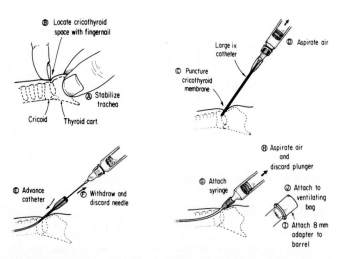

Figure 12-5 Percutaneous cricothyroidotomy. Extend the head in the midline with a rolled towel or folded sheet transversely beneath the shoulders. (A) Stabilize the trachea. (B) The cricothyroid membrane is located with the fingertip between the thyroid and cricoid cartilages. This space is so narrow (1 mm) that only a fingernail can discern it in an infant. (C) A large intravenous catheter (12 to 14 gauge) is inserted through the cricothyroid membrane and (D) air aspirated. (E) The catheter is advanced into the trachea through the membrane, and (F) the needle is discarded. (G) The intraluminal position is reconfirmed by attaching a 3-mL syringe and (H) aspirating for air. (I) The 3-mL syringe barrel without plunger is attached to the catheter. (J) An 8-mm endotracheal tube adaptor is attached to the syringe barrel. (Reproduced with permission. Coté C, Todres DI: The difficult pediatric airway, in Ryan J, Coté C, Todres DI (eds): *A Practice of Anesthesia for Infants and Children.* Orlando, FL, Grune & Stratton, 1986, p 50.)

bag ventilation begun, or jet ventilation may be used. Jet ventilation can be accomplished using wall oxygen by connecting O_2 tubing to a Y connector and attaching it to the hub of the catheter by a Luer-lock or stopcock. Ventilation can then be accomplished by intermittently occluding the open end of the Y catheter. This will provide a short grace period during which a tracheostomy can be placed in a slightly more controlled circumstance.

Tension pneumothorax is a common, lethal complication in the pediatric trauma victim. Do not wait for x-ray documentation to treat this condition. Because the mediastinum is less fixed in children and infants than adults, the overdistention of the hemithorax significantly distorts the mediastinum, compressing the great veins, and decreasing the venous return. The result is a marked decrease in cardiac output. At any time during a resuscitation, a sudden deterioration in a child's ventilatory and circulatory status should alert the physician to the possibility of tension pneumothorax. The patient may be immediately stabilized by use of needle thoracostomy (Fig. 12-6). This is accomplished by threading a small intravenous catheter into the thoracic space and aspirating air. Chest tube placement must follow needle thoracotomy. The site of chest tube insertion is higher in the pediatric patient than in the adult patient, at the fourth intercostal space in the mid or anterior axillary line. This is because the horizontal, distensible pediatric diaphragm may be high in the thorax, and intraabdominal placement of the chest tube may occur. Decompression of the stomach before chest tube placement may help prevent this complication.

Flail chest is uncommon in children because their pliable, cartilaginous ribs are not easily fractured. It usually occurs in patients who are victims of high-speed motor vehicle accidents, auto–pedestrian collisions, and falls from significant heights. Paradoxic motion of the flail segment of the lung leads to impaired ventilation, and early intubation and positive pressure ventilation are usually necessary.

Open pneumothorax is usually caused by penetrating trauma and is, therefore, less common in children. The open wound should be covered with an occlusive dressing. If hemodynamic or respiratory deterioration occurs after occluding the wound, a tension pneumothorax may have occurred, and the dressing should be opened to allow pressure to escape.

Pericardial tamponade is usually caused by penetrating injury and is a rare cause of shock in children. It can also occur after iatrogenic trauma, for example, cardiac surgery, central line placement, and cardiac catheterization. The classic signs of cardiac tamponade are often absent in the child, and unex-

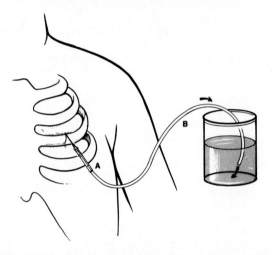

Figure 12-6 Needle thoracostomy. (A) A 20-gauge angiocath-ether is inserted into the chest at the second intercostal space at the midclavicular line. The puncture is made just above the rib to avoid the neurovascular bundle, which lies just beneath the lower border of each rib. (B) Intravenous extension tubing is connected to the catheter after it is threaded off the needle, and the other end is placed under a water seal. This maneuver allows more time for preparation for insertion of a chest tube because the air will remain evacuated.

plained hypotension may be the only finding. Even central line placement and venous pressure monitoring does not completely rule out tamponade if a child is hypovolemic. Likewise, the hypovolemic child may not show neck vein distention or an enlarged cardiac silhouette. Myocardial tamponade should be a suspected cause (albeit rare) in the patient with unexplained hypotension. (Others could include undiagnosed c-spine transsection, septic shock, or undiagnosed tension pneumothorax. Bear in mind that the most common cause for hypotension in the traumatized pediatric patient is hypovolemia, hypovolemia, hypovolemia.) Treatment of tamponade includes emergent stabilization with needle pericardiocentesis (Fig. 12-7) if the child is extremely unstable or a pericardial window under local anesthesia if time permits. Occasionally, a less compromised child may be anesthetized with a rapid-sequence induction and ketamine or etomidate for a pericardial window. This is usually done after the patient is prepared, when the surgeons are scrubbed and ready to proceed.

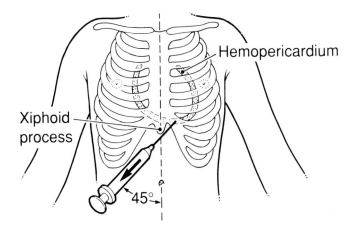

Figure 12-7 Needle pericardiocentesis may be used to aspirate a myocardial tamponade if urgent intervention is needed. It is accomplished by aiming a needle at the tip of the left scapula, 45° laterally and 45° superiorly, and aspirating during needle advancement. Blood aspirated from the pericardial sac does not clot by contrast with blood aspirated from the heart chambers.

Pulmonary contusion may initially show few physical and radiologic findings. Careful observation is necessary because these injuries can progress and result in hypoxia. Provide O_2, elevate the head of the bed, and minimize fluids (unless the patient is in shock).

Myocardial contusion may occur in children who have sustained severe blunt chest trauma. Elevated cardiac enzymes or electrocardiographic evidence of ischemia should alert one to this possibility. A central venous pressure or pulmonary artery catheter may aid in volume replacement and the use of inotropic infusions. Table 12-7 provides a list of normal pediatric hemodynamic values.

Abdominal Injuries

The onset of symptoms of abdominal injuries may be rapid (massive hemorrhage) or delayed (slow hemorrhage or development of peritonitis). The liver and spleen are the most frequently injured abdominal organs, usually from a motor vehicle accident or direct blows to the abdomen. Treatment of these injuries can range from observation and conservative management to emergent surgical exploration and aggressive volume

Table 12-7   Normal Hemodynamic Values in Children

PARAMETER	VALUE
RA	3 mmHg
RV	25 mmHg/3 mmHg
PA	25 mmHg/10 mmHg
LA	8 mmHg
LV	100 mmHg/8 mmHg
AO	100 mmHg/60 mmHg
SVR	15 to 30 units/m^2
PVR	1 to 2 units/m^2 (after age 2 to 4 mo)

RA = right atrium (central venous pressure); PA = pulmonary artery; PVR = pulmonary vascular resistance; AO = aorta; RV = right ventricle; LA = left atrium; LV = left ventricle; SVR = systemic vascular resistance.

resuscitation and transfusion. Usually, CT scan or abdominal examination determine the diagnosis. Diagnostic peritoneal lavage is used when other injuries require emergent treatment, and the presence or absence of abdominal bleeding is in question. A child with a neurologic injury and multiple trauma, in whom cardiovascular status is easily stabilized, will usually have a full neurologic workup first. At the other end of the spectrum, a child with neurologic injury who requires massive volume resuscitation and continues to show signs of shock requires urgent surgical exploration and treatment of internal hemorrhage. Anesthetic care of these patients must take into account the presence or absence of head and neck trauma, the presence of a full stomach, the volume status of the patient, and the possible presence of other undetermined injuries. Induction techniques may range from typical rapid-sequence induction, using thiopental and succinylcholine in the volume-resuscitated, non-head-injured child to the use of only atropine and a Sellick maneuver for the moribund child.

There is no foolproof induction technique for the child who is not completely volume resuscitated. If complete restoration of the circulating blood volume is impossible before induction or if the status of rehydration is not completely clear, intravenous agents that have been used with success include: ketamine, 1 to 2 mg/kg (avoid in head injury); etomidate, 0.2 to 0.3 mg/kg; or fentanyl, 5 to 10 μg/kg. Blood loss varies widely with each individual case, making preparation for rapid transfusion a necessity. This includes adequate large-bore venous cannulas, an apparatus for warming blood products, and the presence of blood products in the room before exploration begins. Urine output is a useful means for measuring the adequacy of fluid replacement during the surgical procedure. A urine output of 2 mL/kg for infants and 1 mL/kg for children is considered evidence of adequate renal perfusion. Central venous catheter placement and measurement of venous pressure may be warranted in some cases. It bears repeating that what seems to be an insignificant amount of blood loss may represent a large proportion of an infant's or small child's blood volume. Care must be taken to ensure adequate volume replacement.

Musculoskeletal Injury

It is easy to underestimate the blood loss that can occur in the fractured hip or femur of a child. Careful assessment and reassessment of circulatory status, as previously discussed, is important. Other considerations include the possibility of fat embolism with manipulation of the long bones and of pulmonary embolism from thrombus formation.

CONCLUSIONS

In conclusion, pediatric trauma is a leading cause of mortality among children. Rapid assessment and treatment of life-threatening injuries, followed by appropriate management of less serious injuries is essential. Space prevents a discussion of the psychological impact of pediatric trauma, but its importance must not be overlooked. Fear, pain, separation from parents, and a frightening, confusing emergency room or operating room environment makes an enduring impression on these patients. Unfortunately, they are poorly equipped to comprehend or express their fears. The importance of a supportive, understanding caretaker who takes the time to establish the child's trust during these trying circumstances cannot be overemphasized.

BIBLIOGRAPHY

Berry FA: *Anesthetic Management of Difficult and Routine Pediatric Patients*. Edinburgh, Churchill Livingstone, 1989.

Berry FA: Perioperative anesthetic management of the pediatric trauma patient. *Crit Care Clin* 1990; 6:147–163.

Cameron C: Paediatric airway management problems: Is there an anaesthetist in the house? *Can J Anaesth* 1991; 38:151–154.

Gerns SL (ed): *The Pediatric Airway*. Philadelphia, WB Saunders, 1991.

Hodge D: Intraosseous infusions: A review. *Pediatr Emerg Care* 1985; 1:215.

Kanter RK, Zimmerman JJ, Strauss RL, et al: Pediatric emergency intravenous access. *Am J Dis Child* 1986; 140:132–134.

Martin SW, Gussach GS: Pediatric penetrating head and neck trauma. *Laryngoscope* 1990; 100:1288–1291.

Mayer TA (ed): *Emergency Management of Pediatric Trauma.* Philadelphia, WB Saunders, 1985.

Mazurah A: Anesthesia for the trauma patient, in Touloukian R (ed): *Pediatric Trauma.* Chicago, Mosby Year Book, 1990, pp 77–89.

Myer CM, Orobello P, Cotton RT, et al: Blunt laryngeal trauma in children. *Laryngoscope* 1987; 97:1043–1048.

Ovassapian A, Dykeks M, Yelich S: Difficult pediatric intubation: An indication for the fiberoptic bronchoscope. *Anesthesiology* 1982; 56:412–413.

Rowe MI, Nakayama DK, Gardner MJ: Emergency endotracheal intubation in pediatric trauma. *Ann Surg* 1990; 211:218–223.

Ryan J, Todres D, Coté C, et al. (eds): *A Practice of Anesthesia for Infants and Children.* Orlando, FL, Grune & Stratton, 1986.

Siegel MB, Wetmore RG, Handler SD, et al: Mandibular fractures in the pediatric patient. *Arch Otolaryngeal Head Neck Surg* 1991; 117:533–536.

Silverman B: *Advanced Pediatric Life Support.* Elk Grove, IL, American College of Emergency Physicians, American Academy of Pediatrics, 1991.

Touloukian RJ (ed): *Pediatric Trauma,* ed 2. Chicago, Mosby Year Book, 1990.

CHAPTER 13

The Difficult Pediatric Airway

Laura Loftis
Trevor G. Pollard

Managing the pediatric airway may be challenging under the most controlled situations, but in emergent situations or when an unanticipated difficulty is encountered, the problems may be life threatening for the patient. Often, the difficult airway can be predicted, allowing for the formulation of several plans of airway management; the unanticipated difficult airway, however, calls for the expedient use of alternate techniques to secure the airway. The anesthesiologist must be skilled in several methods for establishing and maintaining an emergency airway. This chapter is a brief review of difficult airways and of alternate airway management techniques.

ANTICIPATION OF THE DIFFICULT AIRWAY: ANATOMIC CONSIDERATIONS

There are many conditions, congenital and acquired, that make direct visualization of the larynx and intubation difficult or impossible. Alignment of the oral–laryngeal axis may be hindered by any impairment in mouth opening or neck extension, that is, in some trauma victims, patients with Goldenhar's syndrome, patients with fused cervical vertebrae, or patients with congenital temporomandibular joint anomalies. When we refer to "anterior cords" during laryngoscopy, it means that the larynx is relatively anterior to the line of vision because displacement of the soft tissues is impaired for some reason. Anatomically, however, the larynx is no more anterior than in a normal airway. The potential space for displacement, bounded anteriorly by the mentum of the mandible, laterally by the mandibular rami, and posteriorly by the hyoid bone, may be restrictive in a number of situations. The most notable of these are Pierre Robin or Goldenhar's syndrome (Figs. 13-1 and 13-2), but it may be seen with any syndrome in which midfacial hypoplasia is a compo-

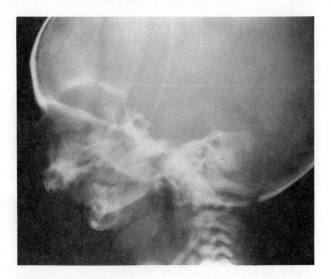

Figure 13-1   Pierre Robin syndrome. Note hypoplastic mandible with resultant decrease in potential displacement space and relatively anterior cords. (Used with permission of Dr. Ewell Clarke.)

nent. Any increase in the soft tissues in this region will have the same relative effect, that is, cystic hygromas (Fig. 13-3), hemangiomas, and tumors of the tongue.

Other causes of upper airway obstruction are infections, such as epiglottitis (Fig. 13-4), membranous croup, or retropharyngeal abscesses (Fig. 13-5). Enlarged tonsillar tissue and other rare congenital anomalies, like ectopic retropharyngeal goiters, may also make visualization of the larynx a problem (Fig. 13-6).

Congenital sublaryngeal anomalies leading to difficult intubation include cricoid ring stenosis, laryngeal webs or vascular rings, subglottic hemangiomas, and acquired lesions, such as foreign bodies, infections (bacterial tracheitis), and trauma.

When attempting nasotracheal intubation, possible malformations in this region, such as choanal atresia, nasal polyps, or juvenile angiofibromas (Fig. 13-7), become relative contraindications to passage of a nasotracheal tube.

Most of these situations may be anticipated from the preoperative evaluation, and the appropriate airway management can be planned. However, we must also be prepared for those situations in which intubation or bag–mask ventilation is not possible, which could result in poor oxygenation and/or ventilation.

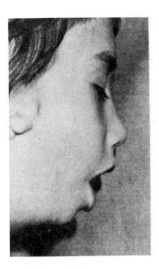 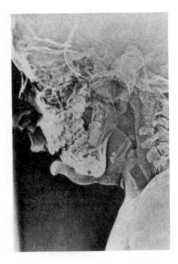

Figure 13-2 Goldenhar's syndrome. Note maldevelopment of mandible, which might not be noted preoperatively unless direct laryngoscopy had been performed. (Reproduced with permission from Berry FA: Anesthesia for the child with a difficult airway, in Berry FA (ed): *Anesthetic Management of Difficult and Routine Pediatric Patients*. New York, Churchill Livingstone, 1990, p 169.)

In this chapter, airway control measures are discussed that might be utilized to secure the airway of the patient with both a known or an unexpected difficult airway. A plan for airway management should be formulated in each case and equipment and supplies made available, such that several options may be exercised should the original plan for airway management fail (Figs. 13-8 and 13-9). These plans should also be discussed by everyone involved in that patient's care before the case begins, including the anesthesiologist, surgeon(s), nurses, and technicians. Advance preparation should be made for surgical intervention in case it is needed.

METHODS OF AIRWAY CONTROL: ANTICIPATED DIFFICULT AIRWAY

In a patient with a known difficult airway, either from a previous anesthetic record, a history from the parents of difficult intubations or postponed operations, or obvious oropharyngeal malformations, careful planning with several options, including surgical intervention, needs to be considered. Ideally, spontaneous ventilation should be maintained. If this is not feasible,

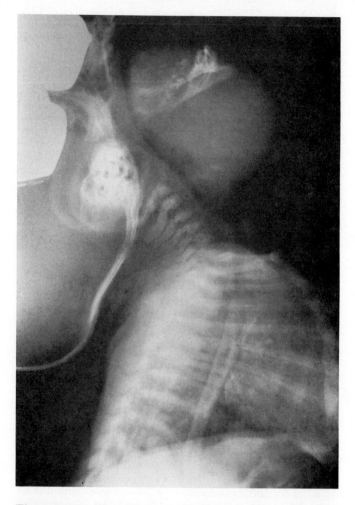

Figure 13-3 Cystic hygroma, resulting in decreased potential displacement space and probable airway obstruction after sedation or muscle relaxants. (Used with permission of Dr. Ewell Clarke.)

we need to be assured that bag valve mask ventilation can be adequately performed before administration of a muscle relaxant. If the airway does prove to be difficult or impossible to intubate and oxygenation ventilation is not guaranteed, it may

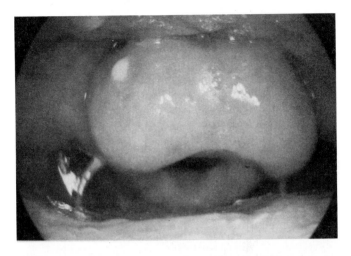

Figure 13-4 Epiglottitis, with resultant inability to adequately visualize by direct laryngoscopy the larynx and vocal cords. (Reproduced with permission from Becker W, Brekingham RA, Hillinger PH, et al: Disease of the larynx, in Becker W (ed): *Atlas of Ear, Nose, and Throat Diseases,* ed 2. Philadelphia, WB Saunders, 1984, p 186.)

be best to awaken the patient and reschedule the procedure for another day.

Blind Nasal Intubation

Blind nasal intubation in infants and young children is much more difficult than in adults for several reasons. Anatomically, the large occiput, more superior location of the larynx, and large tongue cause the tube to be directed toward the esophagus. Also, laryngospasm (which often prevents successful passage of the tube) is much more difficult to control with topical anesthesia unless the drugs are delivered through a bronchoscope or by transtracheal injection. For this method to be successful, the patient must maintain spontaneous respirations and must have adequate anesthesia (topical and intravenous sedation) to depress the protective airway reflexes. Topical anesthesia for the nasopharynx may be produced by 4% cocaine or a combination of 0.25% phenylephrine and 4% lidocaine. Nasal stylets are rarely used in children during blind insertion of the endotracheal tube because of the risk of mucosal damage. However, if used, they must be bent to approximate the anatomic

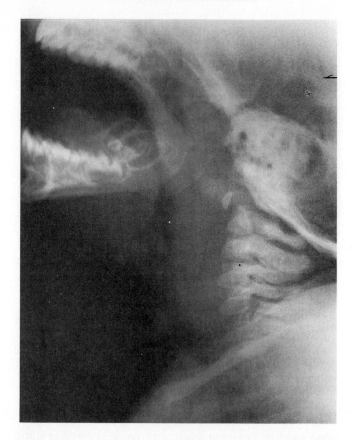

Figure 13-5 Retropharyngeal abscess with extensive soft tissue edema of the retropharynx. Note patient prefers to keep neck extended to improve airway patency. (Used with permission of Dr. Ewell Clarke.)

curve of the airway. As the tube is passed through the nasopharynx toward the larynx, increasing breath sounds indicate that the vocal cords are approaching. A decrease in breath sounds indicates esophageal intubation or lateral displacement of the tube. A withdrawal of the tube until breath sounds are again heard is followed by slow progression. Most children will cough as the tube is passed into the trachea. Inability to vocalize, auscultation of bilateral breath sounds, collapse and reinflation of the anesthesia bag, and presence of end-tidal PCO_2 con-

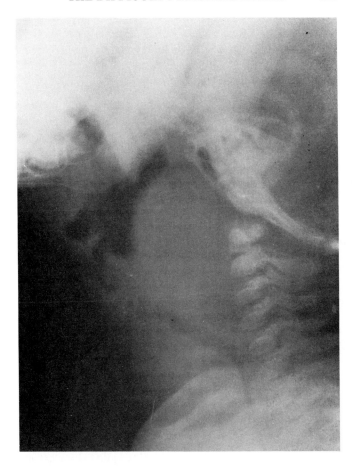

Figure 13-6   Retropharyngeal goiter. Note extensive soft tissue density impinging on upper airway structures and extending into subglottic region. (Used with permission of Dr. Ewell Clarke.)

firm proper placement. Techniques used to secure a difficult airway, such as flexible bronchoscopy and blind nasal intubation, should be well practiced in a controlled normal situation to improve proficiency.

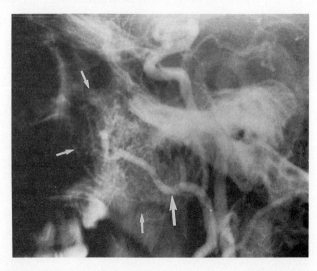

Figure 13-7   Juvenile angiofibroma demonstrated during angiogram would make nasal intubation hazardous. Aberrant feeder arteriole (large arrow), surrounding vascular blush of tumor (small arrows). (Used with permission of Dr. Ewell Clarke.)

Flexible Fiberoptic Bronchoscope (FOB)

This method is a useful adjunct in the nonemergent intubation, allowing for direct visualization to ensure tracheal placement of the endotracheal tube. A 4.5-mm endotracheal tube will accommodate a 3.2-mm pediatric FOB. The tube is placed into the nasopharynx, and the FOB is inserted within the tube. After the larynx is visualized, the FOB is passed into the trachea approximately to the level of the carina because more shallow placement of the FOB in children might allow for displacement of the entire apparatus into the esophagus as the tube is advanced over the FOB through the cords. The disadvantages of this method are the poor suction capabilities caused by the small size of the suction ports, and considerable practice is necessary to become proficient in this maneuver.

Bullard Fiberoptic
Intubation Laryngoscope

This laryngoscope is specifically designed for the difficult-to-visualize larynx and for patients with cervical spinal injuries. It is relatively simple to use in adults after minimal training, but it is considerably more difficult to use in the pediatric patient.

Tactile Intubation

After the patient is deeply anesthetized, the second and third digits are inserted into the hypopharynx, feeling for the epiglottis. After this is palpated, the endotracheal tube is guided along the groove between the two fingers and into the larynx. This procedure requires long, slender fingers and may be difficult in the smaller pediatric patient. Remember that the child is anesthetized, and if laryngospasm were to occur, the patient may be difficult to ventilate and oxygenate.

Laryngeal Mask Airway

The laryngeal mask airway, which is a device only recently approved for use in the United States, has an elliptical, inflatable cuff that slides into position in the hypopharynx with the lumen of the tube opposite the laryngeal inlet. The epiglottis is ideally pressed anteriorly by the cuff, but adequate oxygenation and ventilation can occur with the epiglottis falling posteriorly to the cuff. This device does not provide a watertight seal and should not electively be used in patients at risk of regurgitation (Fig. 13-10). Several case reports in adults show successful ventilation of patients who were impossible to ventilate or intubate in an emergent situation by conventional means. In pediatric patients, various reports show 95 to 99 percent successful placement of this device on the first or second attempt. Therefore, it seems reasonable to attempt ventilation with a laryngeal mask airway briefly when conventional bag valve mask and oral/nasal airways fail. If ventilation and oxygenation improve, then time may be taken to provide a more permanent airway (fiberoptic intubation through the device or surgical tracheostomy). If it fails to improve ventilation, then transtracheal jet ventilation should be instituted immediately.

Several case reports in the literature also support the use of a laryngeal mask airway as a conduit for difficult FOB intubations. After the device is in good position to provide adequate ventilation, its shaft will be well aligned with the laryngeal inlet, and visualization of the glottic opening is much simplified.

Retrograde Wire

Another alternate method for the difficult, but not emergent, airway is the placement of a J-wire or stylet in a plastic catheter

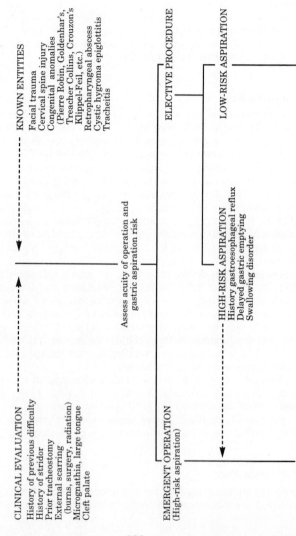

CLINICAL EVALUATION
History of previous difficulty
History of stridor
Prior tracheostomy
External scarring
  (burns, surgery, radiation)
Micrognathia, large tongue
Cleft palate

KNOWN ENTITIES
Facial trauma
Cervical spine injury
Congenital anomalies
  (Pierre Robin, Goldenhar's,
  Treacher Collins, Crouzon's
  Klippel-Feil, etc.)
Retropharyngeal abscess
Cystic hygroma epiglottitis
Tracheitis

Assess acuity of operation and
gastric aspiration risk

ELECTIVE PROCEDURE

LOW-RISK ASPIRATION

HIGH-RISK ASPIRATION
History gastroesophageal reflux
Delayed gastric emptying
Swallowing disorder

EMERGENT OPERATION
(High-risk aspiration)

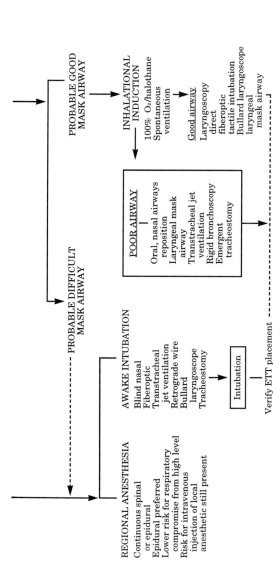

Figure 13-8 Algorithm for a pediatric patient with a suspected difficult intubation.

227

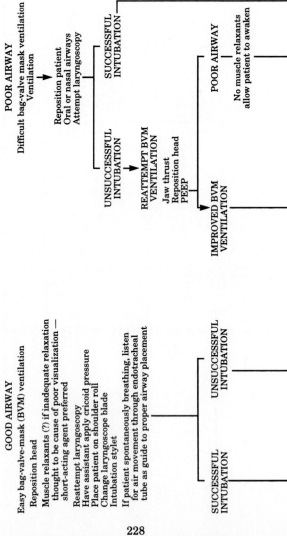

GOOD AIRWAY

Easy bag-valve-mask (BVM) ventilation

Reposition head

Muscle relaxants (?) if inadequate relaxation
thought to be cause of poor visualization —
short-acting agent preferred

Reattempt laryngoscopy
Have assistant apply cricoid pressure
Place patient on shoulder roll
Change laryngoscope blade
Intubation stylet

If patient spontaneously breathing, listen
for air movement through endotracheal
tube as guide to proper airway placement

SUCCESSFUL   UNSUCCESSFUL
INTUBATION   INTUBATION

POOR AIRWAY

Difficult bag-valve mask ventilation
Ventilation

Reposition patient
Oral or nasal airways
Attempt laryngoscopy

UNSUCCESSFUL   SUCCESSFUL
INTUBATION   INTUBATION

REATTEMPT BVM
VENTILATION

Jaw thrust
Reposition head
PEEP

IMPROVED BVM   POOR AIRWAY
VENTILATION

No muscle relaxants
allow patient to awaken

228

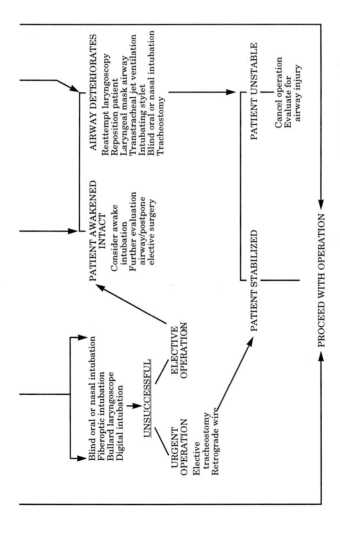

Blind oral or nasal intubation
Fiberoptic intubation
Bullard laryngoscope
Digital intubation

UNSUCCESSFUL

ELECTIVE
OPERATION

URGENT
OPERATION

Elective
tracheostomy
Retrograde wire

PATIENT AWAKENED
INTACT

Consider awake
intubation
Further evaluation
airway/postpone
elective surgery

AIRWAY DETERIORATES

Reattempt laryngoscopy
Reposition patient
Laryngeal mask airway
Transtracheal jet ventilation
Intubating stylet
Blind oral or nasal intubation
Tracheostomy

PATIENT UNSTABLE

Cancel operation
Evaluate for
airway injury

PATIENT STABILIZED

PROCEED WITH OPERATION

Figure 13-9 Algorithm for a pediatric patient with an unsuspected difficult intubation.

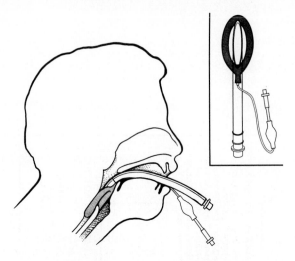

Figure 13-10 Laryngeal mask airway.

through the cricothyroid membrane in a retrograde manner. The wire is hopefully passed through the vocal cords and into the hypopharynx. It may then be used as a stylet over which an endotracheal tube may be passed blindly into the larynx. This would necessitate a cooperative patient who could tolerate regional block of the laryngeal structures or an anesthetized patient with a maintainable airway.

METHODS OF AIRWAY CONTROL: UNANTICIPATED DIFFICULT AIRWAY

When difficulty with intubation is unanticipated, airway management proceeds based on whether or not the patient can or cannot be ventilated by bag and mask. Algorithms for both of these instances are included on the preceding pages (see Figs. 13-8 and 13-9). Presented here are a few methods that can be life saving if ventilation is impossible. These techniques may provide a little extra time during which a more secure, permanent airway can be created either surgically or by the previously mentioned techniques.

Laryngoscopy

Simply lifting the soft tissues out of the airway with the laryngoscope blade may allow gas exchange in some spontaneously breathing patients to prevent hypoxemia and bradycardia.

Cricothyrotomy

Emergency cricothyrotomy, although associated with some morbidity to the patient, may be life saving in the patient who is impossible to intubate and ventilate in a conventional manner. Quite a bit has been written in the adult literature about the internal diameter of the catheter required to allow ventilation and oxygenation, but little data exist concerning pediatric-sized airways. The following should be sufficient: an 18- to 20-gauge intravenous catheter for newborns, 16-gauge for older infants, and 12- to 14-gauge for older children. As seen in Fig. 12-5, the thyroid and cricoid cartilages are palpated and the cricothyroid membrane localized. In infants, this area may be so small that only a fingernail may fit between the two cartilages. The catheter is directed midline, avoiding the two laterally located cricothyroid arteries, which converge superiorly. The catheter is advanced until air is aspirated. Then it is advanced slightly more and the catheter alone is passed into the trachea while withdrawing the needle. Once again, check to make sure that it is possible to aspirate air.

Attach the catheter to a 3.0 mm I.D. endotracheal tube connector, which will then fit into the jet ventilation source, or attach the 3-mL syringe barrel without plunger to the catheter. To the barrel, attach an 8-mm endotracheal tube adaptor. Some jet ventilator attachments will attach directly to the catheter. If there is complete upper airway obstruction, that is, no anatomic pressure vent, then either a second percutaneous catheter needs to be placed or the jet apparatus must be removed after each jet to allow for exhalation through the catheter. Fatal bilateral tension pneumothoraces and/or pneumopericardium can occur if the jet is utilized without venting. Watch for chest movement up and down!

Most operating room anesthesia machines can be equipped with jet ventilation and an adjustable pressure-reducing valve. These values are often calibrated in pounds per square inch (psi). Remember that one atmosphere $= 760$ mmHg $= 58.4$ cmH$_2$O $= 14.7$ psi; therefore, 10 psi $= 40$ cmH$_2$O, which is a good starting point for inspiratory pressure in children.

The anesthesia machine circuit or a handheld bag-valve device will also connect to the endotracheal tube adaptor. As a result of Poiseuille's equation, we will need much higher pressures than usual to achieve enough flow through the catheter because of its relatively high resistance to flow, and it may be very difficult to ventilate in this manner.

Tracheotomy

Many techniques have been described for performing tracheotomies, but as with most airway procedures, adequate anesthesia to maintain spontaneous ventilation is a prime concern. General anesthesia with halothane in conjunction with topical anesthesia is possible in children with stable hemodynamics. Both aspiration and total airway obstruction are possible risks during this procedure in the emergency situation. The oropharynx is anesthetized with lidocaine. The area of the tracheotomy is infiltrated with 0.5% lidocaine with 1:200,000 epinephrine.

An inverted U-shaped incision through the skin and tracheal cartilages (one to two rings below the cricoid cartilage) is made, and an appropriate-sized tracheostomy tube is placed. The skin and tracheal flap may be sutured together, keeping the airway open in the event of accidental tube dislodgment. This procedure should be performed only by skilled personnel.

SUMMARY

There are many difficult airways that may be predicted in view of the physical examination or history and many emergent or semiemergent situations. Planning is always half the battle; however, it is also necessary to have a repertoire of procedures useful to deal with the unexpected. Know the equipment. Know when to call for a backup. Remember the most important thing is to keep the child neurologically intact, even if it means postponing a procedure.

BIBLIOGRAPHY

Benumof JL: Laryngeal mask airway. *Anesthesiology* 1992; 77:843–846.

Berry FA: Anesthesia for the child with a difficult airway, in Berry F (ed): *Anesthetic Management of Difficult and Routine Pediatric Patients*. New York, Churchill Livingstone, 1990, pp 167–198.

Coté C, Todres D: The pediatric airway, in Ryan JF, Coté C, Todres D, Goudsouvian N (eds): *A Practice of Anesthesia in Infants and Children*. Orlando, FL, Grune and Stratton, 1986.

Dallen LT, Wine R, Benumof J: Spontaneous ventilation via transtracheal large-bore intravenous catheters is possible. *Anesthesiology* 1991; 75:531–533.

De Mello WF, Kocan M: The laryngeal mask airway in failed intubation. *Anaesthesia* 1990; 45:689–690.

France NK, Beste DJ: Anesthesia for pediatric ear, nose, and throat surgery, in Gregory G (ed): *Pediatric Anesthesia,* ed 2. New York, Churchill Livingstone, 1989, pp 1097–1147.

Goldman E, McDonald JS, Peterson SS, et al: Transtracheal ventilation with oscillatory pressure for complete upper airway obstruction. *J Trauma* 1988; 28:611–614.

Mason DL, Bungeham RM: The laryngeal mask airway in children. *Anaesthesia* 1991; 45:760–763.

Milner SM, Bennet IDC: Emergency cricothyrotomy. *J Laryngol Otol* 1991; 105:883–885.

Rasch DK, Browder F, Burr M, et al: Anaesthesia for Treacher Collins and Pierre Robin syndromes: A report of 3 cases. *Can J Anaesth* 1986; 33:364–370.

Ross ED: Treacher Collins syndrome: An anaesthesia hazard. *Anaesthesia* 1963;18:350–352.

Rowbottom SJ, Simpson DL, Grubb D: The laryngeal mask airway in children: A fiberoptic assessment of positioning. *Anaesthesia* 1991; 46:489–491.

CHAPTER 14

Diagnosis and Management of Upper Airway Obstruction

Deborah K. Rasch
Susan H. Noorily
Trevor G. Pollard

There are many causes of acute upper airway obstruction in pediatric patients. Anesthesiologists play a key role in the treatment of these airway emergencies. The most common causes of acute airway obstruction in children are infection, foreign-body aspiration, and juvenile papillomatosis. Critical to a safe outcome in these patients is a prompt diagnosis and the appropriate management of the airway. This chapter will review the differential diagnosis of acute upper airway obstruction in children and the clinical management of patients with airway obstruction.

CAUSES OF ACUTE AIRWAY OBSTRUCTION

Stridor is a presenting symptom that can occur with any type of airway obstruction. A patient can be stridorous during inspiration, expiration, or both. The timing of stridor can be useful in determining the location of the airway obstruction. In general, inspiratory stridor is caused by airway obstruction in an extrathoracic location. Airway obstruction in the subglottic or intrathoracic areas can result in inspiratory stridor, expiratory stridor, and wheezing.

Acute Epiglottitis (AE)

AE is a bacterial infectious disease most frequently seen in children 2 to 6 years of age, although it can occur in younger children and adults. In most cases, the responsible organism is *Haemophilus influenza* (*H. flu*), type b. With the advent of the *H. flu* vaccine, there are fewer cases of invasive *H. flu* disease in pediatric patients. Other organisms implicated in epiglottitis

234

include *Streptococcus, Staphylococcus, Pasteurella, Klebsiella, Citrobacter,* and *Enterobacter* species. There is a slight predilection (60 percent) for the male population.

AE is a local manifestation of a pervasive systemic disease. It results in massive inflammatory edema of the supraglottic structures, including the epiglottis, the arytenoid cartilages, the aryepiglottic folds, and the uvula. This inflammatory response can progress to hemorrhagic ulceration and submucosal abscess formation (Figs. 14-1 and 14-2). As a direct result of the inflammatory response, the airway is progressively compromised. This can occur extremely rapidly in children, presumably because the normal airways are smaller.

Classically, the pediatric patient will present to the emergency room during the winter months, particularly October and November and February and March, when the weather is in transition. There will be a history of a brief, mild prodrome (consistent with an upper respiratory tract infection), soon followed by fever (39 to 40°C), malaise, lethargy, and signs of progressive supraglottic swelling. Diaz refers to the signs of progressive supraglottic swelling as the "four Ds," that is, *d*ysphonia, *d*ysphagia, *d*rooling, and respiratory *d*istress.

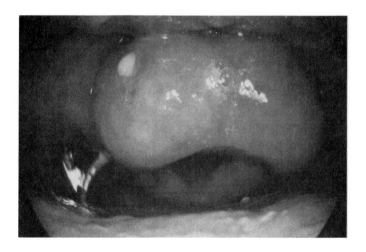

Figure 14-1   The supraglottic structures in acute epiglottitis. Note the enlarged epiglottis and narrow glottic opening produced by inflammation and edema of the supraglottic structures. (Reproduced with permission from Becker W, Brekingham RA, Hillinger PH, et al: Diseases of the larynx, in Becker W (ed): *Atlas of Ear, Nose, and Throat Diseases,* ed 2. Philadelphia, WB Saunders, 1984, p 186.)

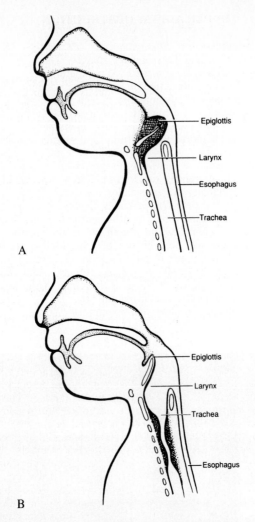

Labels in figure A:
- Epiglottis
- Larynx
- Esophagus
- Trachea

A

Labels in figure B:
- Epiglottis
- Larynx
- Trachea
- Esophagus

B

Figure 14-2 (A) Acute epiglottitis results in edema of the supraglottic structures, resulting in rapid airway compromise. (B) Croup results from edema in the subglottic region and may result in airway compromise.

As the disease progresses, the dysphonia changes from mild hoarseness to a characteristic muffled "hot potato" voice. The child will be reluctant to speak and may even refuse to do so. Dysphagia is the result of both pain and dysfunction caused by inflammation. This leads to the pooling of oral secretions and drooling. Simultaneously, the patient develops respiratory distress from airway compromise. Initially, the patient will have mild subcostal retractions and a slightly increased respiratory rate. The retractions will usually worsen and involve the intercostal, supraclavicular, and suprasternal areas. Because of the four Ds, the child may assume the characteristic AE posture by sitting in a tripod stance, leaning slightly forward, and holding the head and neck in the sniffing position. The facies can vary from expressions of concentration to anxiety, depending on the extent of airway obstruction.

The signs and symptoms just described are accompanied by signs of severe systemic disease. Most patients are markedly febrile and will appear toxic. Bacteremia occurs in up to 95 percent of patients with AE. The inability to take fluids leads to dehydration. The child's sensorium will vary with the degree of airway obstruction and toxemia. Initially, the child will appear irritable. Later, the child may seem disinterested or anxious. In the worst case, the child will become obtunded and lose consciousness.

It is important to remember that, in the child, there is a rapid progression of signs and symptoms, beginning at home and ultimately leading to a life-threatening hypoxic crisis. This can occur within a 4- to 12-h period. The hypoxia and respiratory acidosis caused by the acute airway obstruction is exacerbated by the increased metabolic demands of toxemia, the febrile state, and the profound muscular workload of breathing.

AE in older children and adults tends to be a less severe disease. The most frequent presentation is a patient with a sore throat, mild dysphagia, and tenderness to palpation of the anterior neck. Airway obstruction is infrequent in adults with AE, probably because the normal airway diameter is increased. Acute obstruction can occur, however, and is usually associated with *H. flu* infection.

Laryngotracheobronchitis (LTB)

Viral LTB, or infectious croup, is probably the most common infectious cause of acute upper airway obstruction in children. It is usually seen in children from the ages of 6 months to 3 years, although it can occur in older children. As children grow, the subglottic opening enlarges enough to prevent the critical narrowing responsible for the croupy stridor.

The presentation of viral croup is characteristic. It is slow in onset, beginning as a mild upper respiratory infection. Symptoms of upper airway obstruction appear over the next 1 to 3 days because the infection causes inflammation and edema of the airway mucosa, especially in the subglottic area (Fig. 14-2B). There is usually a small temperature elevation (38 to 39°C), mild retractions, and rhinorrhea. The patient may have a barky cough. Usually, the parents are very worried, but the child may be playful or sleeping peacefully, albeit noisily.

Typical viral croup may be treated symptomatically, although severe cases require hospitalization and possibly mechanical ventilation. The symptoms of croup must be differentiated from those of AE. The salient features of each are summarized in Table 14-1. Unfortunately, often the child's condition will be in a gray area, and clinical judgment will be important in guiding therapy. When in doubt, it is preferable to err on the conservative side, assume the possibility of AE as a diagnosis, and proceed accordingly.

Spasmodic Croup

Spasmodic croup is a recurrent disease of sudden onset, which can present with stridor and respiratory distress. It usually occurs at night and is not accompanied by fever or other constitutional symptoms. The cause of this illness is unknown, but it is thought to be allergic or viral. It is almost always readily treated with warm mists or nebulized bronchodilators (e.g., epinephrine or terbutaline).

Diphtheritic Croup

Diphtheritic croup is caused by infection with *Corynebacterium diphtheria,* which produces a toxin responsible for the observed clinical signs and symptoms. The disease is uncommon today because of current immunization practices. The incubation period lasts 2 to 5 days and is followed by a sore red throat, malaise, and mild temperature elevation. Later in the course of the disease, the temperature may rise to 39°C. The characteristic grayish membrane may be readily visible or might involve only the more posterior structures, thus making it difficult to see. A case severe enough to produce airway obstruction is accompanied by a readily visible pharyngeal membrane, often involving the tonsils and uvula. There is abundant foul-smelling nasal discharge, and the temperature fluctuates widely.

Foreign-Body Aspiration

A child who has aspirated a foreign body will present with an acute onset of coughing during the waking hours. The child,

Table 14-1 Differential Diagnosis of Acute Epiglottitis

DISEASE	SYMPTOMS OTHER THAN STRIDOR	EMERGENT TREATMENT
Acute epiglottitis	Rapid onset. Fever to 40°C, toxic appearance. Drooling, characteristic posture. Occurs in ages 2 to 6 yr. Usually caused by *H. influenzae*.	Oxygen, intubation, antibiotics
Laryngotracheobronchitis or viral croup	Usually slow onset (although may be rapid in smaller children). Upper respiratory infection slowly progressive to stridor (1 to 3 days), cough, rhinorrhea, fever to 39°C. Usually younger than age 2 yr. Caused by viral infection.	Oxygen, mist, racemic epinephrine, steroids, rarely intubation
Spasmodic croup	Sudden onset. Nocturnal. No fever. Viral or allergic cause.	Oxygen, bronchodilators, mist
Diphtheritic croup	Slower onset. Fluctuating fever up to 39 to 40°C. Foul-smelling nasal discharge preceded by sore throat, malaise. Caused by *C. diphtheria*.	Oxygen, antibiotics
Foreign body	Sudden onset of spasmodic cough during waking hours; ages 9 mo to 5 yr.	Oxygen, removal of foreign body under anesthesia

usually between the ages of 9 months and 5 years, will have been previously healthy. There can be varying degrees of respiratory distress, depending on the type and location of the foreign body.

Aspirated foreign bodies located above the level of the cricoid cartilage will generally produce stridor. Those located in the lower trachea or bronchi tend to produce wheezing. Aspirated vegetable material (especially peanuts and popcorn) reacts locally within the airway, producing edema, which worsens the obstruction. Laryngeal and tracheal foreign bodies generally cause more severe symptoms because a larger percentage of the airway is compromised. However, endobronchial foreign bodies can dislodge when the child is agitated or coughing and relocate in the trachea, resulting in severe obstruction.

Evaluation of these patients should include careful auscultation over the trachea and lung fields. Drooling or difficulty swallowing may occur when a foreign body, such as a coin, becomes lodged in the esophagus posterior to the arytenoid cartilages. Radiodense objects are easily identified. The majority of aspirated foreign bodies are radiolucent, but chest x-rays can help locate the object by the particular pattern of airway obstruction that shows up on film. Segmental atelectasis may be the result of total obstruction of a particular bronchus. Hyperinflated lung segments are more common as air trapping occurs. Time is allotted for radiographs of the neck or chest only when the airway obstruction is not severe. Ideally, both inspiratory and expiratory films should be obtained, although the practice of using forced expiratory chest films is controversial when an endobronchial foreign body is suspected. This is because the foreign body is at risk of becoming dislodged and entering the opposite bronchus or the trachea.

MANAGEMENT OF ACUTE AIRWAY OBSTRUCTION

The initial assessment of a child with an acute airway obstruction usually takes place in the emergency room by a primary care physician. Children with acute epiglottitis can deteriorate very rapidly, and therefore, this diagnosis must be considered early on in all patients with acute airway obstruction. There are three questions that must be answered without delay. First, what is the probability that the child has AE? Second, what is the degree of airway obstruction? Third, what is the mental status of the patient? Acute airway obstruction has a wide spectrum of presentations, from mild stridor to cardiopulmonary arrest.

The Patient with Mild Stridor

If the patient clearly does not have AE and is not in acute respiratory distress, further evaluation should be undertaken to make a diagnosis. This process should include a clinical assessment of the extent of the respiratory embarrassment and toxicity, which will be supported by appropriate laboratory studies and radiologic examinations, for example, chest x-ray and/or lateral neck films (Fig. 14-3).

There are classic radiographic signs for differentiating between AE and LTB, but radiographic diagnosis is not 10⁰ percent successful. Usually, as the epiglottis swells, it resembles a thumb on lateral films of the neck (Fig. 14-3A). By contrast, the neck films of a child with LTB demonstrate subglottic narrowing (Figs. 14-3B and 14-3C).

The Patient with Moderate
Airway Compromise

If the diagnosis of AE is unlikely but the child shows signs of respiratory distress, an anesthesiologist should be consulted. The respiratory effort exerted by a child with severe viral croup can lead to exhaustion, respiratory failure, and arrest. A foreign-body aspiration can lead to immediate and profound airway obstruction. There is usually time to pursue laboratory work and/or radiologic studies, but the patient must not be lost in the "emergency room shuffle." If it is deemed necessary to take a look in the child's mouth, the clinician must have a very strong conviction that the patient does *not* have AE.

LTB

In the case of viral croup, treatment consists of oxygen therapy, intravenous hydration, and tracheobronchial humidification. Aerosolized vasoconstrictors and/or bronchodilators can be effective in serious cases. The use of steroids is controversial in the acute phase of viral croup, but they have been shown to decrease the length of the hospital stay. With most cases of viral croup, the physician has adequate time to evaluate a child completely before employing invasive treatments.

A decision to intubate a child with croup is based on the diagnosis of impending respiratory failure (arterial hypoxemia in the face of augmented O_2, hypercarbia, near-complete airway obstruction, and respiratory muscle fatigue) and not on the visual appearance of the hypopharynx and supraglottic structures. Intubation should be accomplished according to the same principles described for patients with AE.

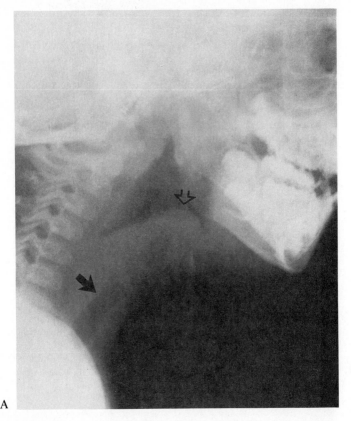

A

Figure 14-3 (A) Epiglottitis. The epiglottis (open arrow) has lost its normal conical contour and is now markedly swollen and rounded. The subglottic trachea (solid arrow) remains normal.

Foreign-Body Aspiration

A foreign-body aspiration in a child is a surgical emergency. Although the patient may appear to be stable, the foreign body is not and can be dislodged at any time to a more compromising location. If the location of the foreign body is known, the child should be kept on his or her side with the involved airway in the dependent position.

The patient with a foreign body is assumed to have a full stomach. Even if the operation is delayed because of the full stomach, it cannot be assumed that gastric emptying times are

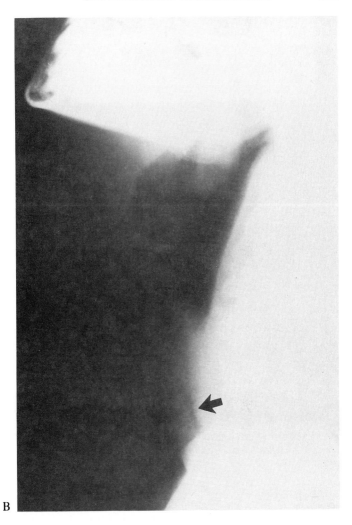

B

Figure 14-3 (continued) (B) Croup. The hypopharynx is overdistended, but the trachea (solid arrow) is narrowed by subglottic edema.

normal. It is recommended that metoclopromide and ranitidine be administered when intravenous (IV) access is available.

The authors advocate inhalation inductions in these patients. Spontaneous respiration is preferred because positive pressure can move a foreign body deeper into the airway. If this tech-

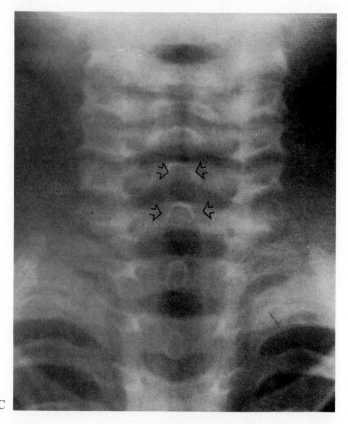

C

Figure 14-3 (continued)   (C) Croup. The "steeple sign" of subglottic edema seen on the frontal view.

nique is used, expect that the induction will take longer than usual. Some anesthesiologists add nitrous oxide to hasten the induction, but this can result in increased airway pressures in areas of obstructive emphysema. Also, the use of nitrous oxide requires that a lower F_{IO_2} be delivered to a child who is at significant risk for airway obstruction. This will allow less time for correction of the problem should complete airway obstruction occur. If nitrous oxide is used, it should be discontinued after the child is asleep. Ideally, cricoid pressure is maintained until the airway is protected.

During the bronchoscopy, deep anesthesia is essential. There are several techniques available to achieve this goal.

Some prefer to maintain continuous spontaneous ventilation throughout the procedure; others routinely employ controlled ventilation and give muscle relaxants.

It is important to keep in mind that the airway can be traumatized during the foreign-body retrieval. Humidified oxygen, racemic epinephrine, and dexamethasone are useful to help decrease subglottic swelling.

The Patient with Severe Airway Obstruction

When a patient presents with severe upper airway obstruction or obvious AE, this is clearly an emergent situation. Management details are carried out most efficiently and safely when a protocol outlining specific procedures is followed. The ultimate goal is safe transport of the patient to the operating room where an artificial airway can be placed under general anesthesia. Communication between all involved medical personnel (the pediatrician, anesthesiologist, otolaryngologist, respiratory therapist, and nurses) is essential and must be maintained.

The pediatrician, anesthesiologist, and otolaryngologist must be notified immediately after the diagnosis of AE is assumed. The operating room should be prepared for the patient and equipped for an airway emergency with a tracheostomy setup available.

The first priority is supportive care and attention to the airway. The child should be given supplemental O_2 if he or she will tolerate it. The child should never be *forced* to do anything because crying could precipitate an immediate airway obstruction. For the same reason, any painful procedures (IV placement or venous or arterial puncture) should be avoided.

Radiologic studies are also contraindicated. They do not help with the diagnosis. The quality of portable films is often inadequate. The amount of hyperextension required for adequate supraglottic visualization can cause an obstructive crisis. Most importantly, the time required may delay life-saving treatment.

The parent(s) are allowed to remain with the child in the hope that their presence will prevent further anxiety. Calm explanation and reassurance should be offered while preparations are being made to transport the child to the operating room. This will help the parent(s), the child, and assisting medical personnel.

The anesthesiologist should not leave the side of a patient with severe acute upper airway obstruction until the airway is proved to be secure. All equipment necessary for emergency endotracheal intubation must be immediately available (including styletted endotracheal tubes, a functional laryngoscope and

various blades, tape, bag-valve device, and oxygen). Muscle relaxants should be *avoided*. Ideally, the otolaryngologist and a
tracheostomy tray should accompany the patient to the OR.
The child may assume the position of maximal comfort during
the transport. The OR personnel should be informed when the
patient is en route.

In the OR, each caregiver should be assigned a specific task
to facilitate a smooth induction. The anesthesiologist should
gently take charge. The OR must be quiet. At some institutions,
a parent is allowed to accompany the child to the OR until the
induction is underway, with the understanding that he or she
will be asked and expected to leave after the child is asleep.
Monitors (especially the pulse oximeter sensor) should be applied to the patient, as tolerated, while the surgeon quickly
scrubs, gowns, and gloves.

When the surgeon is ready, an inhalation induction is initiated with 100% O_2/halothane. The authors avoid nitrous oxide
to provide the highest possible oxygen concentration to the
lungs, anticipating the possible consequences of laryngospasm
or complete airway obstruction. Some anesthetists prefer to begin the induction with an oxygen and nitrous oxide mix. In this
case, the nitrous oxide is discontinued after some halothane is
introduced. The induction may be accomplished with the child
remaining in the sitting position.

Laryngoscopy is performed when the patient is deeply anesthetized. Insertion of a styletted endotracheal tube (usually 1
to 1½ sizes smaller than usual for age) is attempted. If the patient has AE, normal airway anatomy may not be apparent.
Often, all that is visualized is a pinkish-red mass of flesh, perhaps with a dimple where the larynx ought to be. To facilitate
intubation in cases such as this, an assistant is asked to compress the chest while the laryngoscopist looks for a bubble. The
endotracheal tube is placed where the bubble is seen. If this
maneuver is not successful, an anesthesiologist experienced in
airway anatomy may make a blind attempt at intubation. It is
usually best to place an oral endotracheal tube initially to gain
control of the airway. If no difficulty is encountered, a nasal
tube can be placed later for postoperative management. Careful
securing of the endotracheal tube is very important.

During the induction, the patient with severe airway obstruction is at risk for laryngospasm. Unfortunately, laryngospasm may occur suddenly and without warning. Laryngospasm can be precipitated by a seemingly minimal stimulus,
such as IV placement. When this happens, mask ventilation
should be attempted before laryngoscopy. Many of these patients can be oxygenated sufficiently in this manner. However,
mask ventilation will almost always distend the stomach be-

cause the glottic obstruction favors air entry into the esophagus.

An anesthesiologist is usually the physician most experienced with airway management. It is therefore difficult for an anesthesiologist to admit his or her inability to intubate a patient. However, this is one time when a rapid admission of inability may be life saving. If, after a few attempts, the most experienced laryngoscopist present is unable to recognize the laryngeal structures and/or intubate the patient, immediate preparations for cricothyrotomy must begin. Attempts at intubation may continue. If surgical cricothyrotomy is not a viable option, percutaneous cannulation of the trachea through the cricothyroid membrane with a 14- or 16-gauge catheter is indicated (see Chap. 13).

Before or during induction, an intravenous line must be established. Because the child is probably dehydrated, a bolus of balanced salt solution (25 mL/kg) should be administered. Anesthesia can be maintained with low-dose halothane. Narcotics and benzodiazepine may be added for sedation because the patient with AE will remain intubated. Ensure adequate ventilation because the patient is likely to be hypercarbic. Laboratory specimens should be obtained at this time (complete blood count, electrolytes, arterial blood gases, and blood cultures). A culture of the epiglottis is optional because it has a low yield (15 percent). Antibiotics should be started as soon as possible (after blood cultures have been obtained). A chest x-ray is taken in the operating room or in the pediatric intensive care unit (PICU) to document correct endotracheal tube placement and to look for pneumonia.

After all procedures have been completed in the OR, the patient is transported to the PICU, intubated, and monitored. Children should be restrained and sedated so they do not extubate themselves. Sedation can be safely accomplished using narcotics and anxiolytics. Intubation equipment must always be readily available. Many physicians augment ventilation of these patients with continuous positive airway pressure or low intermittent mandatory ventilation rates to prevent atelectasis.

These patients should be extubated as soon as it is safely possible to avoid potential complications (including infection, atelectasis, subglottic stenosis, vocal cord injury, and tracheal granulomas). The indications for extubation include an awake and alert patient, the resolution of fever and toxic appearance, and a marked reduction in the swelling and size of the epiglottis. The epiglottis may be evaluated using direct laryngoscopy or fiberoptic bronchoscopy (both will require sedation). If the patient is able to move air around the endotracheal tube while the tube is momentarily obstructed, the swelling has probably diminished. The patient must be closely observed for signs of respiratory distress for several hours after extubation. Rarely, the airway created by the endotracheal tube will close as a result of edema reaccumulation.

Occasionally, AE will have an unusual presentation. This should be kept in mind during the evaluation and management of patients with acute airway obstruction. For example, AE has presented as uvulitis, progressing to airway obstruction requiring intubation. A case of AE presented with a history of a brief choking spell followed by mild subcostal retractions. Once intubated, this child developed acute pulmonary edema. Pulmonary edema in these patients is noncardiogenic in origin. It responds readily to mechanical ventilation and positive end-expiratory pressure. Cases of epiglottitis caused by Group A β-hemolytic *Streptococcus* result in prolonged fever (mean, 10.5 days) and a protracted intubation (mean, 7.5 days compared with 24 to 72 h with *H. flu*-caused AE).

There exists some controversy about the benefits of intubation versus surgical tracheostomy. Numerous articles, arguing both sides, have been published. Both intubation and tracheostomy allow airway protection and adequate ventilation, and both methods have potential complications. The duration of intubation and hospital stay is significantly shorter with intubation. Currently, the standard of care in the United States favors short-term oral or nasotracheal intubation in patients with AE. Circumstances in Third World countries, however, may dictate a preference for tracheostomy because there are limited material (humidification) and human (nursing) resources in some areas of the world. Certainly, a tracheostomy also may be the airway of choice in other situations.

BIBLIOGRAPHY

Algren WE, Axel J: Epiglottitis, in Bready LL, Smith RB (eds): *Decision Making in Anesthesiology*. Philadelphia, BC Decker, 1992, pp 302–303.

Blackstock D, Adderly RJ, Steward DJ: Epiglottitis in young infants. *Anesthesiology* 1987; 67:97.

Cohen EL: Epiglottitis in adults. *Ann Emerg Med* 1980; 13:620–623.

Diaz JH: Croup and epiglottitis in children: The anesthesiologist as diagnostician. *Anesth Analg* 1985; 64:621–633.

Fisher GC: Management of acute epiglottitis (letter). *Crit Care Med* 1987; 15:182.

Friedman EM, Damion J, Healy GB: Supraglottitis and concurrent *Haemophilus* meningitis. *Ann Otol Rhinol Laryngol* 1985; 94:470–472.

Griffin JA, Perkin RM: Management of acute epiglottitis in pediatric patients (letter). *Crit Care Med* 1987; 15:283.

Hanna GS: Acute supraglottic laryngitis in adults. *J Laryngol Otol* 1986; 100:971.

Lacroix J, et al: Group A streptococcal supraglottitis. *J Pediatr* 1986; 109:20.

Lee SC, et al: Epiglottitis presenting as acute pulmonary edema. *Ann Emerg Med* 1985; 14:60–63.

Lipson A, et al: Group B streptococcal supraglottitis in a 3-month-old infant. *Am J Dis Child* 1986; 140:411.

Loomis JC: Pediatric intensive care, in Gregory G (ed): *Pediatric Anesthesia*. New York, Churchill Livingstone, 1983, vol 2, chap 30, pp 938–940.

Musewe NW, et al: Adult respiratory distress syndrome in a child with acute epiglottitis. *Crit Care Med* 1986; 14:74–75.

Nussbaum E: Fiberoptic laryngoscopy as a guide to tracheal extubation in acute epiglottitis. *J Pediatr* 1983; 102:269–270.

Odetoyinbo O: A comparison of endotracheal intubation and tracheostomy in the management of acute epiglottitis in children in the tropics. *J Laryngol Otol* 1986; 100:1273.

Oh TH, Motoyama EK: Comparison of nasotracheal intubation and tracheostomy in management of acute epiglottitis. *Anesthesiology* 1977; 46:214–216.

Passley NRT, Baxter JD: Acute epiglottitis in children: The morbidity and management by elective tracheostomy. *J Otol* 1977; 6:482–486.

Smith DH: *Haemophilus influenza* infections, in Rudolph A, Grossman M (eds): *Pediatrics*, ed 17. Norwalk, CT, Appleton and Lange, 1982, chap 13, pp 533–538.

Stoelting R, Dierdorf S, McCammon R: Pediatric patients, in Stoelting R, Dierdorf S, McCammon R (eds): *Anesthesia and Co-Existing Disease*. New York, Churchill Livingstone, 1988; pp 807–883.

Tarnow-Mordi WO, Berrill AM, Darby CW: Precipitation of laryngeal obstruction in acute epiglottitis. *Br Med J* 1985; 290:629.

Venturelli S: Acute epiglottitis in children (letter). *Crit Care Med* 1987; 15:86.

Vernon DD, Sarnaik AP: Acute epiglottitis in children: A conservative approach to diagnosis and management. *Crit Care Med* 1986; 14:23–25.

Westerman EL, Hutton JP: Acute uvulitis associated with epiglottis. *Arch Otolaryngol Head Neck Surg* 1986;112:448–449.

Williams PA, Armatase EN, Fisher NG: Precipitation of laryngeal obstruction in acute epiglottitis (letter). *BMJ* 1985; 290:1007.

CHAPTER 15

Anesthesia in the Magnetic Resonance Imaging Scanner

Deborah K. Rasch
Lois L. Bready

Magnetic resonance imaging (MRI) is a relatively new noninvasive imaging technique that uniquely challenges the anesthesiologist providing care to pediatric patients scheduled for this diagnostic procedure. A strong magnetic field with radiofrequency pulses is used to create detailed images of internal organs. The MRI scanner has the ability to reconstruct the images in the coronal and sagittal planes in addition to reproducing horizontal images through the body (Fig. 15-1). For scanning, the child must be positioned within a body-length cylindrical radiofrequency shield (Fig. 15-2). During operation, the MRI unit produces a very loud thumping sound. The combination of close quarters and loud noise may make it difficult for even the most stoic adult patient to lie still for the time required to complete the examination. Pediatric patients almost always require heavy sedation or general anesthesia. No radiation is emitted from the apparatus; thus, the anesthesiologist may remain relatively close to the patient without having to wear heavy lead aprons for protection. However, new problems arise from the fact that all ferrous metals (iron, cobalt, and nickel) are attracted to the magnet. Objects such as safety pins, keys, laryngoscope batteries, unsecured O_2 and N_2O cylinders, intravenous poles, and wheelchairs, may become self-propelled toward the scanner, with the obvious risk of damage to the scanner, patient, and/or anesthesiologist! Because most of the equipment in everyday anesthesia practice consists of or contains ferrous metal, our preparations and monitoring require considerable alterations to care for patients who require anesthesia for evaluation by this new technology.

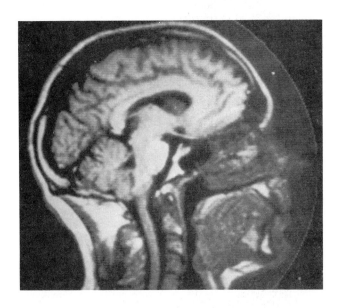

Figure 15-1 The MRI scanner has the advantage of producing images with much greater clarity than the CT scan, and it is able to reconstruct the images in the coronal and sagittal planes. (Reproduced with permission from *Progress in Anesthesiology,* 1991, vol 5, chap. 12, p 158.)

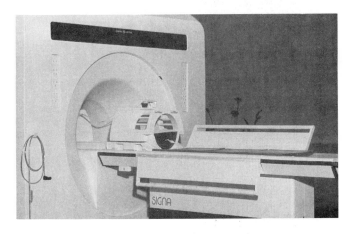

Figure 15-2 Confining cylindrical radiofrequency shield of the MRI scanner can be frightening to even the most stoic adult.

Table 15-1   Contraindications to Magnetic Resonance Imaging

Pacemakers

Ferrous metal vascular clips

Certain joint prostheses

Internal plates, wires, and screws used in orthopedic procedures

---

PREOPERATIVE EVALUATION AND PREPARATION OF THE PATIENT

In addition to the standard preoperative evaluation of patients scheduled to undergo general anesthesia or monitored anesthesia care, specific attention to the previous surgical history is important. A number of objects that may represent a hazard to the child may be located both internal and external to the body (Tables 15-1 and 15-2). Children with cardiac pacemakers are not candidates for MRI because inhibition of pacemaker output may occur, resulting in reversion to an asynchronous mode. The pacemaker also may be subject to programming changes (e.g., altered electrical output or pulse duration), which may not be apparent at the time of the scan. Torque on the pacemaker box and displacement of leads have also been reported. Certain

Table 15-2   Objects That May Present a Hazard in Magnetic Resonance Imaging

Patient Objects
  Clothing snaps
  Safety pins
  Earrings or other jewelry

Monitors and Anesthesia Equipment
  Steel precordial stethoscope
  Laryngoscope

Objects Carried or Worn by the Anesthetist—Check for Ferrous Metal
  Stethoscope
  Blockade monitor
  Eyeglasses
  Hair clips or barrettes
  Metal earpiece connection
  Safety pin
  Ballpoint pen
  Clipboard
  Keys

forms of vascular clips, such as used in patent ductus arteriosus ligation, may vibrate and become dislodged.

Objects external to the patient that may present a hazard include earrings or other jewelry, metal snaps on clothing, and safety pins. A careful search of the bedclothes of the intensive care unit patient should be performed before moving to the magnet room so that all ferrous metal objects are removed. All these items may be drawn forcefully toward the magnet and may injure personnel or patients in their path. If it is not clear whether an object contains ferrous metal, it may be evaluated by holding it close to a strong hand-held magnet. If the object is attracted, it must be removed.

As with other planned anesthetics, patients scheduled to receive sedation or anesthesia should have nothing by mouth for an age-appropriate interval.

PREPARATION OF THE ANESTHESIOLOGIST

Because scheduling of anesthesia services for MRI occurs sporadically, many anesthesiologists may have difficulty establishing a routine. Ferrous metal objects must be sought and not taken into the MRI suite (Table 15-2). In addition, magnetically coded items such as digital pagers, credit cards, audio or video tapes, and digital watches may be altered or erased by the magnetic field. Other ferrous metal objects that are not obvious include the metal connector on a made-to-order earpiece, the safety pin for clipping the earpiece to the anesthesiologist, the metal connectors at the end of the earpiece tubing for connection to a precordial stethoscope, and the spring in a clipboard. The anesthesiologist may be surprised by a sudden tug produced when these objects are brought near the magnet.

MONITORING

Perhaps the most perplexing problem with anesthetic management of these patients is the issue of monitoring. These problems are twofold—most of the monitors we have become accustomed to using in a standard operating room contain ferrous metal and, thus, present a risk to the patient and the magnet and/or distort the images produced. In addition, the radiofrequency signals of the MRI cause significant interference with monitored data.

Electrocardiography (ECG)

The ECG wires serve as antennae for radiofrequency signals originating in the scanner, which result in a distorted tracing on the ECG machine that is often uninterpretable. A wireless

ECG employing a transmitter is available (78100A Telemetry, Hewlett Packard Medical, Waldham, MA, or Saturn Monitor, Spacelab), which decreases the interference produced by the scanner; however, the quality of the ECG tracing is poor compared with the standard ECG. Dimick and associates reported that optimal lead placement in a 1.5-Tesla magnet to maximize QRS clarity and minimize artifact could be obtained by monitoring the V_5 and V_6 leads. Additional maneuvers to enhance the ECG include keeping the electrodes close together, twisting the cables, positioning the electrodes near the center of the imager, and incorporating a 7- to 10-Hz filter into the monitor.

Pulse Oximetry

Pulse oximetry readings are valid within the scanner, and certain oximeters are approved for MRI use (Table 15-3). In our institution, however, we have encountered difficulty using these monitors continuously because they may distort the images produced by the scanner. In addition, the oximeter is susceptible to interference by the changing radiofrequency pulses.

Table 15-3   Monitors for Magnetic Resonance Imaging

Rubber or Brass Precordial Stethoscope
Esophageal Stethoscope
Electrocardiography Equipment
    Hewlett Packard 78100 A Telemetry Unit* (Waldham, MA)
    Sirecust 404*
    Saturn Monitor, SpaceLab Inc*
    Astro-Med Dash II

Pulse Oximetry
    Nellcor N-100*
    Ohmeda Biox 3700
    Biochem 1040
    Criticare System 501+

Blood Pressure
    Manual blood pressure using palpation or auscultation
    Dinamap*
    Dinamap 1846 SK/P
    Omega 1400
    Accutorr 2A

Capnography
    Puritan Bennett 222
    Biochem International: Trimed 511 G or 515 respiratory
        monitor 8800 capnometer

*Tested in magnetic fields of 1.0 Tesla or less.

However, the probe may be positioned on a distal extremity as far from the scanner as possible and turned on during the procedure when the scanner is not being activated. This allows for periodic evaluations of oxygen saturation. Alternatively, we have also had success covering the patient's extremity and the probe with aluminum foil and along the cable for 2 to 3 ft. This maneuver will allow for more continuous readings without distorting the image. Care must be taken to prevent loops in the oximeter cable, which can cause severe burns to the patient where the probe is attached to the extremity. With these problems in mind, patients with an unstable cardiovascular system, respiratory distress, or who are undergoing mechanical ventilation are not candidates for MRI scan. If patients develop airway compromise or cardiac instability while in the scanner, they must be removed from the scanning room for proper resuscitation. Any ferrous metal objects used for resuscitation will be drawn to the magnet (even disposable plastic laryngoscopes contain batteries). Depending on its size, the magnet may take up to 1 h to discharge. During this time, no ferrous metal objects may be brought into the room, and the ECG may be uninterpretable. Physical access to children's airways is also inadequate until they are removed from the scanner because the cylindrical radiofrequency shield encircles the body (Fig. 15-2).

How do we monitor these patients? By contrast with the sophisticated monitoring systems we rely on in the operating room, we must depend on more simple means because few of our "high-tech" monitors are helpful around the magnet. Monitors that can safely be used are listed in Table 15-3. Respirations and heart tones are best evaluated using a rubber precordial stethoscope fashioned from a 60-mL syringe plunger and a length of intravenous tubing (Fig. 15-3). The auditory clarity of transmitted sounds is similar to that obtained with the traditional metal precordial stethoscope but without the attraction to the magnet. However, the rhythmic pulses of radiowaves emitted by the magnet produce a thumping sound similar to heart tones—it is often difficult to discern which beats are heart sounds and which are produced by the scanner. For intubated patients, an esophageal stethoscope may offer better clarity of breath sounds, but the heart sounds will still be obscured by the magnet pulses.

Blood Pressure

For blood pressure monitoring, a diasyst with a hand-pumped aneroid manometer has been the most useful device in our hands because some electronic blood pressure monitors distort

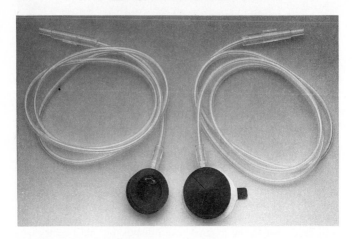

Figure 15-3 A rubber precordial stethoscope allows monitoring of heart and breath sounds with clarity similar to the traditional metal precordial stethoscope, but without attraction to the magnet.

the images produced by the scanner. If an automated blood pressure device (Fig. 15-3) can be used, the electronic portion must be located 12 to 15 ft away from the magnet to prevent attraction, and it should be tested during a dry run of the scanner to evaluate its effect on the images produced. Otherwise, 20 min or more may be wasted with an anesthetized patient in the scanner because it takes 20 to 30 min to collect information before the scans are developed on the screen. Until that time, it is unknown what effect the operation of the monitor has on the quality of the images.

Capnography

Capnography and respiratory gas analysis are now available for use in anesthetized patients in the MRI scanner. Monitors must be interfaced with the airway using long plastic extension tubing. Oxygen analyzers that are essential for monitoring the concentration of oxygen delivered to the patient may also be utilized. Acceptable monitors for use in the MRI suite are listed in Table 15-3, but the electronic portion of these devices must be located as far from the magnetic field as possible to prevent interference with the images. Temperature can be monitored by the use of temperature strips applied to the skin.

Anesthesia Machines

One of the more serious considerations for providing sedative or anesthetic agents in the scanner is the problem of gas supply. The ideal situation would be the provision of permanently constructed supply lines connected to a wall-mounted anesthesia machine. If wall oxygen outlets are not available, oxygen must be provided from cylinders made of aluminum, stainless steel, or other nonferromagnetic alloys. Aluminum tanks are expensive and cannot be refilled because repeated pressurization leads to metal fatigue with a subsequent risk of explosion. Stainless-steel tanks are reusable and MRI compatible.

There are several reports that describe either modification of existing machines or newer MRI-compatible anesthesia machines that are acceptable for use in the MRI suite. Rao and colleagues have published detailed guidelines for alteration of existing machines; however, the major ferromagnetic components are the oxygen and N_2O tanks, the support structures that house the monitors, and the casters. All these components are easily changed to nonmagnetic materials. Alternatively, the Ohmeda Excel 210 has been adapted for MRI use. The vaporizers, inspiratory and expiratory valves, oxygen monitor, and scavenging systems were all found to function properly in the MRI environment. The oxygen analyzer requires lithium rather than the usual zinc batteries. If it is necessary to deliver positive-pressure ventilation to a patient in the scanner, a Jackson-Rees circuit with an aluminum or plastic exhaust valve is most useful. (Remember to arrange for scavenging the waste gases.)

Other technical problems include the cylindrical radiofrequency shield, which is confining and is often disturbing to young children. The apparatus is very noisy during scanning, and the same radiofrequency pulses that interfere with our ability to auscultate heart sounds are often very frightening to the young child. For this reason, sedating children is often very difficult—as soon as a calm, resting state is achieved, the scanner is activated and startles them.

ANESTHETIC CHOICE

Infants and children between 10 months and 3 to 4 years of age are not able to lie still for the full hour required for completion of the scan without considerable sedation or general anesthesia. For good quality imaging, they must lie almost motionless while the scanner is on; however, their relatively small functional residual capacity and the risk for airway obstruction when sedated result in a lowered margin of safety.

Heavy Sedation, Spontaneous Ventilation

Almost any anesthetic technique can be used successfully; however, in our experience, the most satisfactory approach is to maintain spontaneous ventilation, without endotracheal intubation. The reasons for avoiding intubation when possible include difficulty in securing the endotracheal tube and the fact that the anesthesiologist is located several feet away from the airway. Even with rapid recognition of a disconnect or obstructed tube, it would take several minutes, at least, to remove the patient from the scanner and to correct the problem. A technique that we have found to be useful for sedation in children is the use of a pediatric cocktail (meperidine, promethazine, and chlorpromazine) 0.1 mL/kg intramuscularly (Table 15-4). After the child becomes sedated, an intravenous catheter is inserted for access to supplement the sedation with chlorpromazine if the pediatric cocktail is used or ketamine and midazolam if intramuscular ketamine is used as the primary agent. We prefer not to give ketamine after prior administration of the pediatric cocktail, or after other sedative–narcotic mixtures because, in our experience, respiratory depression has been significant and troublesome. The intravenous catheter also provides venous access in case of airway compromise. Additional doses of midazolam are given as 0.025 mg/kg, ketamine as 1 to 2 mg/kg, or chlorpromazine as 0.05 mg/kg. Supplemental oxy-

Table 15-4   Anesthetic Technique*

Heavy Sedation with Spontaneous Ventilation and
   Supplemental Oxygen
  Induction Agents:
    Rectal methohexital 25 to 30 mg/kg
    Intramuscular ketamine 8 to 10 mg/kg
    Pediatric cocktail, 0.1 mL/kg intramuscularly of:
      Meperidine 25 mg/mL
      Promethazine 12.5 mg/mL
      Chlorpromazine 6.25 mg/mL
    Intranasal midazolam 0.2 to 0.3 mg/kg

  Supplemental intravenous doses:
    Midazolam 0.025 mg/kg
    Ketamine 1 to 2 mg/kg
    Chlorpromazine 0.05 mg/kg

General Endotracheal Anesthesia with Spontaneous Ventilation
  Inhaled oxygen /N_2O with intravenous agents
  Inhaled oxygen /N_2O with halogenated agents

*Note dose and route of administration for each agent.

gen can be provided most easily by placing a nasal cannula on the patient after he or she is sedated.

General Endotracheal Anesthesia

If general endotracheal anesthesia is selected, the child must be anesthetized outside the scanner and then carefully inserted into the cylindrical field for scanning. An extralong Jackson-Rees circuit is preferred because the anesthesia machine can then be located 12 to 15 ft from the MRI scanner to prevent any interference with imaging or attraction to the magnet by ferrous parts. If oxygen cylinders are used, flow rates must be reduced to prevent rapid depletion of the oxygen stored in the tanks. A self-inflating bag-valve ventilation device should be available in the scanner room in case oxygen flow is lost so that the patient can be ventilated while the oxygen tanks are being changed.

Anesthetic induction can be accomplished with inhalational agents or a variety of intravenous drugs, depending on the age of the patient and the problems associated with their disease. For example, one of the major uses of MRI scanning is evaluation of the central nervous system. If the patient has elevated intracranial pressure, this must be considered when choosing induction or sedation techniques. It must be remembered that monitoring capabilities in MRI are suboptimal for manipulation of oxygenation, ventilation, or hemodynamic variables (e.g., cerebral perfusion pressure) within a narrow range. The severely compromised patient might be better served by the use of alternate radiologic techniques.

Published experience with anesthesia for MRI from the University of Pennsylvania recommends that the anesthetic approach best suited for MRI is a totally intravenous technique (thiopental, narcotic, and muscle relaxant). Patients are anesthetized outside the MRI and are then transferred to the unit. The pediatric patient may be sedated with chloral hydrate, diazepam, fentanyl, or methohexital. The Cleveland Clinic has also published their system for pediatric anesthesia for MRI. When possible, an intravenous line is started while the child is awake; otherwise, an inhalation induction is performed with O_2/ N_2O/halothane. Intubation follows atropine, thiopental, and succinylcholine. Increments of thiopental are administered according to vital signs and patient movement.

Some institutions have a wall-mounted anesthesia machine located about 3 m from the patient. For general anesthesia, the tubing on a Rees-type modification of the Ayers T-system can be used. Ventilators are available that contain no ferrous metal parts. The 225/SIMV ventilator "MRI compatible" from Monaghan Medical (Plattsburgh, NY) and the Omni Vent Series D/MRI/HBC (Stein-Gates Medical Equipment, Atchinson, KS) are pneumatically driven (by wall oxygen) and volume cycled. Expired tidal volume can be measured with both systems, and we have used the Omni Vent successfully in even small infants.

RECOVERY

After completion of the MRI scan, patients who have been heavily sedated or have required general anesthesia should be observed in a postanesthesia care unit until discharge criteria are met. During transportation from the MRI unit and in the recovery area, more complete monitoring may be instituted as indicated by the patient's condition. Remember that most MRI units are a long distance from the postanesthesia care unit, and airway equipment and portable oxygen should accompany the patient during transport.

BIBLIOGRAPHY

Boutros A, Pavlicek W: Anesthesia for magnetic resonance imaging. *Anesth Analg* 1987; 66:367–374.

Boutros A, Pavlicek W: Anesthesia for magnetic resonance imaging (letter). *Anesth Analg* 1987; 66:367.

Dimick RN, Hedlund LW, Herfkens RJ, et al: Optimizing electrocardiographic electrode placement for cardiac-gated magnetic resonance imaging. *Invest Radiol* 1987; 22:17–22.

Eldemann RR, Shellock FG, Ahladis J: Practical MRI for the technologist and imaging specialist, in Eldeman RR, Hesselink RR (eds): *Clinical Magnetic Resonance Imaging.* Philadelphia, WB Saunders, 1990, chap. 2, pp 39–73.

Fowler JR, Terpenning B, Syverud SA, et al: Magnetic field hazard. *N Engl J Med* 1986; 314:1517.

Geiger RS, Cascorbi HF: Anesthesia in a NMR Scanner. *Anesth Analg* 1984; 63:622–623.

Karlik SJ, Heatherley T, Pavan F, et al: Patient anesthesia and monitoring at a 1.5T MRI installation. *Magn Reson Med* 1988; 7:210–221.

McArdle CB, Nicholas DA, Richardson CH, et al: Monitoring of the neonate undergoing MR imaging: Technical considerations. *Radiology* 1986; 159:223–226.

Nixon C, Hirsch NP, Ormerod IEC, et al: Nuclear magnetic resonance, its implication for the anaesthetist. *Anaesthesia* 1986; 41:131–137.

Patteson SK, Chesney JT: Anesthetic management for magnetic resonance imaging problems and solutions. *Anesth Analg* 1992; 71:121–128.

Plazzo M, Williams RT: Anesthesia in an NMR scanner. *Anesth Analg* 1984; 63:622–623.

Rao CC, Brandl R, Mashak JN: Modification of Ohmeda Excel 210 anesthesia machine for use during MRI. *Anesthesiology* 1989; 71(suppl):A365.

Rao CC, McNiece WL, Emhardt J: Modification of an anesthesia machine for use during magnetic resonance imaging. *Anesthesiology* 1988; 68:640–641.

Roth JL, Nugent M, Gray JE, et al: Patient monitoring during magnetic resonance imaging. *Anesthesiology* 1985; 62:80–83.

Shellock FG: Monitoring sedated pediatric patients during MR imaging. *Radiology* 1990; 177:586–587.

Smith DS, Askey P, Young ML, et al: Anesthetic management of acutely ill patients during magnetic resonance imaging. *Anesthesiology* 1986; 65:710–711.

CHAPTER 16

Diagnosis and Treatment of Malignant Hyperthermia

Lois L. Bready

Malignant hyperthermia (MH) is an inherited disorder of skeletal muscle, which may be a part of a broader subclinical myopathy. These MH-susceptible (MHS) people are usually not incapacitated in their daily lives or activities. However, hypermetabolic crises may be triggered by potent inhalational anesthetics and/or depolarizing neuromuscular blocking agents. Some reports suggest that crises may also be precipitated by nonpharmacologic events, such as severe emotional or physical stress or high environmental temperature. Because the disorder is inherited and most MH crises appear to be brought about by the administration of triggering anesthetic agents, the condition is known as a pharmocogenetic disorder.

The perimeters of MH are blurred; there appears to be significant overlap with other disorders, including primary muscle diseases, hyperthyroidism and thyroid storm, neuroleptic malignant syndrome, and sudden infant death syndrome. The overall incidence of MH crises in the United States has been estimated to be 1 in 15,000 anesthetics in children, 1 in 2,500 anesthetics for strabismus, and 1 in 50,000 to 100,000 in adults. When an MH crisis is triggered, a 1970 survey revealed a mortality of 70 percent. More recently, the mortality rate of an episode was estimated to be 7 percent—a tremendous improvement, which is probably related to increased awareness of this disorder and earlier treatment with the definitive therapeutic agent, dantrolene.

During the past few years, considerable progress has been made in identification of the genetic abnormalities associated with MH. A genetic locus that causes MHS was identified on human chromosome 19q13.1 by two different laboratories. The gene appears to be related to an abnormality of the ryanodine receptor gene, which controls calcium release in skeletal muscle.

Currently, definitive diagnosis of MHS requires caffeine–halothane contracture testing (CHCT) of a freshly biopsied sample of skeletal muscle from the patient. The CHCT is performed at relatively few centers in North America, Europe, and Scandinavia. Various investigators are working to develop non-invasive in vitro tests for the diagnosis of MHS.

PREOPERATIVE DETECTION

The first goal in the management of MH is the preoperative detection of MHS patients, before exposure to anesthetics and an MH crisis occurs. Pending the availability of noninvasive tests, the clinician must rely on history and physical examination to determine which patients are likely to be at risk.

A positive family history is extremely valuable. Although inheritance appears to be dominant, there may be incomplete penetrance. A history of an MH episode or of a positive CHCT in a first-degree relative (parent, child, or sibling) is strong evidence for MHS in a patient. The incidence of MH is higher in the younger age groups (up to 30 years); it occurs more commonly in males, especially in the 15- to 30-year-old age group (e.g., muscular football player). A history of difficulties with temperature control is another clue to the susceptible patient. Mothers of some MHS children may report that the child "gets a fever easily," and there has been at least one report of awake MH attacks, related to physical exertion and emotional stress, in an adult man.

Suspicious previous anesthetic experiences include delayed emergence after previous anesthesia and masseter spasm with halothane or succinylcholine. Many MHS patients have had one or more uneventful anesthetics; one patient in the German literature had 13 anesthetics before the syndrome was triggered! Thus, a history of not triggering with a prior anesthesia is not very helpful.

About one-third of MHS patients are found to have various musculoskeletal abnormalities (Table 16-1). Among the most commonly encountered musculoskeletal disorders are ptosis, strabismus, and muscle cramping.

A number of hereditary myopathies have been associated with MH, including the following: myotonia congenita, central-core disease, Duchenne's muscular dystrophy, King Denborough syndrome (multiple congenital anomalies, including myopathy, short stature, cryptorchidism, thoracic kyphosis, lumbar lordosis, pectus carinatum, hypognathia, low-set ears, webbed neck, and antimongoloid slant of the eyes), and Schwartz-Jampel syndrome (dwarfism, multiple skeletal anomalies, mus-

Table 16-1   Musculoskeletal Disorders Associated with Malignant Hyperthermia

Ptosis	Strabismus
Squint	Ophthalmoplegia
Weakness	Increased muscle bulk
Cramping	Congenital hernias
Recurrent dislocations of joints	Pectus deformities
Scoliosis with thoracic kyphosis	Lumbar lordosis
Scapular winging	Joint hypermobility
Clubfoot deformities	Malalignment of the feet
Limb-girdle muscle weakness	Myelomeningocele
Dental deformities (malocclusion)	Hypognathia
Congenital dislocation of the hip	Spontaneous herniated nucleus pulposus

cular stiffness, and continuous muscle fiber activity using electromyography).

A British investigator, R. J. Smith, described a noninvasive diagnostic index to estimate MH susceptibility in 1988. He found that there was good discrimination among MHS, malignant hyperthermia non-susceptible (MHNS), and control patients using the variables listed in Table 16-2.

LABORATORY DIAGNOSIS OF MH

Creatinine Phosphokinase (CK)

It has long been recognized that the serum CK level is higher than normal in some patients with MH. Similarly, some relatives of afflicted patients also have elevated serum CK levels. It was hoped that CK screening of relatives of patients with MH would provide a simple, cheap, and readily available diagnostic tool. Patients who are MHS by CHCT tend to have higher CKs, but there is a large overlap with the CKs of MHNS people. Thus, unfortunately, CK is considered to be potentially helpful for screening but is not a definitive test.

Muscle Biopsy and CHCT

To date, the most reliable test to detect MHS is in vitro exposure of skeletal muscle strips to caffeine and halothane with measurement of isometric tension and construction of a dose–response curve. When normal muscle is exposed to caffeine, it

Table 16-2   Factors Associated with Malignant Hyperthermia Susceptibility

Previous postoperative problems
   Fever
   Muscle swelling
   Muscle weakness

Personal history
   Squint
   Backache
   Heart disease
   Muscle cramps
   Muscle weakness
   Blackouts
   High fevers
   Febrile convulsions
   Anxiety
   Road accidents

Family history
   Squint
   Foot abnormality
   Congenital abnormality
   Cot deaths
   Muscle, bone, and joint disease
   Diabetes
   Bleeding

Reproduced with permission from Smith RJ: Preoperative assessment of risk factors. *Br J Anaesth* 1988; 60:317–319.

contracts, but the dose required is higher than that required to make MHS muscle contract. When normal muscle is exposed to halothane, usually, no contraction (or a very small one) is observed. The MHS muscle is more sensitive than normal to caffeine-induced contraction, especially in the presence of halothane.

Skeletal muscle for the CHCT study is obtained from the vastus lateralis, quadriceps, or rectus abdominus muscle. This muscle biopsy must be performed in a center where CHCT is done. (Check with the Malignant Hyperthermia Association of the United States at (203) 655-3007 for referral to the nearest testing center.) The tissue cannot be sent through the mail. Anesthesia is necessary for the biopsy, but dantrolene cannot be given because it interferes with the testing. Anesthetic agents that do not trigger MH are employed (e.g., regional anesthesia or nontriggering agents). In the past, some testing centers used one of several nonstandard tests. A patient who has tested positive at a laboratory that employed a nonstandard test may or may not be MHS.

Other Laboratory Indicators

Obviously, it would be advantageous to be able to determine MH susceptibility less invasively than by muscle biopsy or triggering of a MH crisis. A number of investigators are working in this area—development of an accurate, reliable, inexpensive blood test will greatly improve our ability to diagnose MHS preoperatively and to treat these patients appropriately. In the meantime, nontriggering anesthetic techniques are recommended when there is a suspicion of MHS. When MHS is strongly suspected or known, pretreatment with dantrolene (along with avoidance of known triggering drugs) is considered the safest method of reducing the risk of precipitation of a MH crisis.

PATHOPHYSIOLOGY

Altered Calcium Mechanics

The mechanism responsible for the development of MH is thought to be a genetically determined defect in striated (skeletal) muscle. As described earlier, the genetic locus that causes MHS has been identified on human chromosome 19q13.1. It appears to be related to an abnormality of the ryanodine receptor gene, which controls calcium release in skeletal muscle.

In MHS skeletal muscle, the sarcoplasmic reticulum (SR) cannot accumulate calcium normally. This hypothesis explains the basic clinical manifestations of MH, such as the sudden increase in temperature, muscular rigidity, and metabolic acidosis.

During normal skeletal muscle function, contraction begins with the release of acetylcholine by the motor nerve endings in response to an action potential. The postjunctional muscle membrane is depolarized, and a depolarization wave sweeps along the length of the muscle cell. Upon depolarization of the membrane, T-tubules, which are invaginations of the muscle cell membrane (sarcolemma), transmit the signal that initiates the release of calcium from storage sites within the SR. This transmission process is known as "excitation–contraction coupling."

The rise in intracellular Ca^{++} ion concentration triggers the mechanisms involved in contraction. The muscle is kept in a relaxed state by troponin, which prevents actin from attaching to myosin. When Ca^{++} ions are released into the muscle fibers, they bind to troponin and allow myosin and actin to combine. As these filaments slide past one another, contraction occurs. When muscle relaxes, Ca^{++} ions are again taken up by the SR.

The SR of muscle from MHS patients, when exposed to a triggering agent, is unable to accumulate normal amounts of

Ca^{++}. Because the SR cannot take up Ca^{++}, the intracellular Ca^{++} level is elevated. Only a small increase in the free concentration of Ca^{++} within the myoplasm is required to activate phosphorylase kinase, thereby accelerating the catabolism of glycogen to lactic acid, CO_2, and heat. With greater increases in myoplasmic Ca^{++}, other reactions occur as follows:

1. Ca^{++} activates myosin adenosine triphosphatase, which hydrolyzes the conversion of adenosine triphosphate to adenosine diphosphate and inorganic phosphate, with liberation of heat and free energy. This energy is utilized for the interaction of myosin and actin.
2. Ca^{++} induces a conformational change in troponin; myosin and actin slide together but are prevented from relaxing if Ca^{++} remains elevated.
3. When myoplasmic Ca^{++} increases to toxic levels, it is actively accumulated in the mitochondria, where uncoupling of oxidative phosphorylation from electron transport occurs. Adenosine triphosphate formation then ceases and becomes insufficient to supply the needs of the cells. As the O_2 supply is depleted, lactic acid production increases, and metabolic acidosis results.
4. Rising Ca^{++} levels also contribute to the disruption of membranes. This allows K^+, myoglobin, and CK to escape into the circulating blood.

Morphologically, MHS skeletal muscle may have a variety of subtle differences from normal muscle, but these differences may be exceedingly difficult to appreciate. Thus, routine microscopic examination of skeletal muscle is not sufficient to diagnose MHS.

CLINICAL MANIFESTATIONS

The onset of an MH crisis is usually gradual and is heralded by a tachycardia, which is the earliest and most consistent sign (Table 16-3). Unless there is an obvious cause of tachycardia, MH must be suspected. Many fatal cases of MH have occurred when triggering anesthetics were continued despite documented tachycardia. Tachycardia with MH is a response to the slowly developing hypermetabolic state.

Dysrhythmias are also a common early warning sign of MH. A bolus of lidocaine may ameliorate the dysrhythmia for a few minutes, but it does not affect the causative acidosis and rising K^+ level.

Tachypnea may occur in response to increasing CO_2 tension. This would be as common a symptom as tachycardia, except for the frequent use of muscle relaxants in our practice.

**Table 16-3   Signs of Malignant Hyperthermia
(Not All Need Be Present)**

Physical Signs
  Tachycardia
  Tachypnea, if spontaneous ventilation
  Unstable blood pressure
  Dysrhythmias (supraventricular tachycardia, premature
    ventricular contractions, and ventricular tachycardia)
  Dark blood in surgical field despite adequate fraction of
    inspired oxygen
  Cyanotic mottling of skin
  Profuse sweating
  Rapid rise in temperature (1°F/15 min)
  Sustained rise in temperature (to as high as 108°F [42.2°C] or
    more)
  Fasciculations and/or rigidity (may involve total body)
  Trismus of masseter muscles (controversial)
  Anisocoria
  Seizures
Laboratory Abnormalities
  Central venous desaturation
  Central venous and arterial hypercarbia
  Metabolic acidosis
  Respiratory acidosis
  Hyperkalemia
  Myoglobinuria/myoglobinemia
  Elevated creatinine phosphokinase (late)

Hyperthermia is usually a late sign of MH, and the temperature may go down before it increases. The core temperature decreases during general anesthesia, and MH reverses this trend. In some cases, the increase in temperature can be rapid (over a few minutes), but it occurs more commonly at a rate of about 2°F/h. The temperature may be as high as 108° to 115°F if appropriate measures are not taken early. The hyperthermia is caused by the heat of cellular energy. In some fulminant cases of MH, cardiac arrest will precede any marked temperature change.

With controlled ventilation, end-tidal CO_2 may increase.

Arterial blood gases will reveal both metabolic and respiratory acidosis and an increased A-aDO_2. The mixed venous PO_2 will be very low, secondary to an increased oxygen consumption (may be as great as fivefold). If arterial blood gases are not evaluated early, the initial $PaCO_2$ may be as high as 100 to 200 mmHg and the pH, 7.15 to 6.70.

Rhabdomyolysis occurs late in the syndrome and produces gross elevations in serum CK and myoglobin; a complex pattern of electrolyte disturbances, especially hyperkalemia; and

Table 16-4   Suggested Therapy for Malignant Hyperthermia Emergency From the Malignant Hyperthermia Association of the United States, 1993 Revision*

LOOK FOR • tachycardia • muscle stiffness • hypercarbia • tachypnea • cardiac dysrhythmias • respiratory & metabolic acidosis • fever • unstable/rising blood pressure • cyanosis/mottling • myoglobinuria

Emergency Therapy for

Malignant Hyperthermia

* Revised 1993 *

ACUTE PHASE TREATMENT

1. Immediately discontinue all volatile inhalation anesthetics and succinylcholine. Hyperventilate with 100% oxygen at high gas flows; at least 10 L/min. The circle system and CO_2 absorbent need not be changed.
2. Administer dantrolene sodium 2-3 mg/kg initial bolus rapidly with increments up to 10 mg/kg total. Continue to administer dantrolene until signs of MH (e.g. tachycardia, rigidity, increased end-tidal CO_2 and temperature elevation) are controlled. Occasionally, a total dose greater than 10 mg/kg may be needed. Each vial of dantrolene contains 20 mg of dantrolene and 3 grams mannitol. Each vial should be mixed with 60 mL of sterile water for injection USP without a bacteriostatic agent.
3. Administer bicarbonate to correct metabolic acidosis as guided by blood gas analysis. In the absence of blood gas analysis, 1-2 mEq/kg should be administered.
4. Simultaneous with the above, actively cool the hyperthermic patient. Use IV iced saline (not Ringer's lactate) 15 mL/kg q 15 min X 3.
   a. Lavage stomach, bladder, rectum and open cavities with iced saline as appropriate.
   b. Surface cool with ice and hypothermia blanket.
   c. Monitor closely since overvigorous treatment may lead to hypothermia.
5. Dysrhythmias will usually respond to treatment of acidosis and hyperkalemia. If they persist or are life threatening, standard anti-arrhythmic agents may be used, with the exception of calcium channel blockers (may cause hyperkalemia and CV collapse).
6. Determine and monitor end-tidal CO_2, arterial, central or femoral venous blood gases, serum potassium, calcium, clotting studies and urine output.
7. Hyperkalemia is common and should be treated with hyperventilation, bicarbonate, intravenous glucose and insulin (10 units regular insulin in 50 mL 50% glucose titrated to potassium level). Life threatening hyperkalemia may also be treated with calcium administration (e.g. 2-5 mg/kg of $CaCl_2$).
8. Ensure urine output of greater than 2 mL/kg/hr. Consider central venous or PA monitoring because of fluid shifts and hemodynamic instability that may occur.
9. Boys less than 9 years of age who experience sudden cardiac arrest after succinylcholine in the absence of hypoxemia should be treated for acute hyperkalemia first. In this situation calcium chloride should be administered along with other means to reduce serum potassium. They should be presumed to have subclinical muscular dystrophy.

POST ACUTE PHASE

A. Observe the patient in an ICU setting for at least 24 hours since recrudescence of MH may occur, particularly following a fulminant case resistant to treatment.
B. Administer dantrolene 1 mg/kg IV q 6 hours for 24-48 hours post episode. After that, oral dantrolene 1 mg/kg q 6 hours may be used for 24 hours as necessary.
C. Follow ABG, CK, potassium, calcium, urine and serum myoglobin, clotting studies and core body temperature until such time as they return to normal values (e.g. q 6 hours). Central temperature (e.g. rectal, esophageal) should be continuously monitored until stable.
D. Counsel the patient and family regarding MH and further precautions. Refer the patient to MHAUS. Fill out an Adverse Metabolic Reaction to Anesthesia (AMRA) report available through the North American Malignant Hyperthermia Registry (717) 531-6936.

CAUTION: This protocol may not apply to every patient and must of necessity be altered according to specific patient needs.

Names of on-call physicians available to consult in MH emergencies may be obtained 24 hours a day through:

**MEDIC ALERT
FOUNDATION INTERNATIONAL
(209) 634-4917
Ask for: INDEX ZERO**

**For Non-Emergency
or Patient Referral Calls:
MHAUS
(203) 847-0407
P.O. Box 191
Westport, CT 06881-0191**

3/93/12K

*Reproduced with permission.

disseminated intravascular coagulation. Limb–muscle rigidity is a common but late feature of the syndrome.

DRUG THERAPY: DANTROLENE

Dantrolene is a direct-acting skeletal muscle relaxant; it dissociates excitation–contraction coupling in the muscle by inhibiting the release of calcium ions from the SR (through actions on the connections between the transverse tubules and the terminal cisternae of the SR, on the terminal cisternae directly, or both). Although dantrolene's site of action rests in the skeletal muscle, its beneficial effects are far-reaching. By decreasing rigidity and restoring muscle function, dantrolene normalizes all functions associated with muscle hypermetabolism, including cardiac function, respiration, and acid–base balance. As soon as the diagnosis of MH is made, intravenous (IV) dantrolene is indicated at an initial dose of 1 mg/kg. As much as 10 mg/kg IV may be required to treat a crisis. A standard treatment regimen is outlined in Table 16-4.

THE ROLE OF
CALCIUM-CHANNEL ANTAGONISTS

The calcium-channel antagonists inhibit the entry of calcium into cells or its mobilization from intracellular stores. A number of investigators have evaluated their effects in MHS pig models. Verapamil did not inhibit MH development triggered by halothane or halothane and succinylcholine. The time of onset and severity were unchanged. The dose of dantrolene required to treat the MH attack was not affected by verapamil pretreatment, and there was no myocardial depression at a dose of 1 to 2 mg/kg of dantrolene after verapamil. Laboratory animals (dogs and swine) pretreated with verapamil and given IV dantrolene have sustained cardiovascular collapse and hyperkalemia. A human case report details development of hyperkalemia, necessitating therapy with insulin and furosemide. Nifedipine has not been associated with any problematic interactions. Diltiazem appears to prevent and reverse contracture in vitro.

Obviously, the safest course is to avoid the risk of drug interactions by very conservative use of calcium-channel antagonists in patients treated with dantrolene. Based on limited data from animal studies, diltiazem may be the safest of the available agents for use in these patients.

ANESTHETIC DRUGS AND
MALIGNANT HYPERTHERMIA

The syndrome of MH can be triggered by a wide variety of drugs. It is difficult to say which agents are safe with MHS patients because identical techniques of anesthesia, given to the same MHS patient may trigger an MH crisis one time and not another.

The anesthetic drugs that should be avoided in MHS patients include:

1. All volatile anesthetics.
2. All depolarizing neuromuscular blocking agents.

The MH reactions may be aggravated by sympathomimetics, parasympatholytics, cardiac glycosides, and calcium salts.

Among the environmental stress factors that can precipitate a reaction through catecholamine release are emotional excitement, fear, muscle injury, high climatic temperature with high humidity, exercise, and infections.

Anesthetic drugs that are considered to be safe to anesthetize an MHS patient are listed in Table 16-5 and include:

1. Narcotics.
2. Barbiturates (may be protective).
3. Nitrous oxide.
4. Benzodiazepine.
5. Droperidol (may offer some protection).
6. Local anesthetics for local or regional blocks.
7. Nondepolarizing muscle relaxants (antagonism with anticholinesterase should be undertaken with caution).
8. Etomidate (does not trigger MH but does not protect as thiopental does).
9. Propofol.

Table 16-5   Safe Anesthetic Drugs for the Patient With Malignant Hyperthermia

Narcotics
Barbiturates (may be protective)
Nitrous oxide
Benzodiazepine
Droperidol (may offer some protection)
Local anesthetics for local and regional blocks
Nondepolarizing muscle relaxants (antagonism with
    anticholinesterase should be undertaken with caution)
Etomidate (does not trigger malignant hyperthermia but does
    not protect as thiopental does)
Propofol

GENERAL GUIDELINES IN THE
KNOWN MHS PATIENT

Be prepared (cooling blanket, cold IV fluids, and dantrolene)! Anxiety and stress need to be avoided, and the patient should be well sedated preoperatively, using oral premedicants.

Use a clean anesthesia machine, one without residual potent inhalational agents in the breathing circuit. If your facility does not keep a vapor-free anesthesia machine available for these patients, an ordinary anesthesia machine may be rendered sufficiently clean by replacing previously used CO_2 absorbent cannisters and running high flows (10 to 12 L/min) of air/O_2 through the machine for at least 10 to 15 min. Omit atropine to avoid tachycardia. Regional anesthesia is a good choice if it is acceptable to the patient, but if this causes anxiety for the patient, do not force the patient. If possible, the total duration of the anesthetic should not exceed 2 h because reactions are more likely to occur with prolonged anesthetic duration. For the pediatric patient, consider oral midazolam 0.5 to 1.0 mg/kg, oral pentobarbital 3 to 4 mg/kg, or rectal methohexital 15 to 30 mg/kg to induce basal anesthesia, followed by insertion of the IV catheter. A nontriggering intravenous anesthetic should follow. Do not perform an inhalation induction.

PREOPERATIVE DANTROLENE
REGIMENS

Many authorities prefer to treat MHS patients with dantrolene before induction of anesthesia. Others reserve its use for signs of MH activity (Table 16-3). If pretreatment is planned, a dose of 2.5 mg/kg IV dantrolene will provide protection of adequate duration for most surgical procedures. Another dose of dantrolene, 1 mg/kg, should be given after 8 h to provide protection in the postoperative period. If an MH crisis does not occur, no further dantrolene therapy is needed.

CONTROVERSIES IN MH

Masseter Muscle Spasm (MMS)

A rather common clinical scenario is as follows. A child, anesthetized with succinylcholine and halothane, develops MMS after a dose of succinylcholine that should have been sufficient for relaxation. The blockade monitor shows no twitch or tetanus, but the MM is tight, and the mouth may be so tightly closed that it cannot be opened, even for insertion of an oral airway. The incidence of MMS in children anesthetized with halothane and succinylcholine appears to be about one percent, far more common than the prevalence of MHS in the general population.

What percentage of children who develop MMS after exposure to succinylcholine and halothane are found to be MHS when tested by CHCT? Numerous studies suggest that, of patients who were referred for CHCT after MMS, 50 to 70 percent have positive CHCT. This probably represents bias in referral; nevertheless, some patients who develop MMS after exposure to succinylcholine and halothane are MHS. Measurement of CK is not particularly helpful in differentiating MHS from MHNS, although when the CK is measured after MMS, those patients who are subsequently proved to be MHS tend to have higher CK values.

For the clinician, if MMS develops, a decision must be made to continue the anesthetic, using nontriggering agents, or stop the anesthetic, cancel the planned operation, and have the patient evaluated for MHS. This is a controversial area, and individual judgments must be made. If the decision is to continue, it is absolutely mandatory that end-tidal CO_2 and core temperature monitoring be employed and that the anesthesiologist is prepared to treat MH if a crisis occurs.

Management of the MHS Patient in Utero

The fetus of a MHS patient may be genetically MHS, but the incidence of MH crisis in the postnatal period has not been documented. Treatment of the mother results in placental transmission of dantrolene to the fetus, resulting in diminution of muscle tone, a protected but floppy baby.

Treatment of the mother with dantrolene is not without some risk, as exemplified by a recent case report of uterine atony after dantrolene pretreatment, which necessitated an emergency hysterectomy. It was not clearly established that dantrolene was the causative agent for the uterine atony; however, unless there are clear indications for administration of dantrolene to a pregnant patient, it may be safe to manage her labor without its use. The newborn infant of a mother known to be MHS should be observed closely for signs of MH but not treated with dantrolene unless clear indications occur.

MORE INFORMATION

In the treatment of the previously undiagnosed patient with an MH crisis, after the crisis is coming under control and the patient is in the postanesthesia care unit or the intensive care unit, it is important to speak with the family. They will have lots of questions, and you may be viewed with suspicion because MH is a problem of which most lay people (and many medical personnel) are unaware. Helpful resources include the publications of the Malignant Hyperthermia Association of the United

States. Consult this group at (203) 655-3007 for nonemergency or patient referral calls. The emergency number for 24-h MH help is (209) 634-4917 "Index Zero."

At a later, elective time, the anesthesiologist should meet with the family to explain more fully the implications of MHS. The term "malignant hyperthermia" may be confusing to the patient because it is not cancer and there is not always hyperthermia. The patient who had the MH crisis may not need a muscle biopsy—some authorities recommend biopsy, but others suggest that the patient has already demonstrated MHS. Other family members probably should undergo biopsies. Referral to the nearest center that performs CHCT and other valuable guidance can be obtained from the MH experts at the telephone numbers listed previously.

BIBLIOGRAPHY

Brownell AKW: Malignant hyperthermia: Relationship to other diseases. *Br J Anaesth* 1988; 60:303–308.

Byers DJ, Merin RG: Malignant hyperthermia in a renal transplant recipient. *Anesthesiology* 1987; 67:979–981.

Douglas MJ, McMorland GH: The anaesthetic management of the malignant hyperthermia susceptible parturient. *Can J Anaesth* 1986; 33:371.

Ellis FR: The diagnosis of MH: Its social implications. *Br J Anaesth* 1988; 60:252.

Ellis FR, Halsall PJ, Harriman GF: Malignant hyperpyrexia and sudden infant death syndrome. *Br J Anaesth* 1988; 60:28–30.

Gronert GA, Ahern CP, Milde JH: Treatment of porcine malignant hyperthermia: Lactate gradient from muscle to blood. *Can J Anaesth* 1986; 33:729–736.

Gronert GA, Mott J, Lee J: Aetiology of malignant hyperthermia. *Br J Anaesth* 1988; 60:253–267.

Gronert GA, Thomas R, Onofrio B: Human malignant hyperthermia awake episodes and correction by dantrolene. *Anesth Analg* 1980; 59:377–378.

Harriman DGF: Malignant hyperthermia myopathy: A critical review. *Br J Anaesth* 1988; 60:309–316.

Harrison GG: Dantrolene: Dynamics and kinetics. *Br J Anaesth* 1988; 60:279–286.

Heffron JJA: Malignant hyperthermia: Biochemical aspects of the acute episode. *Br J Anaesth* 1988; 60:274–278.

Heiman-Patterson T, Fletcher JE, Rosenberg H, et al: No relationship between fiber type and halothane contracture test results in malignant hyperthermia. *Anesthesiology* 1987; 67:82–84.

Larach MG, Landis JR, Bunn SJ, et al: Prediction of malignant hyperthermia susceptibility in low-risk subjects: An epidemiologic investigation of caffeine halothane contracture responses. *Anesthesiology* 1992; 76:16–27.

Levitt RC: Prospects for the diagnosis of malignant hyperthermia susceptibility using molecular genetic approaches. *Anesthesiology* 1992; 76:1039–1048.

Mauritz W, Sporn P, Steinbereithner K: Malignant hyperthermia susceptibility confirmed in both parents of probands. *Acta Anaesth Scand* 1988; 32:24–26.

Mauritz W, Sporn P, Steinbereithner K: Maligne hyperthermie in Osterreich. *Anaesthesist* 1986; 35:639–650.

MacLennan DH, Phillips MS: Malignant hyperthermia. *Science* 1992; 256:789–793.

Morrell DF, Harrison GG: The screening of atracurium in MHS swine. *Br J Anaesth* 1986; 58:444–446.

Olgin J, Argov Z, Rosenberg H, et al: Non-invasive evaluation of malignant hyperthermia susceptibility with phosphorus nuclear magnetic resonance spectroscopy. *Anesthesiology* 1988; 68:507–513.

Ording H, Hansen U, Skovgaard LT: Age, fiber type composition and in vitro contracture responses in human malignant hyperthermia. *Acta Anaesthesiol Scand* 1988; 32:121–124.

Ording H, Nielsen VG: Atracurium and its antagonism by neostigmine (plus glycopyrrolate) in patients susceptible to malignant hyperthermia. *Br J Anaesth* 1986; 58:1001–1004.

Robinson LK, O'Brien NC, Puckett MC, et al: Multiple pterygium syndrome: A case complicated by malignant hyperthermia. *Clin Genet* 1987; 32:5–9.

Rosenberg H: Clinical presentation of malignant hyperthermia. *Br J Anaesth* 1988; 60:268–273.

Simmons ML, Goldman E: Atypical malignant hyperthermia with persistent hyperkalaemia during renal transplantation. *Can J Anaesth* 1988; 35:409–412.

Smith RJ: Preoperative assessment of risk factors. *Br J Anaesth* 1988; 60:317–319.

Verburg MP, Britt BA, Oerlemans FTJJ, et al: Comparison of metabolites in skeletal muscle biopsies from normal humans and those susceptible to malignant hyperthermia. *Anesthesiology* 1986; 65:654–657.

Weingarten AE, Korsh JI, Newman GG, et al: Postpartum uterine atony after intravenous dantrolene. *Anesth Analg* 1987; 66:269–270.

Williams CH, Dozier SE, Ilias WK, et al: Porcine malignant hyperthermia: Testing of atracurium in MH susceptible pigs. *Anesth Analg* 1985; 64:301.

Yentis SM, Levine MF, Hartley EJ: Should all children with suspected or confirmed malignant hyperthermia susceptibility be admitted after surgery? A 10-year review. *Anesth Analg* 1992; 75:3345–3350.

CHAPTER 17

Transfusion Support and Bleeding Disorders

Chantal R. Harrison

Effective transfusion support of the pediatric patient is dependent on the application of basic knowledge of the blood components available and the expected result of transfusions of these components. Although the surgical procedures performed in pediatric patients requiring blood transfusions are varied, most transfusion decisions are dictated by the volume of estimated blood loss, the child's blood volume, the preoperative hematocrit, and the medical condition. Certain situations, such as the repair of major congenital anomalies in a neonate or the transplantation of the heart, liver, or kidney, may have special requirements. Whereas many surgical procedures could not be performed without the support of blood transfusions, the benefits of transfusion must be weighed against the possible adverse reactions that might occur. The goal of minimizing allogeneic donor exposures is especially applicable to children who usually will have a long life expectancy. Occasionally, a bleeding diathesis, congenital or acquired, may be encountered. In this situation, a combination of careful clinical observation and prompt laboratory evaluation is crucial in obtaining hemostasis.

BLOOD COMPONENT PREPARATIONS

Blood components available for transfusion support usually derive from one unit of whole blood, that is, approximately 450 mL of blood mixed with an anticoagulant–preservative solution, collected from a rigorously screened volunteer blood donor.

Red Cell Preparations

Whole Blood
Whole blood is not routinely available because it is systematically divided into three components: red blood cells (RBC,

often called packed RBC), fresh-frozen plasma (FFP), and platelets. This is done to ensure the maximum effectiveness of each component through storage at optimal temperatures. These temperatures are 1° to 6°C for RBC, less than −18°C for FFP, and 20° to 24°C for platelets. Platelets left in contact with RBC lose their viability in 12 to 24 h, and the factor VIII level in plasma will decrease by one third after 12 h of storage at 1° to 6°C.

RBC

Two different systems of preservative solutions exist and are often available concurrently: Citrate–phosphate–dextrose–adenine (CPDA-1) and additive solutions (AS). When preparing CPDA-1 RBC, the whole blood is drawn into a primary bag containing 63 mL of anticoagulant–preservative solution. Plasma and platelets are removed by differential centrifugation. When preparing AS RBC, the whole blood is drawn into a primary bag containing only anticoagulant. After removal of the plasma and the platelets, the preservative solution is added to the RBC. These two methods result in two RBC preparations with different characteristics described in Table 17-1. The advantage of AS RBC is their longer shelf life and their low viscosity, allowing rapid infusion. The CPDA-1 RBC are very viscous and may require the injection of 50 mL of normal saline into the bag for rapid infusion. On the other hand, CPDA-1 RBC are more effective, volume for volume, in raising the hematocrit of a patient.

FFP

The FFP is separated from whole blood and flash frozen below −18°C within 6 h of collection. When needed for transfusion, it is thawed in a water bath at 37°C. This takes approximately 20 min. For all practical purposes, thawed FFP contains one

Table 17-1   RBC Preparations

	CPDA-1	AS
Volume	260–350 mL	310–400 mL
Hematocrit	70–80%	50–60%
Total RBC	180 mL	180 mL
Total hemoglobin	60 g	60 g
Storage period	35 days	42 days

RBC = red blood cells, CPDA-1 = citrate–phosphate–dextrose–adenine, AS = additive solution.

Table 17-2 Platelet Preparations

	RDP	SDP
Volume	50 mL	200–350 mL
Platelet count	$0.55–1 \times 10^{11}$	$3–6 \times 10^{11}$

RDP = random-donor platelets, SDP = single-donor platelets.

unit of each coagulation factor per milliliter. The average volume of one unit of FFP is 200 mL.

Cryoprecipitate
Cryoprecipitate is prepared by thawing one unit of FFP at 4°C. At this temperature, a white precipitate is formed, which is concentrated into 10 to 20 mL by centrifugation. One unit of cryoprecipitate contains, on average, 100 units of factor VIII, 200 to 250 mg of fibrinogen, 40 to 70 percent of the von Willebrand's factor, and 20 to 30 percent of the factor XIII present in the original unit of FFP.

Platelets
The platelets separated from one unit of whole blood are usually referred to as random-donor platelets (RDP). Platelets can be harvested by apheresis, where only platelets are collected from a donor over a period of 2 h. These are often referred to as single-donor platelets (SDP). Table 17-2 outlines the characteristics of RDP and SDP. One unit of SDP is the equivalent of 6 to 10 units of RDP and has the advantage of exposing the recipient to the platelets of only one donor. Platelets are stored at room temperature for up to 5 days, and fresh platelets provide a significant amount of nonlabile coagulation factors, comparable to FFP, volume for volume.

GUIDELINES FOR THE TRANSFUSION SUPPORT OF A PEDIATRIC PATIENT

The volume of the different blood components administered to a pediatric patient is dependent on the blood volume of the recipient and the desired outcome. The blood volume of a pediatric patient can be calculated from the patient's weight according to the parameters described in Table 17-3. From the blood volume of the child and the preoperative hematocrit, one can calculate the amount of allowable blood loss before a chosen critical hematocrit is reached. For example, if a child who weighs 10 kg and has a hematocrit of 40 percent can be allowed

Table 17-3   Blood Volume in Pediatric Patients

AGE	BLOOD VOLUME (mL/kg)
Premature neonate	90–100
Full-term infant	80–85
Child older than 1 year	70

to bleed to a hematocrit of 25 percent, the following calculation can be made:

1. Blood volume = 10 kg × 70 mL/kg = 700 mL.
2. RBC volume = 700 mL × 0.40 = 280 mL.
3. Minimum RBC volume = 700 mL × 0.25 = 175 mL.
4. Allowable RBC loss = 280 mL − 175 mL = 105 mL.

Considering that the blood loss occurs at a hematocrit averaging at 32.5 percent, the allowable blood loss can be estimated to be 105 mL ÷ 0.325 = 323 mL. Practically, after a blood loss of 300 mL has occurred, to maintain the hematocrit at 25 percent, one should infuse RBC at a rate of one third to one half the volume of additional blood loss, depending on whether CPDA-1 or AS RBC are used, respectively. Although such precise mathematic calculations are not practical to apply strictly in a critical situation, they do give a rational basis for the transfusion of RBC and are a useful exercise to perform preoperatively on any infant or child. From this calculation, an approximate transfusion plan can be devised, which can be adapted according to intraoperative hematocrit values. A rule of thumb in a nonbleeding patient is that a transfusion of 3 mL/kg of RBC will increase the hematocrit by three percent and the hemoglobin level by 1 g/dL in a child whose blood volume is 70 mL/kg. When transfusing AS RBC, the dose should be increased to 4 mL/kg.

In general, no other blood components than RBC are needed intraoperatively unless a bleeding diathesis occurs, manifested by microvascular bleeding, or surgical bleeding is massive and dilutional coagulopathy is impending. If it is determined that FFP administration is indicated, a dose of 10 mL/kg should provide sufficient coagulation factors in the absence of an active consumption. If the coagulopathy is secondary to thrombocytopenia, one unit of RDP per 10 kg will provide a hemostatic dose of platelets and the equivalent of 50 mL of FFP. If consumptive coagulopathy is present and the fibrinogen level is below 100 mg/dL, one unit of cryoprecipitate per 7 kg is an appro-

Table 17-4　Expected Effect of Blood Components

COMPONENT	DOSE	EFFECT (INCREASE)
RBC	3 mL/kg	3% hematocrit or 1 g/dL hemoglobin
FFP	10 mL/kg	Hemostatic dose (30% coagulation factors)
Platelets	1 unit/10 kg	50,000/μL platelet count
Cryoprecipitate	1 unit/7 kg	50 mg/dL fibrinogen

RBC = packed red blood cells, FFP = fresh-frozen plasma.

priate initial dose. This information is summarized in Table 17-4.

SPECIALIZED NEEDS OF THE NEONATE

Although the general principles described apply to neonates, a few additional concerns may need to be addressed. A very small premature neonate whose mother is not seropositive for cytomegalovirus (CMV) antibodies is at risk of acquiring symptomatic CMV infection from blood. This concern only applies to very small premature neonates, weighing less than 1200 g; however, it is common practice to transfuse all premature neonates with blood that is either seronegative for CMV antibodies or has been processed to minimize the risk of CMV infection transmission. A CMV infection is transmitted by white cells contaminating cellular blood components (RBC and platelets) and leukoreduction by the currently available third-generation filters achieve a 99 to 99.9 percent removal of white cells. This appears to be effective in preventing CMV transmission.

Debate is still ongoing whether the preservative materials present in AS RBC have been convincingly proven to be safe for neonates. This concern is most likely not very pertinent if a small amount of RBC is transfused. On the other hand, if entire units are expected to be used, such as in the correction of congenital anomalies, it may be preferable to use CPDA-1 RBC or to have the supernatant preservative solution expressed out from the AS RBC.

In a premature neonate or in a neonate who may have a congenital immunodeficiency, consideration should be given to transfuse irradiated cellular blood components to prevent graft-versus-host disease (GVHD). This can occur when viable T-lymphocytes are transfused into an immunocompromised patient who is unable to destroy foreign lymphocytes. These viable lymphocytes, however, recognize the host as foreign and proceed to reject it. Irradiation will prevent the lymphocytes that contaminate cellular blood components from dividing, thus preventing GVHD. All cellular blood components transfused into an infant with congenital immunodeficiency, such as Di George's syndrome should be irradiated. Although it is standard practice to irradiate blood for intrauterine transfusion, it is undetermined whether a significant risk for transfusion-associated GVHD exists in premature neonates that would necessitate routine irradiation of cellular blood components.

SPECIAL CONSIDERATIONS

Organ Transplantation

A CMV infection is an important cause of morbidity and mortality in organ transplantation. Primary CMV infections, that is, infections occurring in seronegative recipients, are usually the result of the transplantation of a CMV seropositive organ, but they may be secondary to blood transfusions. Most children are CMV seronegative; thus, it is prudent to administer CMV seronegative blood to children receiving an allograft, unless it is documented that the patient is CMV seropositive. An alternative to CMV seronegative blood would be leukoreduced blood.

Repair of Congenital Heart Malformation

Many surgical corrections or palliations of a congenital cardiac anomaly, such as patent ductus arteriosus ligation or Blalock-Taussig shunts, require no blood products or very little blood transfusion. However, some complex congenital cardiac defects now undergo complete repair, often very soon after birth. These procedures are done under cardiopulmonary bypass and sometimes circulatory arrest with hypothermia. Large amounts of blood relative to the blood volume of the child will be used, if only to prime the bypass circuit. A single unit of RBC is the equivalent of one or more blood volumes for an infant who is up to 3 months of age. In this setting, many opportunities exist for the occurrence of an acquired coagulopathy. Children with cyanotic heart disease appear to have an increased risk of excessive bleeding. Hypothermia induces a reversible platelet dysfunction, and extended time on bypass is associated with an increased risk of bleeding. The anesthesiologist must be prepared to detect early, and treat appropriately, any coagulopathy that emerges. A study by Manno and colleagues suggests that whole blood stored for less than 48 h is more effective in controlling postoperative bleeding in children younger than 2 years of age undergoing complex procedures than reconstituted whole blood consisting of RBC, FFP, and platelets mixed together.

This finding has not yet been confirmed by others, and our personal experience is that, if only the RBC and FFP are mixed together in the reconstituted units and the platelets are held and transfused separately, the use of components is just as effective as fresh whole blood.

An important issue in pediatric open heart surgery is the age of the RBC transfused. During storage, metabolic changes occur. Among the most relevant are pH, potassium level, and 2,3-diphosphoglycerate (2,3-DPG) level (Table 17-5). The low pH and high potassium level of older units may increase the risk of arrhythmias, and the low 2,3-DPG level prevents effective oxygen delivery. The 2,3-DPG level will revert back to normal several hours after transfusion, but it seems logical that optimal oxygen delivery should be provided at the crucial time of taking the patient off bypass. The RBC stored for less than 10 days will retain a sufficient 2,3-DPG level. To minimize donor exposures in children, we make every effort to provide RBC, FFP, and platelet units originating from the same donor, which implies that the RBC units must be less than 5 days old (maximum shelf life of platelets).

Massive Transfusion

The definition of massive transfusion is the replacement of at least one blood volume in a 24-h period. In an infant, this may represent as little as one-half unit of RBC. Infants and small children undergoing open heart surgery or children undergoing liver transplantation will automatically experience a massive transfusion. Other surgical procedures that may routinely entail massive transfusion are the excision of large vascular tumors, extensive spinal operations, or traumatic injuries. Specific concerns relating to massive transfusion are dilutional coagulopathy, hypothermia, and citrate toxicity.

When reviewing a study of hemostasis in massively transfused patients, it is important to note whether the RBC support was provided with whole blood or with packed RBC. If whole blood is utilized, there does not appear to be a clinically relevant decrease in coagulation factors correlating with the extent of transfusion. Dilutional coagulopathy is secondary to thrombocytopenia and does not take place until after approximately two blood volume replacements have occurred. However, when RBC support is provided with packed RBC, which is usually the case, the first coagulation abnormality observed is secondary to a deficiency in coagulation factors, which becomes apparent after approximately one blood volume has been replaced. These findings were observed in adults but have been corroborated in children. If an acceptable turnaround time can be obtained, it is preferable to base the decision to transfuse

Table 17-5 Changes in Stored CPDA-1 Whole Blood Over Storage Time

	DAYS			
	0	7	14	21
Plasma K + (mEq/L)	3.3 ± 0.3	12.3 ± 1.7	17.6 ± 2.4	21.7 ± 3.1
pH	7.16 ± 0.03	6.94 ± 0.02	6.93 ± 0.03	6.87 ± 0.03
2,3-DPG* (μmole/g Hg)	13	11	2.5	< 1

2,3-DPG = 2,3-diphosphoglycerate, Hg = hemoglobin.
*Values for RBC and not whole blood extrapolated from graph in Valeri CR, Valeri DA, Gray A, et al. Viability and function of red blood cell concentrates stored at 4°C for 35 days in CPDA-1, CPDA-2 or CPDA-3. *Transfusion* 1982; 22:210–216.

FFP or platelets on the result of the platelet count, prothrombin time (PT), and partial thromboplastin time (PTT). The transfusion goal would be to maintain the platelet count above 50,000/µL and the PT and PTT, below 1.5 times normal. If laboratory monitoring cannot be obtained in a timely fashion, an appropriate plan would be to transfuse FFP after one blood volume has been replaced and platelets, after two blood volumes have been replaced. When estimating the amount of blood infused, it is important to include the number of units of RBC recovered from the cell saver, if one is in use. Each unit of packed RBC or cell saver RBC should be counted as a blood volume replacement of approximately 500 mL since the RBC will be supplemented with crystalloid or colloids. For example, a 20-kg child has a blood volume of 20×70 mL = 1400 mL, and a one blood volume replacement should be considered to have occurred after three units of packed RBC or cell saver blood have been infused. If no consumption coagulopathy is occurring, sufficient levels of coagulation factors can be maintained by transfusing FFP at approximately one half the volume of RBC transfused (i.e., one-half unit of FFP for each packed RBC or cell saver RBC unit). In children undergoing liver transplantation, FFP is needed earlier and in larger amounts as a result of the preoperative coagulation factor deficiency existing in patients with liver disease.

Hypothermia will result from the rapid infusion of large volumes of cold RBC and FFP. With the exception of the patient on cardiopulmonary bypass, where hypothermia is intentional, in most patients hypothermia is deleterious and leads to cardiac dysfunction while contributing to a possible coagulopathy. When large volumes of blood are transfused, the use of blood warmers is recommended, recognizing that the ideal blood warmer for children has yet to be devised.

Citrate toxicity in massive transfusion had been thoroughly reviewed by Dzik and Kirkley. Citrate binds ionized calcium and magnesium. The amount of citrate in various blood components is summarized in Table 17-6. The highest concentration of citrate is found in FFP. Citrate is metabolized by mitochondria, mostly in the liver, kidneys, and skeletal muscle, but it is also excreted nonmetabolized by the kidneys. Although citrate is added to blood for its anticoagulant properties, in vivo hypocalcemia will induce cardiac toxicity before it affects coagulation. Classically, an increase in the QT interval and a depression of ventricular function, resulting in decreased cardiac output, are seen. However, the length of the QT interval cannot be reliably used as a monitor for the need of calcium supplementation. Routine prophylactic calcium supplementation is not recommended because it may lead to dangerous hypercal-

Table 17-6 Citrate Content of Various Blood Components

	CPDA-1 (mg/dL)	AS-1* (mg/dL)	AS-3† (mg/dL)
Whole blood	246	206	274
RBC	76	54	181
FFP, platelets, and cryoprecipitate	384	384	384

CPDA-1 = citrate–phosphate–dextrose–adenine, AS = additive solution.
*AS-1 is an additive solution marketed as ADSOL™ by Fenwall Laboratories.
†AS-3 is an additive solution marketed as NUTRICEL™ by Cutter Laboratories.

cemia after the citrate is metabolized. The best approach is to monitor closely the ionized calcium level measured by an ion-selective electrode method and to administer calcium chloride in repeated doses (5 to 10 mg/kg) with the goal of maintaining the ionized calcium level in the normal range (i.e., 2.5 mg/dL or 1.2 mEq/L). Calcium gluconate can also be used, but it will provide four times less calcium than calcium chloride, weight for weight. We should never administer calcium in the same line where any blood component is being infused because this will cause clotting in the line.

**ADVERSE EFFECTS OF
BLOOD TRANSFUSIONS**

The adverse effects of blood transfusions can be classified as acute, that is, occurring during the transfusion or shortly thereafter, or delayed. A delayed adverse effect may not be detected until years after the transfusion. Most acute adverse effects are immune mediated and are uncommon in children.

Acute Adverse Effects

The most feared acute adverse effect is a hemolytic transfusion reaction. In a child who usually has not been previously exposed to blood, a hemolytic reaction is generally the result of an ABO mismatch. During anesthesia, the only signs of an ABO hemolytic transfusion reaction is the occurrence of dark urine and/or unexplained shock and diffuse intravascular coagulation. Meticulous attention to the identification of the patient and verification that the information on the blood unit to be transfused and the attached paperwork match should prevent such reactions. If a hemolytic reaction is suspected, an immediate check of all identifying information should be performed, and a blood sample should be drawn from the patient and sent to the blood bank for verification of the blood type and examination for hemolysis. Common immune-mediated transfusion reactions in adults are a febrile nonhemolytic reaction secondary to antibodies to white cells and allergic reactions secondary to antibodies to plasma proteins. These reactions are rare in children and usually not detected during anesthesia.

A rare but severe transfusion reaction is caused by bacterial contamination of a blood component, usually RBC or platelets. Septic shock may ensue, evidenced by high fever and intractable shock complicated by diffuse intravascular coagulation. A Gram stain can be performed on the suspected blood component(s) to confirm this diagnosis.

Delayed Adverse Effects

Although alloimmunization and possibly immune dysfunction are potential long-term effects of blood transfusion, the transmission of infectious disease is the greatest concern. All blood components transfused are collected from volunteer blood donors who have been systematically interviewed to determine whether they have an increased risk of transmitting infectious diseases. In addition, serologic testing is performed to detect

Table 17-7   Infectious Disease Tests Performed on Human Blood and Risk of Disease Transmission

INFECTIOUS DISEASE	RISK PER UNIT TRANSFUSED	TEST PERFORMED
Hepatitis	1 in 3000	HBsAg, anti-HCV, anti-HBcAg, ALT
AIDS	1 in 225,000	Anti-HIV 1 and 2
HTLV-I/II	1 in 50,000	Anti-HTLV-1
Syphilis	0	STS
Parasitic infection (malaria, babesiosis, and Chagas disease)	1 in 1,000,000	None

AIDS = acquired immunodeficiency syndrome, HTLV = human T-lymphotropic virus, HBsAg = hepatitis B surface antigen, HCV = hepatitis C virus, HBcAg = hepatitis B core antigen, ALT = alanine transaminase, STS = serologic test for syphilis.

most carriers of hepatitis, human immunodeficiency virus, and human T-lymphotropic virus I. Nevertheless, a residual risk exists for each unit of blood. The infectious disease tests performed on blood and the residual infectious risk per unit transfused are listed in Table 17-7. The risk of infection, while low, can be minimized by minimizing the number of donor exposures to a single patient. Each component transfused, in general, means one donor exposure. Thus, four units of cryoprecipitate will give the same number of donor exposures as two units of RBC given in conjunction with one unit of FFP and one unit of RDP, if no specific effort is made to match the RBC, FFP, and RDP from the same donor. This matching is logistically difficult and generally unrealistic for adults; however, it is worth making this extra effort, if possible, when transfusing children who have a long life expectancy. With advance notice, it is usually possible to assign to a child the RBC and FFP originating from the same donor. Matching the RDP requires greater effort and commitment because platelets have a shelf life of only 5 days and will often have been already transfused or outdated.

BLEEDING DIATHESIS

Excessive bleeding unrelated to surgical complications must be addressed as soon as it is recognized. A good medical history should elicit preoperatively most of the risks for excessive bleeding.

Congenital Bleeding Disorders

Hemophilias
Both hemophilias are X-linked disorders, which affects boys and men, almost exclusively. Hemophilia A is the result of a deficiency in factor VIII and hemophilia B, in factor IX. Both will have an elevated PTT while the PT is normal. A medical and/or family history can usually be elicited, but 30 percent of cases have no family history and may go undetected during the neonatal period. Specific concentrates for both factors VIII and IX exist, which are much more concentrated than FFP. They are heat treated to inactivate viruses and are now considered safe to use. One unit of factor VIII per kilogram will raise the factor VIII level by two percent; one unit per kilogram of factor IX will raise the factor IX level by one percent. If factor VIII is unavailable, cryoprecipitate can be used, which contains approximately 100 units per bag. The only alternative to factor IX concentrate is FFP which contains one unit per milliliter.

Von Willebrand's Disease

Von Willebrand's disease is the most common inherited disorder of hemostasis. Von Willebrand's factor (vWF) is a large multimeric protein produced by endothelial cells and platelets. It serves as a carrier molecule for factor VIII and as a mediator of platelet adhesion to the subendothelium. Von Willebrand's disease is an autosomal dominant inherited disorder, and multiple types exist. Most cases can be attributed to type I, a quantitative defect, or type II, a qualitative defect, where the larger multimers are missing. Von Willebrand's disease is associated with an increased bleeding time and occasionally an elevated PTT if severe. Its exact classification requires complex platelet aggregation and electrophoretic studies. A coagulopathy secondary to type I von Willebrand's disease often responds to the infusion of synthetic vasopressin, desmopressin, at a dose of 0.3 μg/kg diluted in saline and administered intravenously over 15 to 30 min. In type II von Willebrand's disease, cryoprecipitate will provide the missing vWF. A recommended dose is one unit of cryoprecipitate per 5 kg body weight.

Acquired Bleeding Disorders

The most commonly encountered acquired bleeding disorders in children are diffuse intravascular coagulation (DIC) and idiopathic thrombocytopenic purpura (ITP).

DIC

This bleeding diathesis may occur in a variety of circumstances, most often in the surgical patient as a result of severe hypotension and hypoxemia. It is characterized by diffuse microvascular bleeding, an elevated PT and PTT, a low platelet count and fibrinogen level, and the presence of D-dimers and fibrin split products. The cause of the DIC must first be controlled and the consumed coagulation factors (V, VIII, and fibrinogen) and platelets, replaced. This is best done with a combination of platelets, FFP, and cryoprecipitate, with the goal of raising the platelet count to 100,000/μL and the fibrinogen to 150 mg/dL.

ITP

This postinfectious immune disorder of childhood is usually self-limited. Platelets are destroyed through an immune mechanism. Prophylactic platelet transfusions are useless and carry the risk of adverse effects without any benefit. If surgery must be performed on a child with ITP, platelet transfusions may control surgical bleeding, if given at the time bleeding occurs, but they should never be given preoperatively.

Laboratory Evaluation of a Bleeding Diathesis

Unexpected excessive intraoperative bleeding can be evaluated by a simple battery of tests: platelet count and PT, PTT, and fibrinogen levels. From the results of these four tests, a decision can be made on whether the patient's coagulopathy can be best treated with platelets, FFP, and/or cryoprecipitate.

BIBLIOGRAPHY

Boyce NW, Hayes K, Gee D, et al: Cytomegalovirus infection complicating renal transplantation and its relationship to acute transplant glomerulopathy. *Transplantation* 1988; 45:706–709.

Coté CJ, Liu LMP, Szyfelbein SK, et al: Changes in serial platelet counts following massive blood transfusion in pediatric patients. *Anesthesiology* 1985; 62:197–201.

Counts RB, Haisch C, Simon TL, et al: Hemostasis in massively transfused trauma patients. *Ann Surg* 1979; 190:91–99.

Dzik WH, Kirkley SA: Citrate toxicity during massive blood transfusion. *Transfusion Med Rev* 1988; 2:76–94.

Gilbert GL, Hayes K, Hudson IL, et al: Prevention of transfusion-acquired cytomegalovirus infection in infants by blood filtration to remove leucocytes. *Lancet* 1989; 1:1228–1231.

Kang Y, Borland LM, Picone J, et al: Intraoperative coagulation changes in children undergoing liver transplantation. *Anesthesiology* 1989; 71:44–47.

Kang Y, Martin DJ, Marquez J, et al: Intraoperative changes in blood coagulation and thromboelastographic monitoring in liver transplantation. *Anesth Analg* 1985; 64:888–896.

Latham ST, Bove JR, Weirich FL: Chemical and hematological changes in stored CPDA-1 blood. *Transfusion* 1982; 22:158–159.

Leslie SD, Toy PTCY: Laboratory hemostatic abnormalities in massively transfused patients given red blood cells and crystalloid. *Am J Clin Pathol* 1991; 96:770–773.

Manno CS, Hedberg KW, Kim HC, et al: Comparison of the hemostatic effects of fresh whole blood, stored whole blood and components after open heart surgery in children. *Blood* 1991; 77:930–936.

Schulman LL, Reison DS, Austin JM, et al: Cytomegalovirus pneumonitis after cardiac transplantation. *Arch Intern Med* 1991; 151:1118–1124.

Slichter SJ, Harker LA: Preparation and storage of platelet concentrates: II. Storage variables influencing platelet viability and function. *Br J Haematol* 1976; 34:403–419.

Slichter SJ, Counts RB, Hendersen R, et al: Preparation of cryoprecipitated factor VIII concentrates. *Transfusion* 1976; 16:616–626.

Stockman JA: Hematologic manifestations of systemic diseases, in Nathan DG, Oski FA (eds): *Hematology of Infancy and Childhood,* ed 3. Philadelphia, WB Saunders, 1987, pp 1632–1665.

Valeri CR, Feingold H, Cassidy G, et al: Hypothermia-induced reversible platelet dysfunction. *Ann Surg* 1987; 205:175–181.

Valeri CR, Valeri DA, Gray A, et al: Viability and function of red blood cell concentrates stored at 4°C for 35 days in CPDA-1, CPDA-2 or CPDA-3. *Transfusion* 1982; 22:210–216.

Wilson SM, Levitt JS, Strauss RG (eds): *Improving Transfusion Practice for Pediatric Patients.* Arlington, American Association of Blood Banks, 1991.

Yeager AS, Grumet FC, Hafleigh EB, et al: Prevention of transfusion-acquired cytomegalovirus infections in newborn infants. *J Pediatr* 1981; 98:281–287.

CHAPTER 18

Acute Postoperative and Chronic Pain in Children

James Rogers
Michelle Moro

There are few areas in pediatrics more difficult and more frustrating to diagnose and manage than acute and chronic pain. The *Random House Dictionary* defines pain as "physical suffering or distress, as due to injury or illness." We might search for a more scientific definition of pain, but to try to find an understanding of pain and its management by defining it, is not feasible. Pain is a multifactorial syndrome of behaviors that includes neuroanatomic and sensory perception with associated quantitative factors and emotional, motivational, and affective factors, which include guilt, fear, punishment, manipulative behaviors, and helplessness.

Throughout the history of medicine, pain relief has been sought, and the search for new and improved methods of pain relief continues today. For centuries, the main obstacles to surgical intervention for disease processes were pain and infection. Simple surgical procedures were associated with considerable morbidity without the use of anesthetic agents. Until the 1980s, researchers still questioned the need for analgesia and anesthesia in premature infants, term infants, and children. Early research upheld the concept that complete nerve myelination was required for the function of the nerve tracts. Based on this thinking, the widespread assumption was that infants either did not experience or perceive pain as acutely or meaningfully as adults or perhaps did not experience pain at all. It is now clear that even neonates experience pain, and the morbidity and mortality are reduced when pain is adequately treated.

Acute pain, or that pain resulting from tissue damage or disruption, is associated with an increase in small fiber activity and a decrease in large fiber activity. The perception of pain in the acute sense is a protective mechanism that has the obvious benefits of allowing the avoidance or interruption of injury.

Table 18-1   Individual Factors Affecting Pain in Children

Cultural beliefs
Individual pain threshold
Previous pain experience
Anxiety level of child and parents
Intensity of painful experience
Birth order
Sex

Chronic pain consists of two components: one physical and one psychological. The physical component involves the actual neuroanatomic and physiologic transmission of painful stimuli throughout a complex system of pain pathways, which are beyond the scope of this chapter. The psychological component is influenced by a variety of factors, such as the context of pain, prior experience with pain, and many others (Table 18-1).

This chapter will review pain assessment in pediatrics and, with text, tables, and dosage guidelines, will outline practical methods of managing acute and chronic pain.

PEDIATRIC PAIN ASSESSMENT

One of the problems in conducting research to assess pediatric pain is the difficulty in quantifying the intensity of a child's pain. Assessment and management are interdependent; so without adequate assessment of a child's pain, treatment is likely to be ineffective. Selection of a measurement system must take into account the patient's age, sex, ethnic background, and cognitive level, as well as physical and social factors (Table 18-2).

Infants

Behavioral and physiologic changes make up the clinically useful methods available currently for the evaluation of pain in infants. Observations, including changes in body movements, crying, agitation, posture, facial expressions, heart rate, blood pressure, respiratory rate, and diaphoresis, have all been shown to be useful measures of pain.

Table 18-2   Considerations in Pain Assessment in Children

Developmental level
Child's own assessment of pain
Actual stimulus for pain and physical damage to patient
Parents' judgment of their child's pain
Child's language and understanding

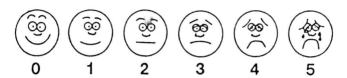

Figure 18-1 Faces Scale. Drawings are presented to the child who is asked to point to the picture that best shows how they feel.

Pre-Schoolers

Many creative ways have been developed to help these children indicate their level of pain. Drawings of facial expressions (Fig. 18-1), pictures of children showing increasing levels of discomfort, color scales, and linear analog scales are being used to evaluate pain levels in these children (Fig 18-2). Behavioral evaluation instruments have also proved to be useful in this age group. The Pain Behavior Rating Scale includes 13 items, such as cry, scream, muscle rigidity, clinging, or flailing, that are in a checklist format. The Children's Hospital of Eastern Ontario Pain Scale system is similar, with behaviors scored for intensity and related distress.

School-Age and Adolescents

Children of school age are capable of concrete thought and are beginning to understand and can communicate abstract thoughts and phenomena. Visual analog scales, pain questionnaires, and the Objective Pain Scale have been successful in assessing pain. It is important to remember that children may regress to an earlier stage of development when ill, and adjustments may be necessary in the use of a particular assessment device.

All current pain assessment devices require further development and testing for accuracy and reliability; however, they

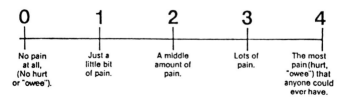

Figure 18-2 A linear analog scale is appropriate for most school-aged children.

Table 18-3   Methods for Assessing Pediatric Pain

Physiologic methods
 Heart rate
 Cortisol levels
 Palmar sweat response
 Transcutaneous oxygen levels
 Blood pressure
 Endorphin levels
 Behavioral methods
 Body movement
 Facial expressions
 Cries
Overt distress scales
 Pain Behavior Rating Scale (revised)
 Observational Scale of Behavioral Distress
 Children's Hospital of Eastern Ontario Pain Scale
Projective methods
 Colors
 Shapes
 Drawings
 Cartoons
Direct report methods
 Interval scales (faces, poker chips, or words)
 Interviews (supplied and generated formats)
Pain questionnaires
 Children's Comprehensive Pain Questionnaire
 Varni-Thompson Pediatric Pain Questionnaire
Visual analog scales
 Pain thermometers
 Oucher scale

can provide useful information in assessing pain in children. The information will be most useful when frequent and systematic assessment is made, similar to the monitoring of vital signs. The information obtained allows the care giver to evaluate the effectiveness of the pain management technique (Table 18-3).

ACUTE PAIN MANAGEMENT

Ideally, medical management of pain should not cause pain or suffering in the patient. The fear of needles may cause a child to deny otherwise obvious pain. Unfortunately, it is not always possible to avoid causing discomfort. Injections and side effects, such as nausea and vomiting, are often unavoidable. Table 18-4 summarizes available treatment for the management of pediatric pain.

Concern about opioid addiction in children had been commonly cited as a reason for not using opioids for acute or

**Table 18-4   Classification of Modalities Useful
for Pain Management**

Pharmacologic
    Narcotics, sedatives, and antidepressants
    Intermittent dosing regimens
    Continuous infusions in intensive care unit
    Patient-controlled analgesia
    Regional anesthetic techniques
    Local anesthetics by infiltration or topical application
Diagnostic and therapeutic nerve/plexus blocks
    Epidurals: caudal, lumbar, and thoracic
    Brachial plexus block
    Lumbar and/or sacral plexus block
    Intraarticular local anesthetic
    Bolus versus continuous infusion
Nonpharmacologic
    Psychological
    Distraction techniques
    Relaxation and music techniques
    Behavior modification
    Family or individual psychotherapy
    Hypnotherapy
    Physical therapy
    Massage therapy
    Transcutaneous electrical nerve stimulation
    Parent participation

chronic pain relief. The fear of addiction may be attributable, at least in part, to a common confusion between the concept of physical dependence and addiction. Physical dependence generally refers to an altered physiologic state that occurs after repeated drug administration and results in the manifestation of withdrawal symptoms on discontinuance of the drug. Addiction is a behavior pattern involving compulsive drug use and obsession with attaining a drug supply. Newburger and Salen summed up this issue well when they stated, "A child undertreated for pain desperately and single-mindedly awaiting his next dose of medication comes closer to the definition of addiction than the properly treated patient at peace to pursue other concerns."

Dependence is common with repeated administration of narcotics but can be fairly easily controlled when necessary through gradual tapering in the hospital. Certainly, the question of narcotic dependence should be irrelevant with regard to the child in pain in a terminal situation. Berde recommends that, when using patient-control and analgesia in those with cancer, basal infusion rates should be considered routine to avoid the peak and trough effects of the narcotic and thus provide better analgesia.

Oral Medication

A wide variety of analgesic agents are available in oral preparations for use in children. Nonopioid agents, such as acetaminophen, aspirin, and other nonsteroidal antiinflammatory drugs (NSAID) are useful in the treatment of mild to moderate pain. Acetaminophen, the most widely used analgesic, has a high therapeutic index in children of any age. Aspirin, although especially useful in pain of inflammatory origin, has a statistical association with Reye's syndrome and side effects of gastritis and platelet dysfunction. The NSAIDs inhibit prostaglandin synthetase and have side effects similar to aspirin. Naproxen, tolmetin, and ibuprofen have been approved by the Food and Drug Administration for use in children.

Intravenous Injections

Opioids are the mainstay of this form of administration. Intramuscular injections should be avoided whenever possible because a shot is almost always terrifying to children.

The opioids produce excellent pain relief but include many other physiologic effects, such as sedation, respiratory depression, pruritus, nausea, vomiting, decreased gastric motility, miosis, biliary spasm, vasodilation, and cough suppression. Doses should be titrated to clinical effect to minimize these side effects. Table 18-5 gives guidelines for the starting doses of opioids.

A useful way to titrate opioids is by using a patient-controlled analgesia pump. The patient receives a small amount of an opioid (for example, 0.02 to 0.03 mg/kg of morphine) when they push a button connected to an infusion pump. In younger patients, the control of the pump can be delegated to properly instructed parents or members of the nursing staff. It has been used successfully in children as young as 3 to 5 years of age. It is important that if someone other than the patient is doing the dosing, they must be taught that dosing should not occur if the patient is sleeping (see Table 18-6). The dose in infants younger than 3 months of age is usually given in increments of one third to one half of the usual dose because there is some evidence of increased risk of developing respiratory depression in this age group.

The NSAIDs are gaining increased acceptance in pediatric analgesic by the oral, intravenous, and rectal routes. Ketorolac is used on a schedule of 0.5 mg/kg q 6 h for 48 h, with empirically reduced doses in pediatric patients with known renal and/

Table 18-5   Starting Doses for Postoperative Analgesia
with Opioids

ROUTE	DRUG	DOSE (AGE > 3 MO)*
Continuous IV	Morphine	0.05 to 0.1 mg/kg/h
	Meperidine	0.5 to 1.0 mg/kg/h
	Fentanyl	1 to 5 μg/kg/h
Intermittent IV	Morphine	0.08 to 0.1 mg/kg q 2 h
	Meperidine	0.5 to 1.0 mg/kg q 2 h
Oral	Codeine	0.5 to 1.0 mg/kg q 4 h
	Morphine	0.2 to 0.4 mg/kg q 4 h
	Methadone	0.1 to 0.15 mg/kg q 4 to 8 h
Intramuscular	Morphine	0.1 to 0.15 mg/kg q 3 to 4 h
	Meperidine	1.0 to 1.5 mg/kg q 3 to 4 h

IV = intravenous.
*Doses in infants younger than 3 mo of age are given in increments
of one-third to one-half because there is some evidence of increased
risk of respiratory depression.

or hepatic dysfunction. Further research on the NSAIDs is
needed for optimal use in pediatric patients.

Transdermal and Transmucosal

Opioids are traditionally very effective in the management of
acute, severe pain, and now they can be found in transdermal
and transmucosal preparations to avoid the dreaded shot. These
do have associated limitations and side effects, such as unpredictable absorption, nausea/vomiting, and sedation. The transmucosal route has been used to provide effective preoperative
sedation and for minor procedure analgesia and sedation, such
as lumbar puncture or bone marrow biopsy. Feld and associates
have shown that oral transmucosal fentanyl (12 to 20 μg/kg)
provided better separation from parents, decreased anxiety, and
smoother induction than placebo. However, Goldstein-Dresner
and associates have found that these benefits are accompanied
by a higher incidence of side effects before induction when 20
to 25 μg/kg of fentanyl was used in conjunction with other
agents, such as meperidine, diazepam, and atropine in patients
with congenital heart disease.

Regional Blockade

Using long-lasting local anesthetics or opioids, regional blockade modulates the transmission of afferent nociceptive impulses

**Table 18-6   Patient-Controlled Analgesia (PCA)
Intravenous Route**

Key Items in Order Writing:
  PCA
    PCA or basal?
    PCA with basal infusion?
    Constant (basal) infusion rate
    Bolus dose (if any) programmed into pump
    4-h limit
    Lock out interval for PCA dose (usually 6 to 12 min)

Side effects and treatment
  Pruritus
    Diphenhydramine (drug of choice), 1.25 mg/kg/dose (IV,
      PR, avoid IM)
    Low-dose naloxone, 0.5 to 1 μg/kg/h IV
    Turn off PCA 15 min before and 15 min after
      diphenhydramine
  Nausea/vomiting
    Ondansetron, 0.15 mg/kg IV over 15 min (caution in severe
      hepatic dysfunction
    Droperidol, 10 to 30 μg/kg IV/IM (may cause dysphasia,
      hypotension, dystonic reactions)
    Metoclopramide, 0.1 mg/kg IV (may cause dysphasia,
      extrapyramidal effects (GI surgery contraindication)
    Low-dose naloxone, 0.5 to 1 μg/kg/h IV
  Urinary retention (most common with continuous epidural
    medications but can occur with PCA)
    Accurate input–output recordings
    Urinary output parameters (call physician if urine output
      less than 1 mL/kg/h, per 4- to 8-h interval)
    Low-dose naloxone infusion as above
    Bethanechol, 0.05 mg/kg subcutaneously
    Urinary catheter orders (indwelling versus as needed)
  Respiratory depression
    Vital signs (specify parameters that require treatment)
    Include beeper or phone number of responsible physician
    Stop PCA pump
    Provide 100% O_2 and assist and maintain airway
    Naloxone, 1–5 μg/kg IV bolus and repeat as needed
    Consider naloxone infusion, 3 to 5 μg/kg/h IV
  Miscellaneous
    Naloxone at bedside with unit dose calculated
    "Call MD if" parameters (include beeper/phone number)
    Consider apnea monitor and pulse oximeter with
      parameters for calling MD
    Consider ketorolac IV/IM as scheduled dose if not
      contraindicated

IV = intravenous; PR = per rectum; IM = intramuscular; MD =
physician.

and results in pain relief with a minimum of side effects. The main disadvantage is that some pain will occur during placement of the block. Regional techniques often provide more complete relief of pain, and the patient can have a higher functional level of activity. With the increased emphasis on ambulatory surgery, especially in the pediatric age group, regional analgesia can provide a smoother transition from hospital to home.

Local anesthetic blockade can be accomplished by local infiltration, individual peripheral nerve blocks, and plexus blockade at brachial or lumbar levels (Table 18-7). Epidural analgesia

Table 18-7   Uses of Regional Techniques for Postoperative Pain Control in Children

TYPE OF BLOCK	APPLICATION
Wound infiltration	Suture of laceration, skin tag removal, central line insertion
Wrist	Removal of extra digits
Penile	Circumcision, hypospadias repair
Ilioinguinal/iliohypogastric	Inguinal hernia repair
Axillary	Colles fracture, plastic procedures
Femoral	Midshaft femur fracture
Intercostal	Lateral thoracotomy, rib fractures
Interpleural	Lateral thoracotomy, nephrectomy
Caudal epidural*	Inguinal hernia repair, complex hypospadias repair, club foot repair, ureteral reimplantation
Lumbar epidural	Orchiopexy, urologic reconstruction, hemipelvectomy
Thoracic epidural†	Thoracotomy, thoracic or abdominal surgery in patients with severe lung disease

*Caudal epidural space can be entered and a catheter inserted into the lumbar or thoracic epidural canal. This method is useful in children up to the ages of 6 to 7 years because they lack septations in the epidural space, making catheter insertion into the thoracic region from either a caudal or lumbar epidural approach easy.

†There is less risk for nerve damage when the needle is inserted at the lumbar or caudal level as opposed to a traditional thoracic epidural.

(caudal, lumbar, and thoracic) is probably the most versatile regional technique, either by single injection or repeated injections through a catheter with a local anesthetic or opioid.

The epidural space can be approached at any level but is commonly performed at lumbar or caudal levels in children. The caudal approach is most commonly used in young infants. Local anesthetics can be useful when postoperative immobilization and/or regional sympathetic blockade will result in surgical benefits. The addition of opioids results in activation of opioid receptors in the dorsal horn of the spinal cord, producing regional analgesia without anesthesia. Numerous studies have demonstrated the safety and efficacy of these techniques in children. Hypotension is unlikely with local anesthetics, especially in younger children, and motor blockade is rarely a problem, especially if they are not yet ambulatory. Fentanyl by continuous infusion may be inadvisable in neonates, especially if premature. Anecdotal reports indicate a higher incidence of respiratory depression compared with morphine administered epidurally. For a more detailed description of how to perform these blocks, please refer to Chap. 10.

Intrapleural administration of local anesthetics has recently been reported by McIlvaine to be effective in children undergoing major unilateral upper abdominal surgery. Epidural analgesia remains more predictable, but interpleural analgesia may prove to be a practical alternative.

CHRONIC PAIN

Although chronic pain in children is not as common as it is in adults, it can lead to physical, cognitive, and social developmental problems in affected children. The complex psychological variables, such as fear, anxiety, magical thinking, and the parental response to the child's pain, can have an impact on the child's behavior in a self-perpetuating manner. The child in pain can be a most uncooperative patient, which adds to the management challenge. The clinical team approach advocated by Bonica, which includes the primary care physician, anesthesiologist, physical therapist, and psychologist, can prove to be advantageous in the design and delivery of a customized, effective treatment plan.

Children's reactions to painful stimuli are contingent on their age and level of cognitive and social and emotional development. Older children may be more capable of understanding the discomfort associated with procedures, for example, if there is the possibility of a positive outcome. On the other hand, because of increased communicative and cognitive skills, older children have the ability to report more discomfort than younger children who have similar pathophysiology.

Infants tend to react to chronic pain by withdrawal and difficulties with eating, sleeping, and social interactions. Preschoolers may lose motor and toilet training milestones or have increased activity. School-aged children can become increasingly aggressive, withdrawn, and out of control. In adolescents, depression, oppositional behavior, and withdrawal are frequent findings. Physical activity is one coping technique that children use to distract themselves from unpleasant stimuli. Children at all stages may respond to continuous pain by withdrawal and regression to earlier developmental stages.

It must also be remembered that children are experts at magical thinking, attributing cause-and-effect relationships to events that are correlated in time. Sick children may assume that their pain is punishment for some bad thought or misdeed. Chronic pain in children represents a truly biobehavioral phenomenon that usually cannot be optimally treated in an isolated or unilateral manner by medical or mental health professionals.

The diagnostic evaluation should include a detailed history from patient and parent, including the onset, history of injury, severity, and aggravating and mitigating circumstances. A thorough physical examination is necessary, and invasive testing, including blood studies, thermography, electromyography, x-rays, CT and MRI, and nuclear scans, are done as indicated by the history and physical. Psychological testing can also be of assistance in evaluating the patient's pain.

Common types of chronic pain in children are listed in Table 18-8. Headaches and chest and abdominal pain are the most common and can result in a great deal of anxiety to the parents. Many of these cases prove to be functional and can be diagnosed on the basis of the history and selected laboratory and radiographic tests.

Table 18-8   Types of Chronic Pain

Headache
Chest pain
Recurrent abdominal pain
Myofascial pain
Muscle spasm
Low-back pain
Phantom limb pain
Collagen vascular disease
Arthritis and hemophilia (articulations)
Cancer (tumors and metastasis)

Reflex Sympathetic Dystrophy (RSD)

Although regarded as rare in children, RSD is being recognized with increasing frequency in children after sprains, fractures, and surgery. It is frequently confused with psychiatric conditions, such as conversion reaction and malingering, but RSD should always be considered in the differential diagnosis of persistent limb pain because early recognition and treatment can prevent potentially crippling sequelae. In many cases, RSD is mild and self-limited, but it can, in its more severe forms, cause severe pain and marked disability. Classically, RSD includes painful swelling in an extremity with sympathetic hyperactivity, resulting in fluctuating vasomotor changes and dystrophic skin, bone, and muscle changes. The involved area often does not conform to nerve pattern distributions.

Although severe RSD is usually easily diagnosed, less severe cases are frequently misdiagnosed. There is little to no correlation between the amount of pain and the severity of the initial injury. Pain relief with sympathetic blockade, thermography, and triple-phase bone scans can be helpful in making the diagnosis.

There are three stages in the course of RSD (Table 18-9). In the acute stage, early treatment by interrupting sympathetic pathways and restoring normal function and mobility can improve or eliminate the pain. Mild forms may resolve spontaneously. In the dystrophic stage, a series or a prolonged sympathetic block may be required to reverse the dystrophic

Table 18-9   Reflex Sympathetic Dystrophy Syndrome (RSD)*

Acute stage
Intense pain, hyperesthesia, and edema associated with vasodilation and vasoconstriction. A causalgic personality develops—all priority goes to protecting the limb from pain. Immobility follows.

Established RSD (dystrophic stage)
After 1 month or more, pain diminishes, but the edema spreads. The joints thicken, and muscle wasting occurs. The limb is not being used.

Sequelae (atrophic stage)
Pain may or may not be present; the limb is cold and cyanotic, with diminished subcutaneous tissue. Wasted muscles and smooth glossy atrophic skin are present. Complete loss of limb function and bone atrophy (osteoporosis) occur at the end stages.

*Mild forms of RSD may resolve spontaneously. The more severe forms may not leave sequelae if recognized and treated early.

changes. By the time atrophic changes are present, intense physical therapy, psychological counseling, and sympathetic and somatic nerve blockade may be necessary to restore some degree of function.

Therapy should focus on encouraging normal limb mobility with physical therapy. Sympathetic and somatic blockade help break the pain cycle and provide a pain-free environment to assist in the mobilization. Psychotherapy is indicated in patients with dysfunctional behavior. Severe conditions may require hospitalization for intensive therapy and rarely sympathectomy.

Myofascial Pain Syndromes

The recognition of specific muscular pain syndromes in children is increasing but remains controversial because of problems with nomenclature, classification, and pathogenesis. A primary fibromyalgia syndrome has been described in children, which closely matches myofascial pain syndrome in adults.

Exquisite trigger point tenderness with radiating pain is a common finding during physical examination. A history of overt trauma may be present but is not consistently so. The diagnosis is corroborated by the relief of pain after injection of a local anesthetic into the trigger point. Thus, trigger point injection can serve as both diagnostic and therapeutic techniques, although precise localization of the primary trigger points is required. The therapeutic response to the local anesthetic along with directed physical therapy is usually sufficient to reverse the pain process.

Cancer Pain

Acute and/or chronic pain will be experienced by 40 to 80 percent of children with cancer, either from the disease itself or from the treatment. The chronic pain is usually long standing and intractable and is associated with behavioral changes, such as sleep disturbances, anorexia, withdrawal, anxiety, depression, and somatic preoccupation. Although the pain may originally have an organic cause, other factors can influence and exacerbate the pain. The child's reaction and perception of pain is dependent on the developmental age, type of cancer (organ system tumors more painful than blood tumors), and terminal disease (painful experiences not associated with getting better).

The ultimate goal is to decrease or eliminate the cause of pain. When improvement is delayed or unlikely, then other modalities must be used.

Psychological intervention is probably the most widely used modality and can relieve the fear and anxiety, especially associated with acute medical procedures. Hypnosis, positive reinforcement, breathing exercises, and biofeedback have been

Table 18-10   Regional Techniques for Chronic Pain in Children

Trigger point injections
Motor point injections
Peripheral nerve blocks
Plexus limb blocks
Ganglion blocks
Sympathetic blocks
Intrapleural analgesia
Caudal analgesia
Epidural analgesia
Subarachnoid analgesia
Systemic analgesia (usually intravenous or oral)
Patient-controlled analgesia

used successfully to reduce behavioral stress. Education and involvement of the parents can provide therapy for both the child and the family.

Narcotics and/or sedatives may be necessary for a number of patients, especially the terminally ill child. Sedation before painful procedures may also be beneficial. The goal is to relieve pain with a minimal reduction in activity or conscious level of functioning and should be coupled with physical and behavioral therapy.

Regional nerve blocks and epidural narcotics, extensively used in adult cancer pain, are a relatively new approach in children (Table 18-10). They avoid the systemic effects of narcotics and often provide more complete relief of pain and an improved functional level of activity. Implantable devices are available that would allow the parents to participate in the administration of medications through a catheter at home.

The approach to the management of cancer pain should be a progression from relatively low-risk, noninvasive techniques to higher risk, more invasive procedures that are reserved for situations in which other modalities have failed.

SUMMARY

Pain in children truly exists and the treatment of pain in children should not be withheld on the basis of myths and misconceptions. The management of pain in children can be improved with the active participation of anesthesiologists with their knowledge of the pharmacologic effects of drugs and their skill and knowledge in regional anesthesia techniques. This should result in an improved understanding and better application of effective and safe therapies to minimize the suffering of the child in pain.

BIBLIOGRAPHY

Anand KJS, Hickey PR: Pain and its effects in the human neonate and fetus. *N Engl J Med* 1987; 317:1321–1329.

Anand KJS, Sippell WG, Aynsley-Green H: Randomized trial of fentanyl anesthesia in pre-term neonates undergoing surgery: Effects on the stress response. *Lancet* 1987; 1:243–248.

Bell C, Hughes CW, Oh TH: *The Pediatric Anaesthesia Handbook: Department of Anesthesiology, Yale University School of Medicine*. Boston, Mosby Yearbook, 1991.

Berde C: *Acute Postoperative Management in Children: 1992 ASA 43rd Annual Refresher Course Lectures*. New Orleans, ASA. Lecture 125.

Bonica JJ: Cancer pain: A major national health problem. *Cancer Nurs* 1982; 1:313–316.

Cousins MJ, Bridenbaugh PO: Neural blockade, in *Clinical Anesthesia and Management of Pain*. Philadelphia, JB Lippincott, 1980.

Desparmet J, Meistelman C, Barrey J, et al: Continuous epidural infusion of bupivacaine for postoperative pain relief in children. *Anesthesiology* 1987; 67:108–110.

Dodd E, Wang JM, Rauck RL: Patient-controlled analgesia for post surgical pediatric patients ages 6-16 years. *Anesthesiology* 1988; 69:A372.

Feld LH, Champeau MW, Van Streennis CA, et al: Preanesthetic medication in children: A comparison of oral transmucosal fentanyl citrate versus placebo. *Anesthesiology* 1989; 71:874–877.

Foley GV: Care of the child dying of cancer. *CA Cancer J Clin* 1990; 40.

Goldstein-Dresner MC, Davis PJ, Kretchman E, et al: Double-blind comparison of oral transmucosal fentanyl-citrate with oral meperidine, diazepam, and atropine as preanesthetic medication in children with congenital heart disease. *Anesthesiology* 1991; 74:28–33.

Mather L, Mackie J: The incidence of postoperative pain in children. *Pain* 1983; 15:271–282.

McGrath PA: An assessment of children's pain: A review of behavioral, psychological and direct scaling techniques. *Pain* 1987; 31:147–176.

McGrath PA, Johnson G, Goodman JT, et al: The Children's Hospital of Eastern Ontario Pain Scale (CHEOPS): A behavioral scale for rating postoperative pain in children, in Fields ML, Dubner R, Cerveno F (eds): *Advances in Pain Research and Therapy*. Proceedings of the 4th World Congress on Pain. Vol 9. New York, Raven, 1985, pp 395–402.

McIlvaine WB: Perioperative pain management in children: A review. *J Pain Symptom Management* 1989; 4(4):215–229.

Means LJ, Allen HM, Lookabill SJ, et al: Recovery room initiation of patient-controlled analgesia in pediatric patients. *Anesthesiology* 1989; 69:A772.

Newburger PF, Salen SE: Chronic pain: Principles of management. *J Pediat* 1981; 98:180–189.

Olkkola KT, Maunuksela EL: The pharmacokinetics of postoperative intravenous ketorolac tromethamine in children. *Br J Clin Pharmacol* 1991; 31:182–184.

Random House Dictionary. 2nd ed unabridged. New York, Random House, 1987, p 1394.

Rosen KR, Rosen DA: Caudal epidural morphine for control of pain following open-heart surgery in children. *Anesthesiology* 1989; 70:418–421.

Ross DM, Ross SA: *Childhood Pain: Current Issues, Research and Management.* Baltimore, Urban and Schwarzenberg, 1988.

Schecter NL: Acute pain in children. *Pediat Clin North Am* 1989; 36:4.

Schecter NL: Report of the consensus conference on the management of pain in childhood cancer. *Pediatrics* 1990; 86(suppl).

Schecter NL, Berde CB, Yaster M: *Pain in Infants, Children, and Adolescents.* Baltimore, Williams & Wilkins, 1993.

Part III

Neonatal Problems

CHAPTER 19

The Premature and Ex-Premature Infant

Amy C. Benedikt
Deborah K. Rasch

Prematurity is defined as birth before 38 weeks of gestation and, physiologically, does not depend on actual weight. Adjusted age (actual age minus prematurity) must also be calculated for premature infants up to the age of 1 year. Resuscitation of infants as young as 24 weeks of gestation, improved survival rates of low birth weight infants, and the advent of surfactant therapy have increased the number of premature infants and neonatal intensive care unit (NICU) graduates that present to the anesthesiologist for a variety of procedures, of which inguinal herniorrhaphy is the most common. The problems specific to these "preemies" and "ex-preemies" include retinopathy of prematurity (ROP), apnea of prematurity, bronchopulmonary dysplasia (BPD), intraventricular hemorrhage, and subglottic stenosis. Special preoperative, intraoperative, and postoperative care must be directed toward these infants.

PREOPERATIVE ASSESSMENT

The initial assessment of these infants should include a determination of their gestational age and associated disorders. In a premature infant, these disorders include hyaline membrane disease, apnea, bradycardia, hyperbilirubinemia, hypoglycemia, hypocalcemia, hemolysis from Rh or ABO incompatibility, and congenital anomalies. Five systems require evaluation: respiratory, cardiovascular, metabolic, neurologic, and hematologic (Table 19-1).

The primary assessment of the respiratory system includes the duration of oxygen therapy (with or without intubation) and possible residual lung damage (bronchospasm or cor pulmonale). A recent arterial blood gas or oxygen saturation level and a baseline chest x-ray are indicated. Postpone elective surgery if there is any question of active respiratory infection. Chronic

Table 19-1 Complications of Prematurity

Respiratory
   Hyaline membrane disease
   Bronchopulmonary dysplasia
   Apnea, periodic breathing
   Reactive airway disease
   Subglottic stenosis

Cardiovascular
   Patent ductus arteriosus
   Cor pulmonale
   Renal artery thrombosis (with hypertension from UAC)
   Physiologic anemia (hematocrit, 26 to 32 percent)

Neuromuscular
   Intraventricular hemorrhage
   Hydrocephalus
   High degree of vagal tone
   Gastroesophageal reflux
   Retinopathy of prematurity
   Cerebral palsy

UAC = umbilical artery catheter.

mild hypoxemia (PaO_2 50 to 60 mmHg) and hypercarbia ($PaCO_2$ 45 to 50 mmHg) are not absolute contraindications to surgery.

An evaluation of the cardiovascular system includes a detailed history for evidence of congenital heart disease, cor pulmonale, or patent ductus arteriosus (PDA). Premature infants have a greater incidence than age-matched term newborns of left to right shunting through a PDA. Hepatomegaly is an early sign of right heart dysfunction, whereas rales may not occur until severe dysfunction is present. Therefore, if hepatomegaly and tachypnea are present, chest x-ray and possible adjustments of medications are necessary before proceeding with elective operations. Infants receiving digoxin may outgrow their digoxin dose and require evaluation for uncompensated congestive heart failure. These infants may also be receiving chlorothiazide or furosemide; therefore, their fluid and electrolyte status warrants evaluation.

Premature infants are susceptible to metabolic abnormalities; therefore, serum electrolyte levels should be available to exclude hypoglycemia, hypocalcemia, and dehydration. For example, a premature infant with necrotizing enterocolitis may experience significant intravascular volume depletion with metabolic acidosis. A review of the clinical examination of the infant, laboratory values, and discussion of recent changes in the hemodynamic and respiratory status with the neonatologist is also helpful. Aspiration prophylaxis with 1 mL/kg of sodium citrate and 0.5 mg/kg of ranitidine is recommended. For infants undergoing semielective procedures, the fasting period should be equivalent to one feeding interval (3 to 4 h), and sodium citrate should also be given to these patients.

The infant's neurologic state (seizures, motor and mental retardation, deafness, and obstructive hydrocephalus) should be reviewed and anticonvulsant therapy continued throughout the perioperative period. Neurologic deterioration warrants evaluation with cranial sonography or computer tomography to exclude hydrocephalus, intraventricular hemorrhage, and congenital anomalies. Some anticonvulsants (phenobarbital and clonazepam) will increase the hepatic clearance of many drugs used for general anesthesia; others (valproic acid and phenytoin) may cause abnormalities in liver function, which lead to unpredictable actions of hepatically metabolized drugs.

The hematologic assessment should include a complete blood count. Anemia is common at 2 to 4 months of age. For emergent procedures, transfuse the anemic preemie or ex-preemie (hematocrit less than 25 percent) to a hematocrit between 33 and 37 percent if there is pulmonary compromise. Alternatively, whenever possible, postpone elective surgery and treat the infant with iron therapy (6 mg/kg/day of elemental iron). Clotting studies (prothrombin and partial thromboplastin times) and platelet counts are appropriate for the septic infant.

Some surgical procedures may be performed in the NICU such as PDA ligation or central venous catheter placement. This practice reduces the risk of hypothermia and extubation of the infant associated with transport (see Table 20-1). Good hand washing on entry and return to the NICU and the use of sterile precautions are extremely important because these premature infants are not immunocompetent.

Prolonged recovery room or ICU care may be needed postoperatively, particularly for patients with BPD or infants with a history of previous central nervous system hemorrhage.

ANESTHETIC MANAGEMENT

The choice of an anesthetic technique depends on the procedure to be performed, the health status of the infant, and whether there will be a need for postoperative mechanical ventilation. All drug doses and fluid requirements should be calculated in advance and duplicate syringes, labeled with the drug name and concentration, prepared. Battery-operated pumps on intravenous and arterial lines help prevent run-away intravenous fluids. When possible, use one line for drugs and another (with the injection port beyond a bubble filter) for fluids and blood. Neonatal requirements include a warm environment, a radiant warmer (or warming mattress and heat lamps), and 10 to 12.5% dextrose intravenous fluid. A heater–humidifier in the anesthesia circuit and a warm operating room are critical to help maintain body temperature in these neonates (see Table 20-2). Monitors in all preemies and ex-preemies should include blood pressure, electrocardiography, precordial stethoscope, and temperature. Transcutaneous oxygen (PtO_2) or oxygen saturation should be measured in all infants, but it is particularly important in those with ROP and those still at risk (younger than 45 weeks postconceptual age) to develop retinal disease. The PtO_2 should be maintained in the range of 60 to 80 mmHg or the oxygen saturation, 92 to 96%. A PaO_2 of 150 mmHg for only 1 to 2 h may cause ROP in infants younger than 44 weeks of gestational age.

All preemies and ex-preemies should have an intravenous line inserted intraoperatively and, in certain cases, before induction of anesthesia. Premedication of the infant with atropine 0.01 mg/kg (minimum vagolytic dose, 0.1 mg) intravenously just before induction is recommended by some anesthesiologists for vagolytic effect. If pancuronium is used, this may not be necessary.

Patients with BPD are at risk for gastroesophageal reflux and may benefit from antacids, rapid sequence induction, or awake intubation. Except in very ill infants or those likely to have a full stomach, the infant should be anesthetized before intubation to avoid hypertension and increased intracranial pressure. Anesthesia may be induced with fentanyl 10 to 20 μg/kg intravenously or thiopental or halothane 0.3 to 0.75 MAC (minimum alveolar concentration). Narcotic induction may be chosen for hemodynamic stability and when postoperative mechanical ventilation is anticipated. Controlled ventilation is most often preferred if general anesthesia is employed because spontaneous respiration is inefficient as a result of diminished respiratory muscle mass, decreased lung compliance, and bronchospasm.

The muscle relaxant of choice at our institution is pancuronium 0.1 mg/kg, although other agents are equally acceptable. The appropriate endotracheal tube size for most prematures will be 2.5 to 3.0 mm. Secure the tube carefully and periodically recheck the bilateral breath sounds because the length of the premature infant's trachea is only 2 to 3 cm. Only slight repositioning of the patient can lead to inadvertent extubation or mainstem migration of the tube. Ventilate by hand to assess the changing lung compliance, and select a fraction of inspired oxygen that maintains PaO_2 at 60 to 80 mmHg (oxygen saturations, 92 to 95%).

Mask anesthesia in an ex-preemie may be difficult because of airway secretions and irritability. Glycopyrrolate 10 μg/kg intravenously may reduce oral secretions. Inhalational anesthesia for maintenance at approximately 1 MAC with supplemental muscle relaxants avoids intraoperative hypotension and provides an awake vigorous infant after reversal of muscle relaxant at the conclusion of the procedure.

The blood volume of a preemie is 90 mL/kg, and in a term infant, it is 85 mL/kg. Replace blood loss greater than 10 percent of the blood volume. Treat lesser degrees of hypovolemia with colloid (plasma protein fraction or 5% albumin) or balanced salt solution at a ratio of 2 to 3 mL of replacement fluid for each 1 mL of blood loss (see Chap. 9).

Regional anesthesia (caudal epidural, penile nerve block, spinal, or axillary block) is an option for these infants to avoid the central nervous system depression caused by general anesthesia (see Chap. 10). The incidence of postoperative apnea is less with caudal epidural anesthesia than it is with general anesthesia. Regional anesthesia for postoperative pain control in infants with existing lung disease may prevent further pulmonary compromise (atelectasis or pneumonia) secondary to pain and splinting.

EXTUBATION AND POSTOPERATIVE CARE

Airway reflexes are immature, and gastric emptying is delayed in premature infants. Suction the stomach before extubation to reduce gastric distention and the risk of regurgitation and aspiration. Prolonged recovery room or ICU care may be needed postoperatively particularly for patients with BPD or infants with a history of previous central nervous system hemorrhage. The sick infant should be ventilated for several hours or days postoperatively, and almost all premature infants should be transported to the NICU intubated to allow for observation in case of postoperative apnea or hypoventilation from the effects of general anesthesia on their immature respiratory center.

Ex-preemies should be observed closely during the immediate postoperative period for episodes of apnea, periodic breathing, or apnea with associated bradycardia. General anesthesia has been shown to exacerbate apnea in infants at risk. It has also been our experience that ex-preemies up to 1 year of age who have received surfactant can have lung compromise during general anesthesia without baseline pulmonary dysfunction. Additionally, patients with BPD are at increased risk for sudden infant death syndrome. Premedication with caffeine 10 mg/kg orally or intravenously has been shown to be effective in decreasing the incidence of postoperative apnea. One intravenous dose after induction also achieves a therapeutic caffeine level in these infants. Ex-premature infants are also at increased risk for postextubation croup from airway damage caused by previous intubations. Care must be taken to insert an endotracheal tube that has an air leak between 15 to 20 cmH$_2$O pressure to prevent exacerbation of an old tracheal injury. Stridor can be treated with nebulized racemic epinephrine 0.05 mL/kg in 3 to 5 mL of saline. Bronchospasm on emergence can be difficult to manage. Treatment with terbutaline 0.01 mg/kg subcutaneously or 0.1 mg/kg of albuterol by nebulizer can improve pulmonary function.

Narcotics should be used very sparingly but titrated to make the infant comfortable when regional anesthesia has not been utilized. Oral fluids should be withheld for 1 to 2 h postoperatively in those patients in whom general anesthesia or sedative medications were administered because residual anesthesia may lessen their ability to protect the airway. All premature infants younger than 6 months of adjusted age should be admitted for overnight observation.

BIBLIOGRAPHY

Abajian JC, Mellish P, Browne AF, et al: Spinal anesthesia for surgery in the high-risk infant. *Anesth Analg* 1984; 63:359–362.

Baum JD: Retrolental fibroplasia. *Dev Med Child Neurol* 1979; 21:385–389.

Dierdorf SF, Krishna G: Anesthetic management of neonatal surgical emergencies. *Anesth Analg* 1981; 60:204–210.

Gregory GA: Anesthesia for premature infants, in Gregory GA (ed): *Pediatric Anesthesia*. New York, Churchill Livingstone, 1983, pp 579–606.

Robinson S, Gregory GA: Fentanyl-air-oxygen anesthesia for ligation of patent ductus arteriosus in preterm infants. *Anesth Analg* 1981; 60(5):331–334.

Steward DJ: Preterm infants are more prone to complications following minor surgery than are term infants. *Anesthesiology* 1982; 56:304–306.

Welborn LG, DeSoto H, Hannallah RS, et al: The use of caffeine in the control of post-anesthetic apnea in former premature infants. *Anesthesiology* 1988; 68:796–798.

Welborn LG, Hannallah RS, Fink R, et al: High-dose caffeine suppresses postoperative apnea in former preterm infants. *Anesthesiology* 1989; 71:347–349.

Welborn LG, Rice LJ, Hannallah RS, et al: Postoperative apnea in former preterm infants: Prospective comparison of spinal and general anesthesia. *Anesthesiology* 1990; 72:838–842.

Werthammer J, Brown ER, Neff RK, et al: Sudden infant death syndrome in infants with bronchopulmonary dysplasia. *Pediatrics* 1982; 69:301–304.

CHAPTER 20

Newborn Emergencies

Deborah K. Rasch
Rajam S. Ramamurthy
Mary Ann Gurkowski

Most infants undergoing surgery within the first month of life have life-threatening illnesses requiring surgery that cannot be delayed until they are older and larger. Therefore, care of the sick neonate is a challenging problem for the anesthesiologist. The anatomic and physiologic differences between the infant and adult require significant modification of anesthetic techniques to optimize care (see Chap. 2). The following chapter will describe special considerations for the most common emergencies (excluding cardiac malformations) encountered during the newborn period and discuss the transport of the sick neonate.

TRANSPORT

From the time of transport (Table 20-1), a warm environment must be provided to prevent cold stress, which can lead to hypoglycemia, acidosis, and arrhythmias. In intubated patients, the endotracheal tube (ETT) position must be verified by auscultation of the peripheral lung fields and, whenever possible, a review of a recent chest x-ray. Many chronically intubated infants may have copious secretions, and it is helpful to suction the ETT and, if necessary, replace it before transport. Always carry masks, spare ETTs, and a working laryngoscope in case of an airway problem before arrival in the operating room (OR). Very often the operating suites, with all the standard resuscitation equipment, are located "miles away" from the neonatal intensive care unit. Monitors for transport will vary, based on the infant's hemodynamic and ventilatory status. Stable neonates who are either not intubated or on minimal ventilator settings may be transported with a precordial stethoscope, electrocardiography (ECG), pulse oximeter, and a manometer to measure peak airway pressure. The unstable patient with high oxygen requirements and ventilatory support will require more

Table 20-1   Checklist: Transport of the Premature Infant and Neonate

1. *General*

   Review the infant's most recent laboratory results (hematocrit, glucose, and electrolytes), arterial blood gases, oxygen saturations, ventilator settings, medications, intravenous (IV) access, and invasive monitors (locations and trend values).

2. *Endotracheal Tube (ETT)*

   Check the depth (centimeter mark where tube is taped at the gums).

   Check the adequacy of the tape.

   Check the size of the ETT.

   Check the most recent chest x-ray for location of the ETT tip. (If the tip is too proximal or distal, reposition before transport.)

   Check to make sure there is a spare ETT, stylet, laryngoscope handle, and blade available.

3. *Oxygen*

   Check the tank to make sure it is at least half full ($\geq$ 1000 psi for E-cylinders).

   Transport the infant using a fraction of inspired oxygen (FiO_2) that will keep the PaO_2 between 92 to 95 percent whenever possible. If pulse oximetry is not available, transport at a FiO_2 of 1.0.

4. *IV Access*

   Check to make sure the infant has a good functioning IV. The other IVs and arterial line (if not monitored) may be disconnected and placed on a heparin lock.

5. *Temperature*

   It is important to transport the infant in a prewarmed transport especially designed for infants. On arrival to the operating room, make sure the Isolette is plugged in so it will stay warm for transport at the end of the case.

6. *Monitors*

   These vary with the severity of the infant's illness.

   Minimally, electrocardiography, pulse oximeter, pressure gauge (peak airway pressure), and precordial stethoscope.

7. *Drugs*

   Depending on severity of the infant's disease, resuscitation drugs may be necessary.

   Some infants will benefit from sedation to reduce agitation during transport; fentanyl may be useful if the infant's ventilation is controlled.

   Nondepolarizing muscle relaxants may be beneficial for some infants who have poor lung compliance to improve ventilation during transport invasive monitoring, such as continuous arterial pressure and central venous pressure. Some neonates may benefit from sedation and paralysis before transport, and in all cases, atropine and perhaps succinylcholine must be available should reintubation be required.

PREPARATION OF THE OR

Table 20-2 summarizes the general preparation of the OR for the premature infant and neonate. Warming lights, a warm room, and a heating blanket are essential for every neonatal case. For short cases (< 1-h duration) with minimal blood loss, a heat–moisture exchanger may be substituted for a heated humidifier, provided the infant has healthy lungs. Covering the head with a cap and warming the intravenous (IV) fluids, particularly if they must be given rapidly, are important adjuncts to maintaining temperature!

Fluid replacement in the neonate should be given as warmed colloid or crystalloid in a ratio of 2 to 3 : 1 for blood loss until estimated allowable blood loss (EABL) is reached or hemodynamic changes indicate the need for transfusion. For every case, EABL must be calculated preoperatively, and transfusion therapy in the stable patient is always best guided by measuring the hematocrit. Blood replacement formulas are discussed in Chap. 9. Maintenance fluids in neonates, by contrast with those in older infants and adults, should contain glucose to prevent hypoglycemia. Saline-filled syringes that may be used to flush medications are preferable because inadvertent fluid overload of the infant is more easily avoided when a known amount of fluid is given each time a drug is administered. IV pumps or syringe pumps should be used to provide a constant infusion rate.

IV access in the neonate is critical and may be extremely difficult at times. Do not be rushed to begin surgery if satisfactory access is not present. When the IV site is in the femoral region or lower extremity, a low-volume extension set allows small volumes of flush to be used to administer drugs. T-connectors on upper extremity or central lines also allow medications to be given with minimal dead space. An arterial line may be necessary, particularly if the operation involves the thorax or abdomen, or if significant blood loss is expected. The radial artery is preferred; however, collateral circulation should be confirmed as in adults. Lower extremity arterial lines (especially dorsalis pedis) are often unreliable because of compression of the aorta during abdominal procedures or dampening of the pattern should the foot position be altered under the drapes.

Drugs should be aspirated into syringes and labeled with the name of the agent, concentration, and a notation of dos-

Table 20-2 General Preparation of the Operating Room for the Premature Infant and Neonate

TEMPERATURE	FLUIDS	MONITORS	DRUGS	VENTILATION AND AIRWAY EQUIPMENT	ACCESS
Warming lights	Colloid (prewarmed 10 to 20 mL syringes)	A-line	Atropine	Mask	Low-volume extension set if the IV will be out of reach
Warm room		Pulse oximeter with appropriate probe	Succinylcholine	Laryngoscope blade	T-connectors
Warming blanket	Packed erythrocytes in room (filtered and warmed)	Oscillometric blood pressure device or manual readings with radial Doppler	Nondepolarizing relaxant (pancuronium)	Laryngoscope handle	IV equipment: several IV catheters (sizes 22 and 24 gauge)
Humidifier			Rapid induction agent	Endotracheal tubes	
Fluid warmer					
Head cover					

IV fluids (10% dextrose with electrolytes)	Electrocardiography	Narcotic	Stylets (make sure they withdraw easily from the endotracheal tubes)	Infusion pumps for infants < 5 kg or 150-mL burettes for older infants
Saline flush (10 mL syringes)	FiO_2 monitor	Pressor (epinephrine or phenylephrine)	Oral airways	Ether screen
	Mass spectrometer or end-tidal CO_2	Epinephrine, $CaCl_2$, $NaHCO_3$ in the cart	Tongue blade	
	Temperature probe		Precordial stethoscope and esophageal stethoscope	
			Neonatal intensive care unit ventilator or pediatric bellows in selected cases	

IV = intravenous.

319

age in milliliters. Many anesthesiologists prefer single-dose syringes because this leaves less room for error in an emergency situation. For all cases, atropine and succinylcholine should be available. Other anesthetic medications will be dictated by the individual case. For pressor activity, ephedrine is not as effective in hypotensive or bradycardic neonates; therefore, epinephrine is the drug of choice.

Carefully checked airway equipment is essential when dealing with neonates because hypoxemia or hypoventilation, even for short periods, is not well tolerated. Various sized face masks, oral airways, laryngoscope blades, and ETT should be readily available. Stylets should be inserted carefully to be sure they do not protrude from the Murphy's eye or the end of the ETT. They should also be tested before intubation to be certain they can be easily withdrawn without extubating the infant.

Monitors, just as for transport, depend on the surgical procedure planned and severity of the neonate's disease. Minimally, a precordial stethoscope, ECG, pulse oximeter end-tidal PCO_2, temperature probe, fraction of inspired oxygen (FiO_2) monitor, and blood pressure monitor are needed. Invasive monitoring of central venous or arterial blood pressure will be warranted in some cases.

SPECIFIC NEWBORN EMERGENCIES

Congenital Diaphragmatic Hernia

Congenital herniation of the abdominal viscera through the diaphragm is associated with varying degrees of pulmonary hypoplasia, which determines the prognosis in patients with congenital diaphragmatic hernia. The most common location is left posterolateral, but either side may be affected. Elevated pulmonary vascular resistance may result in persistent pulmonary hypertension (PPH) of the neonate, which may be encountered both pre- and postoperatively. PPH consists of arterial desaturation from right to left shunting at the level of the ductus arteriosus or foramen ovale. Simultaneous sampling of arterial blood from the right radial artery (preductal) and umbilical artery (postductal) will help differentiate arterial desaturation from primary lung disease and pulmonary hypertension. When PPH exists, the right radial artery PO_2 will be at least 10 mmHg higher than blood drawn from the umbilical artery. Treatment of PPH includes hyperventilation, sedatives with or without muscle relaxants, and elevation of the mean systolic blood pressure with inotropic agents, such as dopamine or dobutamine to reduce the right to left shunting. Pulmonary vasodilators, such as tolazoline or nitroglycerin, are rarely used by neonatologists. Use of high-frequency ventilation has been very successful, and, in selected patients, extracorporeal membrane oxygenation has proven beneficial. Perioperative mortality is high (33 to 66 percent) and is primarily caused by complications of ventilatory support. Little notice may be given for surgical scheduling because this anomaly has been considered a true surgical emergency. More recently, this premise has been challenged, and some centers are stabilizing the infant's cardiopulmonary system first and delaying surgery for 48 to 72 h. Their results suggest a slightly lower mortality rate.

Preoperative Assessment
The infant with diaphragmatic hernia is born with a scaphoid abdomen and barrel chest. On occasion, bowel sounds may be heard over the chest, and respiratory distress may or may not be present. Chest x-ray may show mediastinal shift and bowel in the chest cavity (Fig. 20-1). If preoperative ventilatory support is required, awake intubation is preferred because bag and

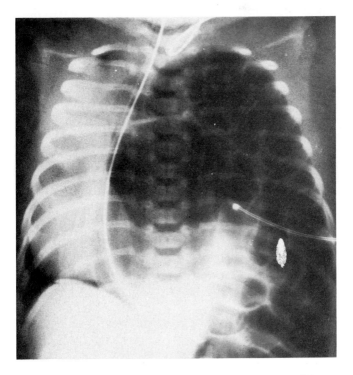

Figure 20-1   Congenital diaphragmatic hernia. Bowel loops fill the left hemithorax, displacing the heart and mediastinum to the right.

mask ventilation distends the stomach, thus further compressing the ipsilateral hypoplastic lung. Insertion of a gastric tube to decompress the stomach may also lower ventilatory resistance. High airway pressure may cause pneumothorax on either side (Fig. 20-2). The infant should also be evaluated for associated anomalies; cardiovascular defects occur in 23 percent and intestinal malrotation in 50 percent.

Anesthetic Management

Anesthesia equipment and the OR should be prepared with neonatal considerations as discussed previously. Monitors should include ECG, temperature, blood pressure, blood gas (right radial arterial line is preferred for preductal samples), oxygen saturation, and end-tidal CO_2 when available. Transcutaneous PCO_2 may be more accurate because only one lung may be ventilated, and therefore, a higher PCO_2 may be present in arterial blood compared with end-tidal sampling. In addition, if there is a large intracardiac or ductal right to left shunt, end-tidal PCO_2 may not be accurate. A manometer inserted in the anesthesia

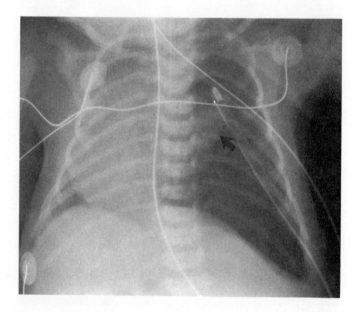

Figure 20-2 Pulmonary hypoplasia secondary to congenital diaphragmatic hernia. The left lung is diminutive (arrow) and surrounded by a pneumothorax after hernia repair.

circuit will allow measurement of ventilating pressures and a heater humidifier for gases will protect against desiccation of secretions.

If not already intubated, the infants should be preoxygenated, given 0.02 mg/kg of atropine, and intubated awake. General anesthesia is most often accomplished using 10 to 15 µg/kg of fentanyl, and the infant is paralyzed with a nondepolarizing relaxant. This provides stability to the cardiovascular system. Oxygen should be administered at an FiO_2 of 1.0 initially and decreased in small increments (a sudden drop may lead to pulmonary vasoconstriction). Check arterial blood gases and acid–base status frequently. Inhalational anesthetics may lower systemic vascular resistance, which can result in arterial hypoxemia from promotion of right to left shunting at the level of the ductus arteriosus or foramen ovale. Inhalational agents may also produce myocardial depression which, in combination with an enhanced pulmonary to systemic pressure gradient, may produce acute cardiovascular compromise. Omit nitrous oxide to avoid bowel distention. Hand ventilation is usually preferred, maintaining the airway pressure below 25 to 30 cmH_2O whenever possible. This will allow immediate changes in ventilation because compliance is altered by closure of the abdomen. Sudden deterioration may be a sign of pneumothorax on the normal side.

The abdominal cavity is underdeveloped and may not accommodate the viscera that is reduced from the thorax. Primary closure may result in increased intraabdominal pressure, cephalad displacement of the diaphragm, diminished functional residual capacity (FRC), and vena caval compression. Hypotension may result from impaired venous return and high pulmonary vascular resistance, ventricular failure, and low cardiac output. Third-space and blood losses are usually minimal, and dopamine support is preferable to large volumes of fluid or colloid. When available, central venous pressure measurements may help guide fluid replacement. Occasionally, primary abdominal closure is impossible. A silastic pouch will be created similar to an omphalocele, and closure will be planned a few days later.

Postoperative Care

A honeymoon period may follow surgery, in which oxygenation is good, but deterioration may occur from increasing right-to-left cardiac shunts through fetal channels. Pulmonary vasodilation with tolazoline, nitroprusside, or nitroglycerin may be helpful. Alveolar-arterial oxygen gradient may be a predictor of survival. Postoperative ventilation should be continued with relaxants, narcotic sedation, and vasopressor support.

Omphalocele and Gastroschisis

Omphalocele, a hernia through the umbilicus, and gastroschisis, eventration of abdominal contents through a defect in the anterior abdominal wall, are different disorders embryologically, but they have similar anesthetic considerations. During the 6th week of life, the midgut herniates into the body stalk because of inadequate space in the abdomen. During the 10th week, the intestines return to the abdominal cavity, and the body stalk constricts to become the umbilical cord. An omphalocele is believed to result from persistence of the body stalk and concomitant failure to develop the lateral wall. The size of the defect is related to the timing of the insult. It contains representative portions of small and large bowel, spleen, stomach, and liver. Gastroschisis, on the other hand, results from a localized abdominal wall defect. This defect is often above the umbilicus. In most cases, an omphalocele is covered with intact peritoneum (Fig. 20-3), whereas in gastroschisis, the bowel is not covered by any membrane. The intestines should be covered immediately with sterile saline-soaked sponges to preserve moisture and help prevent any further contamination of the abdominal contents. Table 20-3 lists other congenital anomalies that occur commonly in these patients (76 percent of patients with an omphalocele will have an associated defect). These patients have a perioperative mortality rate of 30 percent, which is largely the result of cardiac anomalies and prematurity. Gastroschisis is rarely associated with other anomalies, but more

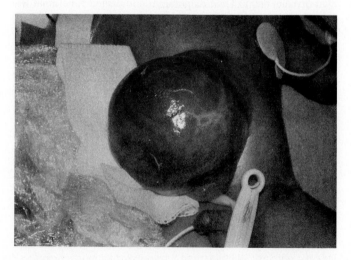

Figure 20-3 An omphalocele has an intact peritoneum.

Table 20-3   Congenital Anomalies Associated with Omphalocele

Congenital heart disease both cyanotic and acyanotic defects
Renal anomalies, for example, Wilms' tumor
Beckwith-Wiedemann syndrome
Adrenal cysts
Malrotation of the intestinal tract
Meckel's diverticulum
Intestinal atresias

infants are premature (58 percent). A similar mortality rate (28 to 30 percent) is caused by intestinal malrotation or atresias and wound complications. The size of the hernia and the intactness of the peritoneal covering determine the urgency of surgical correction.

Preoperative Assessment
Determination of the gestational age and the presence of associated anomalies is very important. For example, Beckwith-Wiedemann syndrome (omphalocele, organomegaly, macroglossia, and hypoglycemia) is a rare defect that can be associated with omphalocele. Life-threatening intraoperative hypoglycemia, which can lead to cardiac dysfunction and seizures, may occur if not treated expectantly with a higher concentration of intravenous glucose and close monitoring of blood glucose values perioperatively. Therefore, preoperative assessment of serum glucose, electrolytes, hematocrit, and acid–base status are important. Infants with gastroschisis and ruptured omphalocele have tremendous protein loss and third-space fluid losses, which lead to hemoconcentration, hypoperfusion, oliguria, and metabolic acidosis. Adequate perfusion to vital organs should be maintained by monitoring blood pressure and urine output and replacing volume losses with isotonic solutions (Normosol, lactated Ringer's, and 5% albumin) or blood depending on the hematocrit values and hemodynamics. Under most circumstances, transfusion is begun in newborn infants after the hematocrit reaches 35 to 40 percent, although such conditions as severe lung disease or cyanotic congenital heart disease may warrant earlier transfusion. Significant evaporative heat and fluid losses occur from exposed bowel. Therefore, exposed intestine should be kept moist with sterile warm saline-soaked pads, and the infant should be placed in a thermoneutral environment. A nasogastric tube is placed to decompress the stomach.

Visual examination of the sac contents may provide information regarding the difficulty of the repair, which can prolong anesthetic time and indicate other possible congenital anomalies. If the sac is intact, notice whether it contains viscera other than the intestines, such as liver and spleen (Fig. 20-4). The presence of the liver may complicate the repair because of angulation of the vena cava when the liver is reduced into a position beneath the abdominal muscles. The intestine should be inspected closely through the sac. The presence of dilated and tiny unused bowel suggests obstruction. If the visualized intestine is completely collapsed and underdeveloped, it may suggest duodenal atresia. An absence of the xiphoid process suggests the presence of diaphragmatic and intracardiac defects.

Anesthetic Management

The infant's body temperature should be maintained and fluid resuscitation continued. A manometer in the breathing circuit to monitor inflation pressure should be used. Monitors should include temperature, transcutaneous PO_2 or pulse oximeter, end-tidal CO_2, and direct arterial blood pressure through an indwelling catheter. In most cases, blood gases, acid–base, and electrolyte status should be followed at least every 20 to 30 min intraoperatively. Also, aspirate the nasogastric tube frequently.

The stable infant with a small hernia covered with peritoneum requires less aggressive management and monitoring. If there is no tension on the abdominal wall after closure of the

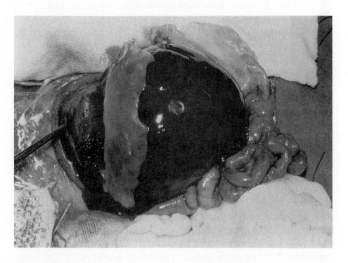

Figure 20-4 Omphalocele sac contents should be examined for presence of organs (in this case, the liver), which can complicate the repair.

defect and profound muscle relaxation is not required to facilitate the return of abdominal contents to the abdominal cavity, there may not be significant respiratory difficulty postoperatively, and extubation in the OR or after transport to the neonatal intensive care unit is feasible. Less stable infants, with large hernias or exposed abdominal contents require emergency repair. These patients are usually intubated awake after volume replacement has been instituted, and small doses of narcotics (fentanyl 10 to 20 μg/kg) and muscle relaxants are used. Babies with moderate defects and stable hemodynamics may be induced using a rapid-sequence protocol under cricoid pressure. Recommended agents at our institution are atropine 0.01 mg/kg in addition to thiopental 4 to 6 mg/kg or etomidate 0.3 mg/kg and succinylcholine 1.5 to 2 mg/kg. However, these patients will have a reduced FRC and a high cardiac output, placing them at greater risk for desaturation during the apneic period prior to intubation. Nitrous oxide should be avoided because of its potential for bowel distention. The anesthesiologist and surgeon work closely to determine whether primary closure can be accomplished. Closure with maximal relaxation may result in excessive intraabdominal pressure, obstruction of the inferior vena cava, lowered cardiac output, hypotension, and elevation of the diaphragm with respiratory embarrassment. After closure, muscle relaxants and ventilatory support are then gradually withdrawn over a period of several hours to days after the infant is returned to the neonatal intensive care unit.

Extubation and Postoperative Care
Postoperative care varies according to the magnitude of the defect, the type of repair, and the associated pathologic findings. In healthy patients whose defect is small and in whom total repair is done easily, the ETT may be removed when the infant is awake, vigorous, and normothermic; adequate reversal of muscle relaxant has been achieved; and good spontaneous respirations are present. Infants with large defects, especially in those who have a complete closure performed, will usually need to remain intubated and ventilated postoperatively for at least 24 h. Some authors recommend maintaining muscle relaxants until abdominal pressure has been reduced to the point at which circulatory and respiratory embarrassment does not exist.

Weaning from the ventilator may take several days. If the infant has a Teflon bag or silo, it will take several days of gradually reducing the size of the pouch until the viscera are returned to the abdominal cavity. After complete reduction has occurred, the infant will be taken back to the OR where the pouch is removed and the major fascial defect repaired. Often, the infant will remain intubated until after the final repair.

Tracheoesophageal Fistula and Esophageal Atresia

Tracheoesophageal fistula is a congenital malformation of the distal trachea and esophagus that occurs in 1 per 3000 live births and is often associated with other organ system defects (Table 20-4). About 35 percent have a major cardiovascular anomaly, such as ventricular septal defect, tetralogy of Fallot, atrial septal defect, or coarctation of the aorta, and 30 to 40 percent are premature. The VATER syndrome (*v*ertebral, *a*nal, *t*racheo-esophageal fistula, *e*sophageal atresia, and *r*enal or *r*adial anomalies) may also be suspected in patients with tracheoesophageal fistulas who have associated vertebral anomalies or imperforate anus. The embryologic origin of esophageal atresia is uncertain, although there are two hypotheses. The first is that the atresia occurs because of localized pressure by an anomalous vessel, such as an anomalous right subclavian artery or persistent right descending aorta passing across the esophagus during the 3rd to 6th week of fetal life. The second is that there is incomplete separation of the tracheal and esophageal portion of the foregut. The normal laryngotracheal tube grows faster than the esophagus. If the separation of the esophagus and trachea is slightly

Table 20-4　Associated Anomalies with Esophageal Atresia and Tracheoesophageal Fistula (Overall Incidence, 30 to 50 percent)

ANOMALY	INCIDENCE (%)
Cardiovascular 　Atrial septal defect, ventricular septal 　defect, patent ductus arteriosus, 　tetralogy of Fallot, coarctation of the 　aorta	35
Musculoskeletal 　Butterfly vertebra, radial aplasia, 　polydactyly, wrist and knee 　malformations	30
Gastrointestinal 　Imperforate anus, malrotation, 　duodenal atresia, annular pancreas, 　pyloric stenosis	20
Genitourinary 　Renal agenesis/dysplasia, ureteral 　anomalies, hydronephrosis, 　hypospadias	10
Craniofacial 　Cleft lip, cleft palate	4

delayed, the rapidly growing trachea causes separation of the proximal and distal esophagus.

Several types of esophageal atresia are well known. The anesthesiologist should be aware of the different esophageal variants because management differs according to the particular lesion involved. It is important to know if there is a fistula present between the trachea and distal esophagus and where the fistula connects. The most common defect is a blind upper esophageal pouch and a fistulous tract between lower esophagus and trachea (Fig. 20-5). The diagnosis may be made during the initial evaluation of a cyanotic infant by failure of the suction catheter or gastric tube to pass into the stomach, by the presence of coughing and cyanosis during feeding, or by x-ray with a radiopaque catheter in the blind pouch about 10 cm from the gumline (Fig. 20-6). Aspiration of secretions or feedings causes pulmonary compromise and possibly injury; therefore, it is important to make the diagnosis before institution of feedings to improve prognosis.

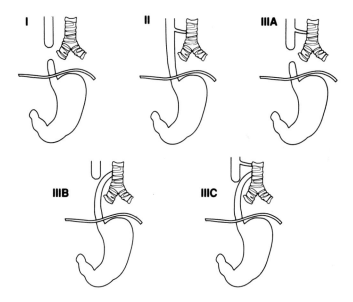

Figure 20-5 Types of tracheoesophageal fistulas. Type IIIB is the most common, and Type II is the most difficult to diagnose. [Reproduced with permission from Rasch DK, Ramamurthy R: Tracheoesophageal fistula, in Bready LL, Smith RB (eds): *Decision Making in Anesthesiology*. Toronto, BC Dekker, 1987, p 92.]

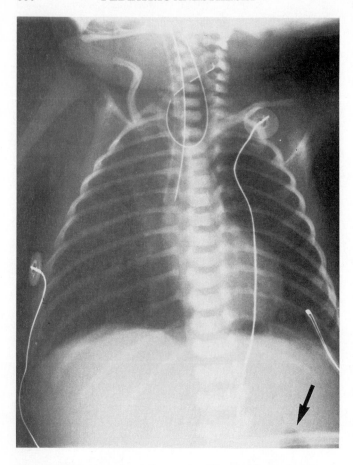

Figure 20-6 Esophageal atresia. The esophageal tube is curled back on itself in the proximal blind pouch. Air in the stomach (arrow) suggests a distal tracheoesophageal fistula.

Preoperative Assessment

After the diagnosis of esophageal atresia is suspected, the infant receives nothing by mouth. A tube is passed into the proximal esophageal segment and placed on continuous suctioning to prevent aspiration of oropharyngeal or nasopharyngeal secretions. The infant is placed in a semiupright position to minimize regurgitation of gastric juice through the fistula. Some authors recommend a head-up prone position so oral secretions can drain.

The gestational age is determined, and the patient is evaluated for the presence of other congenital anomalies. If there is a question of cyanotic congenital heart disease, cardiac evaluation either with echocardiography or catheterization and angiography should precede the surgical repair. Radiographs should be examined for abdominal air (to confirm the location of the fistula from the trachea to the lower esophagus). Pulmonary infiltrates, if present, suggest aspiration pneumonia.

An evaluation for lung disease should be performed. This includes clinical examination, chest radiograph, and arterial blood gases. Placement of an arterial catheter is recommended, and repeated arterial blood gases should be performed to keep a close watch on the pulmonary status. If the child is hypoxemic, supplemental oxygen will be needed. If refractory hypoxemia or hypercarbia occurs, intubation and mechanical ventilation will be required. The acid–base status should be evaluated and corrected preoperatively.

Emergency gastrostomy may occasionally be performed under local anesthesia in the neonatal intensive care unit to relieve the gastric distention and respiratory compromise, should cardiopulmonary stabilization be required. The blind upper pouch should be continuously suctioned.

Anesthetic Management

The operating room is prepared for management of the sick neonate (Table 20-2). Direct measurement of arterial blood pressure using an indwelling catheter, transcutaneous PO_2 or oxygen saturation, end-tidal or transcutaneous PCO_2, and urinary output should be measured. Heart tones and breath sounds can be auscultated with a precordial stethoscope (not esophageal) positioned in the left axilla.

Type I tracheoesophageal fistula (no communication between esophagus and trachea) may be induced with inhalational agents or using an intravenous technique, but all other types are intubated awake after atropine and preoxygenation. The fistula is usually located in the posterior wall of the trachea, close to the carina. Various techniques are recommended to achieve satisfactory tracheal intubation with neither endobronchial intubation nor excessive distention of the stomach. Generally, if the bevel of the ETT is aimed anteriorly, the longer edge of the tube tip will tend to occlude the fistula, and there will be less gastric distention (Fig. 20-7). Maintaining some spontaneous ventilation instead of controlling respiration will also reduce the volume of air forced into the stomach. Also, the right lung will be compressed during the right thoracotomy for fistula repair. If right endobronchial intubation occurs, hypoxemia will develop rapidly.

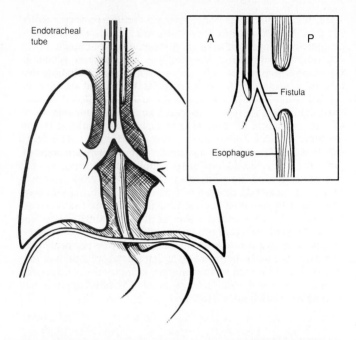

Figure 20-7 Positioning of the endotracheal tube for trans-esophageal fistula. The bevel is aimed anteriorly, such that the posterior fistula will be better occluded and less air should enter the stomach. A = anterior; P = posterior.

The goal of early intraoperative anesthetic management is to prevent gastric distention, which may lead to gastric rupture, ventilatory impedance, and cardiac arrest. Gastrostomy may be needed if distention is unavoidable. Ventilation by hand to assess changing lung compliance and avoidance of muscle relaxants until the chest is open will enhance ventilation. An ETT obstruction by bloody secretions or aspirated material and tracheal obstruction by surgical manipulation should be anticipated and corrected.

Intraoperative arterial blood gases, hematocrit, glucose, and electrolytes should be monitored. Ideally the FiO_2 should be adjusted to keep the PaO_2 between 60 to 90 mmHg or keep the saturation between 92 to 96 percent to avoid unnecessary exposure to high oxygen for prolonged periods.

Extubation and Postoperative Care
The postoperative management of these infants is determined by the degree of preoperative pulmonary dysfunction, the se-

verity of the associated anomalies, and the degree of prematurity. In vigorous, otherwise healthy term infants, the ETT can be removed soon after surgery, providing their temperature is normal, muscle paralysis is reversed, and there is adequate spontaneous ventilation and oxygenation. After extubation, the infants should be given supplemental humidified oxygen as needed to keep a PaO_2 of 60 to 90 mmHg. The most frequent complications in the early postoperative period is pneumonia or atelectasis from retained secretions. This may require frequent nasopharyngeal suctioning, which should be done with a catheter that has been marked to indicate the depth of insertion to prevent disruption of the esophageal anastomosis.

Postoperative ventilation should be planned for sick infants, particularly those with preoperative lung disease. Bloody tracheal secretions often continue to be a problem during the early postoperative period. Esophageal suction and extension of the neck should be avoided to protect the surgical repair. Postoperative complications, such as tracheomalacia or recurrent laryngeal nerve injury, may cause upper airway obstruction immediately after extubation.

Necrotizing Enterocolitis (NEC)

NEC is a complex disease affecting the small bowel and colon, which is seen in three to five percent of newborn infants admitted to a neonatal intensive care unit. Several clinical factors have a high association with the development of NEC, but an exact causal relationship between these clinical parameters and bowel injury has not been determined. Some of these factors are listed in Table 20-5, and there is some controversy over their importance in the production of the illness.

However, of the many factors implicated in predisposing the infant to develop NEC, most investigators agree that hypoperfusion of the intestine (either from a generalized problem, such as hypovolemia or low cardiac output, or a local deficit of per-

Table 20-5   Factors Associated with an Increased Risk of Necrotizing Enterocolitis

Premature or small-for-gestational-age infant
Administration of bicarbonate
Asphyxia (low Apgar score)
Polycythemia
Institution of feeds < 72 h after an asphyxial episode
Placement of a nasojejunal tube
Rapid advancement of feeding volume
Administration of Ca^{++} gluconate as a bolus by umbilical artery or venous catheter

fusion, as in asphyxia or shunting of blood flow away from the intestine) is the major insult that leads to the development of NEC. During hypoxemia, the diving reflex may occur as a result of the infant's adaptive measures against birth asphyxia. Perfusion to the brain and heart are maintained while blood flow to the intestines and kidney are shunted away. In 1969, Lloyd noted that 80 percent of affected babies had at least one documented prior asphyxial episode. The pathophysiology of NEC is multifactorial and has been associated with the following problems.

Premature or Small-for-Gestational-Age (SGA) Infants

These children have host defense impairments related to an immature hematopoietic system. These alterations affect the infant's ability to contain certain bacteria within the intestinal lumen, especially when muscosal insults occur in the bowel wall. In addition, there is an increased incidence of birth asphyxia in the SGA infant and chronic deprivation of oxygen from hypoventilation, respiratory distress, and/or nutritional deficits. These babies also have a higher incidence of requiring instrumentation of the umbilical vessels for blood pressure measurement and sampling of arterial blood gases and of feeding tubes in the gastrointestinal tract.

Administration of Bicarbonate

This has been implicated as a risk factor in NEC because hypertonic solutions if given by a low umbilical venous catheter have been shown to injure the liver directly and also may injure other vascular structures.

Asphyxia

This causes stimulation of the diving reflex in infants. Reduction in arterial oxygen tension, occurring during labor, delivery, or the early postnatal period, may be a trigger. Poor oxygen delivery to the gastrointestinal tract, which has a very limited ability to sustain anaerobic metabolism before permanent damage is done, is the source of the immediate injury. Diminished perfusion promotes further mucosal damage by gram-negative bacteria and anaerobes residing within the intestine.

Placement of Umbilical catheters

Almost 90 percent of arterial catheters used for umbilical artery catheter placement can be demonstrated to have thrombus formation near the tip after 3 days' duration. Up to 50 to 60 percent of infants with proven NEC have such catheters in place at the time of the diagnosis. However, there is no proven correlation between umbilical artery catheters and NEC. Those infants who have umbilical artery catheters placed are the small preterm infants who are also very ill and prone to develop NEC. All the major vessels that supply the gastrointestinal tract leave the abdominal aorta at or above the level of L3. Therefore, placement of the tip of the umbilical arterial catheter at or below L4 is thought to reduce the instance of thrombus formation near the orifice of the inferior mesenteric artery (Fig. 20-8).

Use of Hypertonic Feedings

Hypertonic feedings draw water from the extracellular fluid compartment into the gastrointestinal tract. Bowel distention and also depletion of intravascular volume occurs, making perfusion of the bowel wall diminish. This type of injury is especially likely to occur after an asphyxial episode, in which case the damage from hyperosmolar feedings is often additive. Direct mucosal injury may occur from these formulas, and they provide substrate for anaerobic bacterial growth. Neither the osmolality of the feedings, the timing of first feeding, nor the mode of feedings have been proved to increase the incidence of NEC. However, rapid advancement of volume may have a detrimental effect. In countries where infants are exclusively breast fed, NEC is practically never seen.

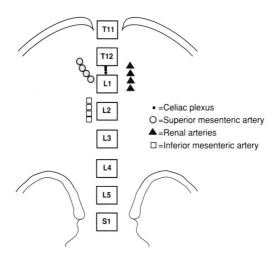

Figure 20-8 Location of various structures in relation to lumbar vertebra. The tip of an umbilical arterial catheter should be placed at or below L4 to reduce the incidence of thrombus formation near the orifice of the inferior mesenteric artery.

Polycythemia
A peripheral venous hematocrit of Hct 65 percent or more, which increases blood viscosity, has been implicated. The neonate may be at greater risk of sludging and poor perfusion of the intestinal wall because of poor red blood cell deformability as a result of fetal hemoglobin.

Administration of Ca^{++}
This can cause problems because of its vasoconstrictor properties. In radiographic studies, a bolus of dye injected at L4 can reflux retrograde and enter the inferior mesenteric artery or from an improperly placed umbilical artery catheter can enter the superior mesenteric artery or renal arteries. Circumstantial evidence regarding intestinal bleeding has been demonstrated by several investigators after bolus Ca^{++} therapy through an umbilical artery catheter.

The relationship between intestinal colonization with specific pathogens and the development of NEC is not known. However, one third of infants with NEC have positive blood cultures at the onset of their illness. In experimental situations, only animals colonized with gram-negative organisms that had an asphyxial episode developed the disease. Epidemics of NEC have been associated with *Escherichia coli, Klebsiella, Pseudomonas, Salmonella,* and *Clostridium* in the nursery environment.

The diagnostic workup depends on the stage at which the infant is suspected of having NEC. The most common early signs are abdominal distention and an increase in residual from gastric aspirate (Table 20-6). The problem with these criteria is that almost all preterm infants have slow gastrointestinal motil-

Table 20-6   Diagnostic Signs of Necrotizing Enterocolitis

EARLY	LATE
Increased volume of gastric aspirate, vomiting	Abdominal erythema or tenderness
	Gross gastrointestinal bleed
Guaiac-positive stools	Petechiae or spontaneous bleeding from other sites
Glucose-positive stools	Shock from sepsis
Lethargy, hypothermia, apnea	
Abdominal distention	

ity from an immature nervous system and frequently become somewhat distended.

After NEC is suspected, the following diagnostic studies should be performed:

1. Complete blood count with differential and platelet count every 12 h to watch for thrombocytopenia.
2. Flat plate (KUB) and crosstable lateral x-ray of the abdomen to look for ascites, pneumatosis intestinalis, free air, or portal vein gas, all of which indicate that operation is necessary (Fig. 20-9).
3. Prothrombin time, partial thromboplastin time, and fibrinogen levels should be done, especially if clinical bleeding is apparent.
4. Arterial blood gases to detect acidosis and serum electrolytes to look at the potassium level, blood urea nitrogen concentration, and bicarbonate value.

Medical Management

If NEC is highly suspected, then aggressive therapy should be started to avoid progression of the ischemic insult. This includes stopping enteral feedings. Intravenous hyperalimentation to support nutritional needs, gastric decompression with a nasogastric tube, and abdominal x-rays as frequently as clinically indicated to monitor bowel gas pattern and the presence of free air are equally important. Hematologic parameters should be followed closely. Often a fall in the platelet count is the first sign of an intestinal perforation. These patients may need large volumes of intravascular expansion fluids (20 to 30 mL/kg or more over a 2- to 4-h period) to maintain stable vital signs. Electrolytes and acid–base parameters should be followed because acidosis, hyperkalemia, hyponatremia, and hypocalcemia may occur. Antibiotics (to provide gram-negative infection coverage) should be started.

Surgery is usually indicated if any of the following occur:

1. Clinical deterioration with sepsis.
2. Unrelenting acidosis.
3. X-ray evidence of intestinal perforation.
4. Clotting abnormalities that are resistant to medical therapy.
5. Development of peritonitis.

Preoperative Evaluation

This should be very detailed in these patients.

1. Volume and electrolyte status are very important variables in the infant suspected of having NEC. Infants

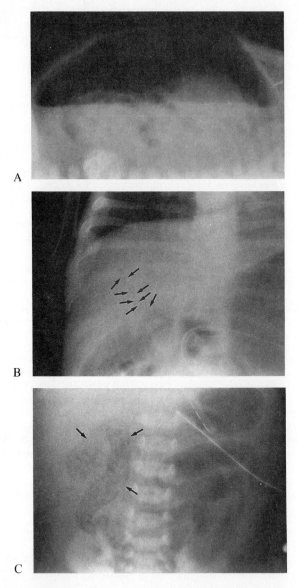

Figure 20-9 (A) Cross-table lateral radiograph of the abdomen demonstrating free air in the peritoneal cavity. (B) KUB radiograph of the abdomen showing accumulation of gas in the portal venous system also indicative of intestinal perforation. (C) KUB radiograph of the abdomen showing pneumatosis intestinalis, which represents air in the bowel wall from an ischemic event (arrows).

should be examined carefully for peripheral perfusion, urine output, and vital signs. Ideally, capillary refill should be brisk ($<$ 1.5 s) with urine output of 1 mL/kg/h or more, and mean arterial pressure normal for age and weight (approximately, 40 to 45 mmHg). Weight is a less reliable measure of volume status in these infants because enormous weight gain can occur from sequestration of fluids in the bowel or peritoneum. Acid–base abnormalities and hypovolemia should be treated with volume expanders before transport to the OR.

2. Hematologic parameters should also be evaluated. Evidence for clotting abnormalities should be sought on examination (excessive oozing from puncture sites, bruising, or petechiae). Important laboratory studies include hematocrit, clotting profile, and platelet count. Infusion of one unit of platelets should be started preoperatively in patients with a rapidly falling platelet count and clinical signs of abnormal bleeding. If volume overload is a concern, the platelets may be concentrated to a volume of 10 to 15 mL before infusion.

3. Respiratory distress is common in these infants, and they are at risk for development of pulmonary complications; therefore, a review of the most recent chest x-ray, arterial blood gases, and physical examination of the lung fields are important.

Several precautions need to be taken to provide optimal care of these infants, both in transport to and from the OR and during the operative procedures. Caution must be exercised:

1. To maintain an adequate PaO_2 to deliver sufficient oxygen to ischemic bowel without making the infant hyperoxic, that is, a PaO_2 between 80 to 100 mmHg (O_2 saturation, 94 to 97 percent). Note: these levels of recommended oxygen tension are slightly higher than those for healthy preemies.

2. To remove air bubbles from all IV tubing leading into the patient to reduce the risk of paradoxic venous air embolism.

3. To provide a thermoneutral environment to prevent cold stress, which has been shown to worsen existing lesions.

4. To humidify and warm inhaled gases administered through the ETT to prevent respiratory fluid and heat loss.

On arrival in the OR, both fresh-frozen plasma and packed red blood cells should be readily available because opening of the abdominal cavity will result in losses of large volumes of protein-containing fluids. The calculations of intraoperative fluids depend on the estimations presented in Table 20-7, but they must be governed by the clinical response, the most sensitive parameter of which is the heart rate.

Anesthetic Management
In addition to the usual preparation for a neonate, a calculation of resuscitation drug doses (including dextrose 25%, calcium chloride, and sodium bicarbonate) should be done preoperatively. Dopamine infusion should be available, and the infusion rate should be calculated. A peripheral arterial line will allow direct monitoring of blood pressure and access for the measurement of glucose, hematocrit, and blood gases. Umbilical arterial lines are usually removed in infants suspected to have NEC; hence, a peripheral arterial catheter may be necessary. Blood warmers and heater–humidifier should be set up. A suction trap should be inserted in the surgical suction and the sponges weighed so that a better idea of blood loss may be achieved.

These patients are most often intubated awake because of their debilitated state, borderline hemodynamics, and potential for regurgitation and aspiration. Rarely, a rapid-sequence induction may be indicated. Rapid fluid resuscitation is often necessary as the abdomen is opened; therefore, two functioning IV lines are necessary.

Induction of general anesthesia in the unintubated infant with stable hemodynamics but questionable intravascular volume may be accomplished with etomidate 0.3 mg/kg or ketamine 1 to 2 mg/kg IV and a muscle relaxant. Fentanyl 10 to 20 μg/kg may be chosen in hemodynamically stable patients who are already intubated. Oxygen and air are mixed to produce a PaO_2 of 80 to 100 mmHg. Avoid N_2O because it may increase the size of the gas bubbles in the bowel wall and hepatic portal

Table 20-7   Intraoperative Fluids

Maintenance
 4 mL/kg/h of 10% dextrose with electrolytes

Ongoing losses
 7 to 10 mL/kg/h for an open abdomen. Blood loss should be replaced at a ratio of 1 mL of packed erythrocytes to 2 mL of blood loss to maintain hematocrit around 40 to 45 percent.

Deficit
 This should be replaced rapidly and, if possible, before the abdomen is open to prevent hypotension when ascitic fluid is lost.

system. Pancuronium 0.1 to 0.2 mg/kg provides good surgical relaxation. Controlled ventilation by hand allows assessment of the changing compliance. If pressor support is needed, dopamine (starting at 5 μg/kg/min and titrated to effect) is the choice. For each one-third blood volume replaced, consider giving calcium chloride 10 to 20 mg/kg IV for prevention of hypotension and arrhythmias caused by a low ionized Ca^{++} from ionic binding by the citrate buffer used as an anticoagulant in blood products.

Frequent measurement (every 15 to 30 min) of pH, glucose, and hematocrit is important because septic infants are very susceptible to rapid development of acidosis and hypoglycemia.

Postoperative Care
These patients should remain intubated and maintained on mechanical ventilation. Postoperative abdominal distention, massive fluid resuscitation, and persistent acidosis may cause respiratory compromise for several days.

Occasionally, a large segment of the bowel is necrosed, which is incompatible with survival. The surgeon may decide to close the abdomen without any further intervention. The infant should then be transported to the neonatal intensive care unit where proper parental preparation is done before withdrawal of support.

BIBLIOGRAPHY

Bloss RS, Aranda JV, Beardmore HE: Congenital diaphragmatic hernia. *Pathophysiology and Pharmacologic Support Surgery.* April 1981, pp 518–524.

Caplan MS, MacGregor SN: Perinatal management of congenital diaphragmatic hernia and abdominal wall defects. *Clin Perinatol* 1989; 16:917–938.

Dierdorf SF, Krishna G: Anesthetic management of neonatal surgical emergencies. *Anesth Analg* 1981; 60:204–215.

Greenwood RD, Rosenthal AM, Nadas AS: Cardiovascular malformations associated with omphalocele. *J Pediatr* 1974; 85:818–821.

Hazebroek FW, Tibboel D, Bos AP, et al: Congenital diaphragmatic hernia: Impact of preoperative stabilization: A prospective pilot study in 13 patients. *J Pediatr Surg* 1988; 23:139–146.

King DR, Saurin R, Boles T: Gastroschisis update. *J Pediatr Surg* 1980; 15:553–557.

Kliegman RM: Neonatal necrotizing enterocolitis. *Pediatr Clin North Am* 1979; 26:327–344.

Kliegman RM, Fanaroff AA: Necrotizing enterocolitis. *N Engl J Med* 1984; 310:1093–1096.

Levin DL: Congenital diaphragmatic hernia: A persistent problem. *J Pediatr* 1987; 111:390–392.

Lloyd JR: The etiology of gastrointestinal perforations in the newborn. *J Pediatr Surg* 1969; 4:77–81.

Manthei U, Vaucher Y, Crowe CP Jr: Congenital diaphragmatic hernia: Immediate preoperative and postoperative oxygen gradients identify patients requiring prolonged respiratory support. *Surgery* 1983; 93:83–87.

Morray J: Anesthesia for thoracic surgery, in Gregory GA (ed): *Pediatric Anesthesia.* 2nd ed. New York, Churchill-Livingstone, 1989, Vol 2, pp 908–927.

Phillippart AI, Canty TG, Filler RM: Acute fluid volume requirements in infants with anterior abdominal wall defects. *J Pediatr Surg* 1982; 7:553–558.

Quain L, Smith DW: The VATER association: Vertebral defects, anal atresia, tracheoesophageal fistula with esophageal atresia, radial dysplasia. *Birth Defects* 1972; 8:75–78.

Spear RM: Anesthesia for premature and term infants: Perioperative implications. *J Pediatr* 1992; 120:165–176.

Thein RMH, Epstein BS: General surgical procedures in the child with a congenital anomaly, in Stehling LC, Zauder HL (eds): *Anesthetic Implications of Congenital Anomalies in Children.* New York, Appleton-Century-Crofts, 1980, pp 87–109.

Towne H, Peters G, Chong JT: The problems of giant omphalocele. *J Pediatr Surg* 1980; 15:543.

CHAPTER 21

Newborn and Pediatric Resuscitation

Dawn E. Webster
Alice Gong
Deborah K. Rasch

Cardiopulmonary arrest in infants and children is usually not a sudden event but is the result of prolonged deterioration in respiratory and circulatory function. After cardiac arrest occurs, the prognosis is very poor. For this reason, the emphasis on resuscitation of infants and children must be on rapid recognition of impending arrest and swift intervention. The goal of this chapter is to review the components of a rapid cardiopulmonary assessment, the basics of cardiopulmonary resuscitation, and resuscitation algorithms for the neonate, infant, and child.

RAPID CARDIOPULMONARY ASSESSMENT: THE ABCs

A: Airway

Assess the ability of the child to exchange air, and evaluate the airway for the presence or absence of obstruction. If obstruction is present, the most common cause is the tongue falling back on the soft palate. The airway can be opened using either the jaw thrust or chin lift–head tilt maneuver. In a trauma patient, always stabilize the neck in a neutral position and avoid flexion or extension of the neck. The airway in a trauma patient should be opened with a jaw thrust maneuver. Any child with a significant injury above the clavicles or any unconscious child with major trauma should be assumed to have a possible neck injury requiring neck stabilization during initial care and radiologic examination as soon as is practical (see Chap. 12). The airway should be suctioned of secretions, vomitus, and debris, which may be interfering with ventilation. An oral or nasal airway may be used to improve ventilation. The choice of the correct size of the airway is important because incorrect size or placement of an airway can produce further obstruction. New-born infants are frequently obstructed by mucus and amniotic fluid, making bulb syringe suctioning an important aspect of obtaining an airway.

B: Breathing

Assess the rate of respiration and the adequacy of the air exchange by chest wall movement, the presence or absence of breath sounds (best assessed in the upper lung fields and axilla), stridor, or wheezing. Note the mechanics of ventilation, that is, the use of accessory muscles, retractions, grunting, and nasal flaring. These are important indicators of respiratory distress. Evaluate the child's color; cyanosis, mottling, or a pale or gray color are important clues of impending cardiopulmonary decompensation.

C: Circulation

The heart rate is one of the most sensitive measures of cardiovascular function in the infant or child. The carotid, femoral, brachial, and umbilical artery pulses can all be used. The brachial pulse may be the easiest to palpate in the neonate or infant. Blood pressure measurements can be misleading. Do not assume that a normal blood pressure means a normal circulatory status! The older infant and child are capable of maintaining a normal blood pressure simply by peripheral vasoconstriction even in the face of a loss of 25 percent of the circulating blood volume. Assess the presence or absence of peripheral pulses and whether they feel weak or full. The best indicator of circulatory status is end-organ perfusion, particularly of the central nervous system, kidneys, and skin.

1. CNS perfusion. Check recognition of parents, muscle tone, pupil size, and response to vocal and painful stimulation.
2. Skin perfusion. Check capillary refill (normal is 2 seconds), temperature, and color.
3. Renal perfusion. Check urine output.

BASICS OF RESUSCITATION

The most important resuscitation measure in the infant and child is ventilation. Open the airway using a jaw thrust or chin lift and attempt ventilation if the patient is not breathing adequately. In neonates or small infants, an oral or nasal airway may be necessary. If ventilation is not successful, a small shoulder roll may be necessary to position the airway properly. The correct tidal volume is the one that makes the chest wall move.

Table 21-1 Basics of Resuscitation: Ventilation and Chest Compressions

	NEONATE	INFANT (< 1 YR)	CHILD (> 1 YR)
Chest compression rate	100 to 120/min	100/min	80 to 100/min
Depth	0.5 to 0.75 in.	0.5 to 1 in.	1 to 1.5 in.
Technique	2 fingers	2 fingers	heel of hand
Respiratory rate (breaths/min)	40 to 60	20	15

In newborns, considerable pressure may be necessary to accomplish adequate ventilation. After ventilation is established, the presence or absence of a pulse should be determined. If there is no pulse, chest compressions should begin, following the depth and rate guidelines listed in Table 21-1. Proper hand positioning for chest compressions is one finger breadth below the nipple line, using two fingers in the neonate or infant and the heel of the hand in the child older than 1 year of age.

Indications for intubation include inability to ventilate with a bag and mask, the need for prolonged ventilation, the need for hyperventilation, and airway protection against aspiration.

Endotracheal tube selection is made according to the patient's size and age. The choice of an appropriate tube size is important to prevent postresuscitation iatrogenic airway complications. Guidelines for the choice of face masks, airways, and endotracheal tubes have been discussed elsewhere in this handbook.

Gastric distention is a common complication of bag–mask ventilation in children and can contribute significantly to inadequate ventilation. An orogastric tube should be used to decompress the patient's stomach if gastric distention is present, if prolonged bag–mask ventilation is needed, or if the patient is intubated and likely to remain intubated for a period of time.

NEONATAL RESUSCITATION

Newborn resuscitation differs from that of the older infant and child in some important ways. Neonates come from a wholly different environment. The maternal uterus provides all the nutrition, gas exchange, and warmth that is needed for growth and development of the fetus. The birth process also offers many opportunities for the development of fetal asphyxia, even if the pregnancy is term and establishment of an adequate placental gas exchange has taken place. The process of changing from a parasite to independent survival makes the neonate more frequently in need of resuscitation than any other age group. The way that those first few critical minutes are handled can alter the quality of life for that patient. The use of the inverted pyramid (Fig. 21-1) is a visual reminder of the order in which the neonate should be resuscitated.

The initial steps on the pyramid (drying, warming, positioning, suctioning, and tactile stimulation) will be all the resuscitation that the majority of infants require. Drying and warming are extremely important to prevent the neonate from becoming cold stressed. Neonates are extremely susceptible to heat loss, and they are particularly limited in their ability to produce heat. Hypothermia can complicate resuscitation efforts by increasing the metabolic rate and oxygen consumption and, thus, creating more acidosis. After delivery, the baby should be placed on his/her back or side with the neck slightly extended. Suctioning is done first through the mouth and then the nose with a bulb sy-

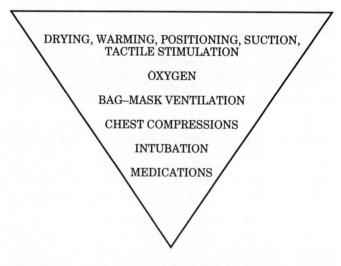

Figure 21-1 The inverted pyramid. (Reproduced with permission, *Textbook of Pediatric Advanced Life Support,* 1988. Copyright American Heart Association.)

ringe or a soft suction catheter connected to low wall suction (100 mmHg). Tactile stimulation includes rubbing the back or flicking the soles of the feet. Two attempts at tactile stimulation are all that are recommended. After these initial steps, the infant needs to be evaluated for respiratory effort, heart rate, and then color. If the infant is apneic or if the heart rate is less than 100 beats/min, further intervention is needed in a timely manner. More vigorous stimulation is to be discouraged.

The need for further resuscitation should be based on the rapid cardiopulmonary assessment of the airway, breathing, and circulation and never on the 1-min Apgar score. Positive-pressure ventilation with bag and mask and 100% oxygen is indicated if the infant is apneic or if the heart rate is less than 100 beats/min. Chest compressions should be started if the infant has a heart rate less than 60 beats/min, or if the heart rate is between 60 and 80 beats/min and is not improving. Indications for intubation are if tracheal suctioning is necessary (i.e., meconium), if prolonged positive-pressure ventilation is required, if bag–mask ventilation is ineffective, or if a diaphragmatic hernia is suspected. Medications are required if the infant's heart rate remains below 80 beats/min despite adequate ventilation with 100% oxygen and chest compressions for a minimum of 30 s, or if the heart rate is zero. An algorithm summarizing this information is available in Fig. 21-2.

The exception to the inverted pyramid rule is the child born with thick meconium staining. This infant requires intubation and suctioning of meconium before stimulation and, hopefully, before the first breath.

Thin, watery meconium may not require suctioning, particularly if the infant is vigorous and does not appear depressed. The full diameter of the endotracheal tube is required for suctioning of thick meconium. This may be accomplished with endotracheal intubation and continuous suction applied to the tube as it is withdrawn. Suction can be applied to the endotracheal tube by the use of an adaptor and a regulated wall suction device. Reintubation followed by suctioning should be repeated until returns are free of meconium. A smaller suction catheter should never be inserted down the endotracheal tube for suctioning of meconium. The size required to fit through an endotracheal tube in the newborn is too small to remove meconium adequately.

The drug of choice for neonatal resuscitation, if the heart rate does not improve with adequate ventilation and chest compressions, is epinephrine, 0.1 to 0.3 mL/kg of a 1:10,000 solution. The American Heart Association has updated its drug dosage for naloxone, to be used in the case of severe respiratory depression *and* a history of maternal narcotic administration

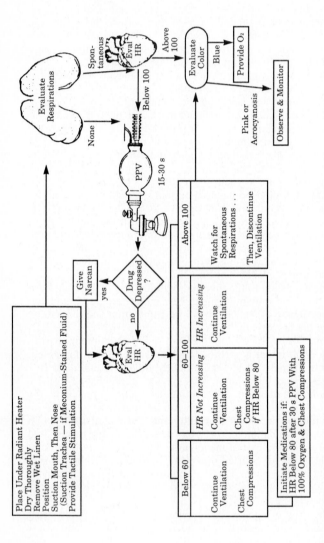

Figure 21-2 Overview of resuscitation in the delivery room. (Reproduced with permission, *Textbook of Neonatal Resuscitation*, 1987, 1990. Copyright American Heart Association.)

within the past 4 h, to 0.1 mg/kg. Both epinephrine and naloxone can be given through the endotracheal tube. Although the American Heart Association has increased the second dose of epinephrine given to children to 0.1 mg/kg (0.1 mL/kg of 1:1000 epinephrine), there has been no such change in neonates because of the risk of intraventricular hemorrhage.

Postresuscitation concerns for the neonate include hypothermia, hypovolemia, acidosis, and hypoglycemia. A heat source, such as a radiant warmer, should always be used for resuscitation. Sometimes, a heating blanket may be needed to add warmth underneath the baby. As will be discussed, the endotracheal tube may be used for instillation of certain drugs during resuscitation. However, the umbilical vein or peripheral veins may be cannulated for other medications. In the delivery room, the most common and accessible vascular route is the umbilical vein, and it may be easily catheterized with 3.5- or 5.0-French umbilical catheter with a single end hole. The catheter should be inserted into the vein until the tip is just below the skin level and free flow of blood is present. Volume expanders, such as whole blood, 5% albumin, normal saline, or Ringer's lactate, are indicated during resuscitation when there is evidence of acute bleeding with signs of hypovolemia. An infant with 10 to 15 percent loss of total blood volume may show no other signs than a slight decrease in systolic blood pressure. With 20 percent or greater blood loss in total volume, the following signs may be apparent: (1) pallor persisting after oxygenation, (2) weak pulses with a good heart rate, (3) poor response to resuscitation, and (4) decreased blood pressure. The dose for the volume expanders is 10 mL/kg given over 5 to 10 min intravenously. Metabolic acidosis that is documented or presumed may be treated with sodium bicarbonate. However, effective ventilation must precede or accompany the administration of sodium bicarbonate. Because of the risk of intraventricular hemorrhage in the neonate, a 4.2% (0.5 mEq/mL) solution of sodium bicarbonate must be used and infusion must be done slowly, at least over 2 min. The dose is 2 mEq/kg given intravenously. After an extensive resuscitation requiring medications, a neonate should have his/her blood sugar level checked and then be supported with a 10% glucose solution. Should a neonate deteriorate suddenly after a successful resuscitation, we should think of airway complications, particularly endotracheal tube obstruction, accidental extubation, endobronchial intubation, and pneumothorax.

PEDIATRIC RESUSCITATION

Again, the most important aspect of resuscitation of the infant and child is early recognition and intervention in the child in respiratory or circulatory distress to prevent cardiopulmonary arrest. The most important resuscitation intervention is providing an airway and ensuring adequate ventilation. If a child has required intubation to provide an airway, the adequacy of ventilation must still be assessed carefully to ensure against the complications of intubation, that is, esophageal intubation, endobronchial intubation, occlusion of the endotracheal tube by secretions, and barotrauma to the lungs resulting in pneumothorax. Likewise, if a child comes in from the incident site or from another hospital intubated, the position of the endotracheal tube and the adequacy of ventilation must be reassessed. If there is doubt about the endotracheal tube placement, direct visualization of the tube through the vocal cords is required. If this is impossible, it is clear that the child is not receiving adequate ventilation through the endotracheal tube, and there is no mechanical problem with the oxygen delivery system, the endotracheal tube should be removed and bag–mask ventilation resumed. Any resuscitation attempt begins with ensuring the adequacy of ventilation, with chest compressions, if appropriate, occurring either simultaneously or rapidly after the airway is secured. Figures 21-2 through 21-4 provide algorithms for various different cardiopulmonary resuscitation scenarios in the child.

Bradycardia

The first maneuver in response to pediatric bradycardia is to ensure adequate oxygenation and ventilation. The drug of choice for hemodynamically significant bradycardia is epinephrine. Careful auscultation of the lung fields to ensure the proper position of the endotracheal tube and adjustment of ventilation to improve oxygenation will treat most pediatric patients with bradycardia. If adequate oxygenation and ventilation fails to improve heart rate, then alternate causes (e.g., cardiac, vascular, or central nervous system causes, or acidosis) should be sought and treated (Fig. 21-3).

Asystole

This is the most common pediatric arrest rhythm. The most recent recommendations from the American Heart Association are to use "high-dose" epinephrine, 0.1 mg/kg (or 0.1 mL/kg of a 1:1000 solution), for the second dose should an initial dose of 0.1 mL/kg of a 1:10,000 solution fail to provide adequate results. Use of a volume bolus, 20 mL/kg of isosmotic nonglucose-containing fluid, is also recommended if resuscitation attempts are unsuccessful. Bicarbonate is useful if blood gas analysis demonstrates acidosis or if severe acidosis is suspected. Calcium is indicated if hyperkalemia, hypocalcemia, hypermagnesemia, or calcium channel overdose is suspected. Atropine is rarely help-

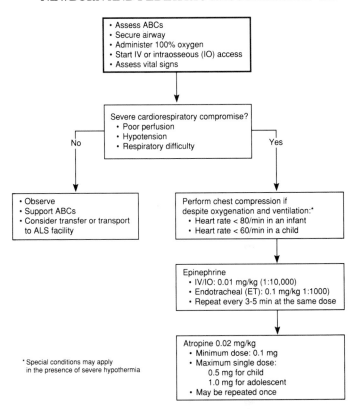

Figure 21-3 Bradycardia decision algorithm. (Reproduced with permission, *Guidelines for Cardiopulmonary Resuscitation and Emergency Cardiac Care,* 1992. Copyright American Heart Association.)

ful. Frequent reassessment of ventilation and adequacy of chest compressions is necessary (Fig. 21-4).

Ventricular Fibrillation

This is an uncommon pediatric arrest rhythm but may occur in postoperative cardiac patients. The algorithm for treatment is the same as for the adult, with immediate defibrillation required (see Fig. 21-4).

Electromechanical Dissociation

This is an ominous rhythm in which the heart displays electrical activity on the electrocardiograph but the patient has no pulse.

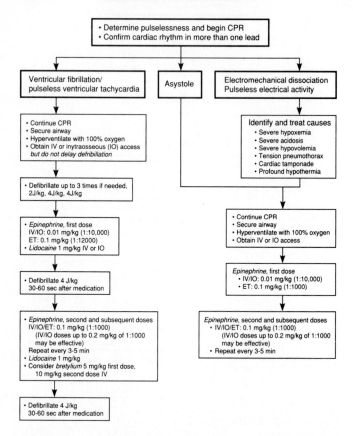

Figure 21-4 Asystole and pulseless arrest algorithm. (Reproduced with permission, *Guidelines for Cardiopulmonary Resuscitation and Emergency Cardiac Care,* 1992. Copyright American Heart Association.)

It is treated the same as asystole, with one important difference. There are some treatable causes, including tension pneumothorax, severe hypovolemia, pericardial effusion, and severe hypoxia and acidosis. Attempts should be made to diagnose and treat these problems if they exist.

Supraventricular Tachycardia

This is characterized by a heart rate of greater than 220 beats/min. If the child is stable, consult a cardiologist. If the child is unstable, the treatment is cardioversion with 0.5 J/kg, which may be increased to 2 J/kg if needed. Adenosine 0.1 mg/kg rapid intravenous bolus may also be used. If there is no effect, the dose may be doubled (maximum dose, 12 mg). In some cases, it is difficult to differentiate from sinus tachycardia resulting from hypovolemia. The history may be helpful. If cardioversion does not work, consider that the child may be hypovolemic and may benefit from a fluid challenge.

FLUID AND DRUG THERAPY

The child with adequate ventilation who is suffering from shock needs aggressive fluid therapy to prevent cardiac collapse. Appropriate resuscitation fluids include nonglucose-containing, isosmotic crystalloid or colloid. Fluid boluses are 10 mL/kg in the neonate and 20 mL/kg in the older infant and child. Fluid administration is guided by clinical signs of continuing hypovolemia (e.g., tachycardia, slow capillary refill, possibly poor blood pressure, or a diminished central nervous system perfusion) versus signs of fluid overload (rales or large heart on chest x-ray). When in doubt, the child with early or impending shock needs volume! The use of inotropes should be considered only after adequate volume replacement is accomplished or definite signs of volume overload are present, and perfusion is still poor.

Vascular Access

In children younger than 6 years of age, an intraosseous catheter should be placed after 90 s or three failed attempts at peripheral intravenous cannulation (see Chap. 12). Until this time, certain drugs may be given down the endotracheal tube. Under no circumstances should prolonged attempts to secure venous access delay the placement of an intraosseous cannula. In children older than 6 years of age, intraosseous cannulation, surgical cut down to a peripheral or central vein, or percutaneous central venous access may all be used, depending on the skill of the practitioner. If cardiopulmonary resuscitation is in progress, the femoral vein is probably the most accessible of the central veins.

The following drugs can be given down the endotracheal tube until intravenous access is established.

L: lidocaine.

E: epinephrine.

A: atropine.

N: naloxone.

Epinephrine administered down the endotracheal tube should be given in high dose of 0.1 mg/kg to ensure adequate drug levels. Other endotracheally administered drugs, naloxone, lidocaine, and atropine, should be given in slightly higher than their usual intravenous doses. (Exact endotracheal doses of other resuscitation drugs are unestablished; we use two to three times the intravenous bolus.) These drugs should be diluted in 1 to 2 mL of normal saline and followed with positive-pressure ventilation to ensure delivery to the distal airways. If intravenous or intraosseous access is available, this is the preferred site for drug administration because absorption from the endotracheal tube may be erratic.

POSTRESUSCITATION CARE

The child, immediately postresuscitation, is still in critical condition and needs frequent reassessment of respiratory and cardiac status. Any sign of deterioration requires immediate attention, with airway complications being considered first. Attention to the patient's temperature, blood glucose level, and blood gas or electrolyte abnormalities is important at this time. The patient should be transported when stabilized. Transport is a critical time, requiring that the patient have a secured airway, secure vascular access, an oro- or nasogastric tube, a Foley catheter (usually), and appropriate monitors. It is important that personnel be in attendance who are trained in pediatric resuscitation. Good communication between the referring and the accepting teams and complete medical records are essential for optimal postresuscitation care of the critically ill child.

CONCLUSIONS

In conclusion, early intervention in the child in respiratory distress or cardiovascular compromise may prevent cardiorespiratory arrest. After cardiorespiratory arrest occurs, the prognosis is markedly worse, and skilled emergent care is needed. Ventilation is the most important resuscitation maneuver in the pediatric population. With the increase in research in the field of emergency cardiac care, new recommendations are being made, questioned, and revised frequently, making it both necessary and challenging for the practitioner to stay up-to-date in this important subject.

BIBLIOGRAPHY

Bloom R, Cropley C: *Textbook of Neonatal Resuscitation*. Dallas, TX, American Heart Association and American Academy of Pediatrics, 1987.
Chameides L (ed): *Textbook of Pediatric Advanced Life Support*. Dallas, TX, American Heart Association and American Academy of Pediatrics, 1990.

Emergency Cardiac Care Committee and Subcommittees of the American Heart Association: Guidelines for cardiopulmonary resuscitation and emergency cardiac care: I. Introduction. *JAMA* 1992; 268:2172–2183.

Emergency Cardiac Care Committee and Subcommittees of the American Heart Association: Pediatric basic life support. *JAMA* 1992; 268:2251–2261.

Emergency Cardiac Care Committee and Subcommittees of the American Heart Association: Pediatric advanced life support. *JAMA* 1992; 268:2262–2275.

Emergency Cardiac Care Committee and Subcommittees of the American Heart Association: Neonatal resuscitation. *JAMA* 1992; 268:2276–2281.

Hazinski M, Chameides L: Interim training guidelines for pediatric resuscitation, in Neuman M (ed): *Currents in Emergency Cardiac Care*. Vol 3, No 4, Winter 1992, pp 20–25. Newsletter.

Keenan W, Raye J, Schell B: Interim training guidelines for neonatal resuscitation, in Neuman M (ed): *Currents in Emergency Cardiac Care*. Vol 3, No 4, Winter 1992, pp 25–26. Newsletter.

Part IV

Specialty Anesthesia

CHAPTER 22

Pediatric Orthopedics

Deborah A. Nicholas

PATIENT PROFILES

The patients evaluated and treated surgically in the practice of pediatric orthopedics are varied and range from the premature infant with a septic joint needing drainage to the infant with congenital hemivertebrae requiring emergency spinal cord decompression to the normal child with a fracture. A particular challenge to the anesthesiologist is to manage all these situations and others too numerous to discuss adequately in this chapter.

Certain patients with unusual congenital syndromes will require multiple surgical interventions to treat adequately the orthopedic manifestations of their disorders. These individuals frequently present the anesthesiologist with unique challenges. The following patient profiles are among those unusual disorders most commonly encountered by the pediatric orthopedist.

Arthrogryposis Multiplex Congenita (AMC)

Any large pediatric orthopedic service will evaluate and treat patients with AMC (multiple congenital contractures). This is a rare clinical disorder occurring in 1 in 3000 births. By contrast, 1 in 200 infants is born with dislocated hips, and 1 in 500 infants is born with clubfoot. Really, AMC is a descriptive term because there are more than 150 conditions in which multiple congenital contractures may occur. All cases of the disorder have in common a severe limitation of fetal intrauterine movement; therefore, any disease associated with a decrease in fetal intrauterine movement may result in contractures.

Etiology

The reasons for depressed fetal movement can be divided into four categories: (1) neuropathic, resulting from both central or peripheral neurogenic causes; (2) myopathic, caused by muscular degeneration or dystrophy; (3) connective tissue or joint abnormality; and (4) restrictive, in which there is decreased space in which the fetus can move. Affected children are typically born with joint rigidity, fusiform or cylindrical extremities, multiple joint fixations and muscle contractures, and possibly additional involvement (Fig. 22-1).

Classification
Children with AMC can be divided into three categories: (1) primarily limb involvement, (2) limb plus other body areas, and (3) limb plus severe central nervous system dysfunction. It should be emphasized that these children have a normal intelligence and can be expected to live a nearly normal life span.

Subtypes
There are the following subtypes: (1) amyoplasia—primarily limb, with a specific limb position of internal rotation of the

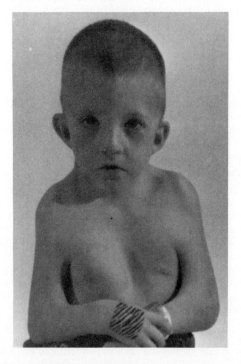

Figure 22-1   Child with arthrogryposis and Klippel-Feil syndromes. Note the short fused neck and small mouth that may contribute to a difficult intubation.

shoulders, fixed extended elbows, flexed wrists, and severe equinovarus deformities of the feet, typically severe contractures and (2) multiple pterygium (webbed joints)—includes a lethal form in which survival is rare past the neonatal period.

Anesthetic Implications
Intravenous access can be particularly difficult. The fusiform deformity and lack of skin creases creates a cylindrical extremity in which veins are hard to visualize and palpate. The underlying defects in the subcutaneous tissues cause the operator to feel false sensations as if the intravenous catheter were entering vascular structures. Craniofacial involvement can be severe, and intubation can be difficult. Head and neck involvement tends to become progressively more severe as the patient ages. In addition to craniofacial anomalies, airway compromise resulting from dysphagia and achalasia with the potential for aspiration exists in those patients with otolaryngologic manifestations. Muscular myopathies and dystrophies can be coexisting, and a careful workup should be done. Malignant hyperthermia has been said to be a risk factor, although Baines and associates reviewed cases over a 32-year period that included 67 patients having 398 anesthetics and concluded that it remains to be proven that patients with AMC are at greater risk for malignant hyperthermia.

Klippel-Feil (KF)

Originally described in 1912, KF syndrome consists of the triad of low hairline, short neck, and decreased cervical motion (Fig. 22-2). This rare disorder is estimated to occur in 1 of 40,000 births. Individuals typically seek surgical consultation for scoliosis or symptoms of cervical spinal stenosis.

Etiology
The etiology of KF has been proposed to be a disruption in the vascular supply of the subclavian artery around the 6th week of fetal life, producing predictable patterns of defects. The decreased blood supply leads to malformations of the cervical vertebrae.

Classification
Feil originally described the disorder according to the site and number of vertebrae affected (Table 22-1). The original patient described by Feil was said to have a short neck, low hairline, and severely restricted neck movement. Feil's classification has not proven to be clinically useful, and a more clinically useful classification describes the disorder as having either spondy-

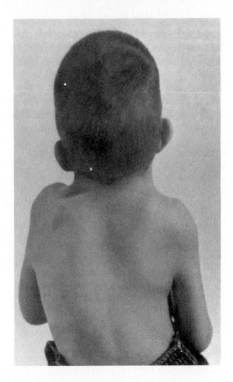

Figure 22-2 Child with classic triad of Klippel-Feil: (1) short neck, (2) low hairline, (3) severely restricted neck movement.

losis, hypermobility, or both. The patient with minimal involvement can be expected to live a normal life span and have normal intelligence. Additional abnormalities have been recorded with frequency in this syndrome. Those associated anomalies of interest to the anesthesiologist are listed in Table 22-2.

Table 22-1   Classification of Klippel-Feil Cervical Disease

Type I	Extensive cervical and thoracic spine fusion
Type II	One or two interspace fusions often associated with atlantooccipital fusion and hemivertebrae
Type III	I or II with fusion in the lower thoracic or lumbar spine

Table 22-2   Additional Abnormalities Found in Klippel-Feil Syndrome

MUSCULOSKELETAL	NEUROLOGIC	CARDIOVASCULAR	URINARY
Scoliosis	Extraocular muscle palsies	Ventricular septal defect	All types
Sprengel's	Congenital deafness		
Spina bifida occulta			

Anesthetic Implications

The anatomic cervical abnormalities and the potentially unstable neck present an anesthetic challenge for intubation. Preoperative flexion and extension cervical neck films are essential in evaluating the degree of instability. Case reports in the adult literature describe awake fiberoptic laryngoscopy as the technique of choice for securing a safe airway. This method is often unfeasible in the child, who cannot cooperate for such an invasive procedure. In the infant, fiberoptic intubation is very nearly impossible to perform because of technical limitations in the size of fiberoptic scopes and the size of the endotracheal tube required; so that other means and precautions must be relied on. Our approach to these difficult problems depends on the age of the patient. The preschool-aged patient is carefully induced with an inhalation technique, and intubation is done with an assistant holding the head and neck in a neutral position. The older school-aged child also undergoes an inhalation induction, but anesthetized fiberoptic intubation is possible in these patients. Insufflation using an endotracheal tube in one nostril provides a means of ventilation during fiberoptic intubation. The mouth is clamped shut with the left hand, which also supports the endotracheal tube. The fiberoptic laryngoscope is then passed via the other nostril into the trachea, and a second endotracheal tube is threaded over the fiberoptic scope into the trachea. An alternative is to perform anesthetized fiberoptic intubation orally through an intubation mask airway. Another option is retrograde passage of a wire guide through the cricothyroid membrane. All of these maneuvers require considerable skill. Careful intraoperative positioning of the head and neck is mandatory.

Osteogenesis Imperfecta (OI)

Etiology

This is a heritable disorder of connective tissue. It is a rare group of syndromes resulting from a defect in Type I collagen genes or protein. This group of disorders is manifest in a variety of ways, including abnormalities in bones, teeth, sclera, and ligaments. The patient may be mildly or severely afflicted (Fig. 22-3).

Classification

The most definitive and quoted classification scheme comes from Sillence and colleagues who divided the syndrome into four groups (Table 22-3).

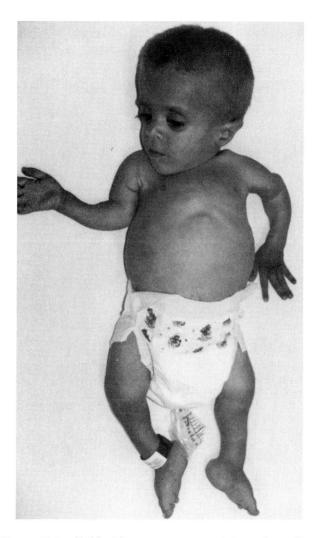

Figure 22-3 Child with severe osteogenesis imperfecta. Note bony deformities characteristic of multiple pathologic fractures due to fragile bones.

Table 22-3   Sillence Classification of OI Syndromes

TYPES	CLINICAL FINDINGS
I.	Mild bone fragility, blue sclerae, hearing loss, easy bruising
II.	Extreme fragility, perinatal death
III.	Severe fragility, fractures heal with deformity and bowing
IV.	Skeletal fragility, normal sclerae

Used with permission from Sillence DO, Senn A, Danks DM: Genetic heterogeneity in osteogenesis imperfecta. *J Med Genet* 1979; 16:101–116.

Anesthetic Implications

Hyperthermia

Patients with OI are known to have a hypermetabolic state. This can be manifested in acute episodic temperature elevations, diaphoresis, and increases in oxygen consumption. Under anesthesia, these phenomena can be misinterpreted as malignant hyperthermia. It is important not to be aggressive in usual methods to prevent intraoperative hypothermia, such as warming blankets, heated cascade humidifiers, plastic coverings, and other means of conserving body heat. In fact, it is not unusual to require some means of cooling the patient as a result of a temperature rise, especially if intraoperative tourniquets are used. The intraoperative hyperthermia of OI is not typically associated with recognized features of malignant hyperthermia, such as muscle rigidity, metabolic acidosis, hyperkalemia, clotting defects, or vascular instability. Several case reports of patients with OI and malignant hyperthermia reactions do exist, however, and OI has been stated to be a disease that can be associated with malignant hyperthermia. Careful vigilance for its symptoms is important, but avoidance of triggering agents is probably unnecessary, and the preoperative administration of dantrolene is not recommended. It may be wise to avoid anticholinergics because of the abnormal energy state.

Coagulation

Some patients with OI have easy bruising but rarely have actual problems with bleeding or hemorrhage. However, there are case reports of significant postoperative bleeding after open heart procedures. Platelet dysfunction has been stated as the cause, but the exact nature of the problem is undefined. Approximately 30 percent of patients with OI will exhibit abnormal bleeding times, enhanced capillary fragility, a reduction in factor VIII, and decreased platelet retention. The preoperative evaluation should include tests of bleeding time. The availability of platelets, fresh-frozen plasma, and cryoprecipitate may be important if clinical bleeding becomes a significant problem.

Fractures

Bone fragility is recognized as the hallmark of OI, and fractures are the primary reason patients come to the operating room. It is of extreme importance to prevent intraoperative fractures resulting from positioning, automated blood pressure devices, and other manipulation. Careful transfer of the patient from the stretcher to the operating room table, gentle face mask application and intubation, manual blood pressure determination, and even direct measurement of arterial pressure using an indwelling catheter is indicated in the most fragile patients. The use of succinylcholine could result in fractures in particularly fragile patients.

Kyphoscoliosis

Patients with OI have a high incidence of scoliosis and kyphoscoliosis. These patients can present a challenge during anesthesia for spinal surgery. Pulmonary restrictive lung disease and cor pulmonale may be present from the spinal pathology. Difficult intubation from cervical scoliosis and unstable cervical spine and problematic line insertion caused by deformities resulting from frequent fractures can complicate the anesthetic. Careful positioning is vital.

Cerebral Palsy

Cerebral palsy is one of the most common disorders presenting to the pediatric orthopedist for evaluation and treatment. It is estimated that as many as 1 in 500 school-aged children are affected. The term is used to describe a variety of disorders in which motor dysfunction or abnormal movement resulting from developmental delay is associated with perinatal injury or developmental problems in the central nervous system. These lesions are static, and although the nature and location of brain damage is variable, the disability by definition must be fixed and nonprogressive. A primary etiology is prematurity. Hemiplegia, spastic diplegia, and quadriplegia are common manifestations. There is a large spectrum of disease, and mild or severe mental and motor delay can be present.

Anesthetic Implications

Special Considerations

The child with cerebral palsy may be significantly mentally delayed, but there are those children with major physical delay and only mild or moderate mental delay. These children frequently have communication problems, secondary to their motor dysfunction. Special efforts should be made to ensure that these patients can relate their needs and questions. Teen-agers are especially sensitive to their problems in communication. Family involvement is often extremely helpful.

Seizures

Patients with global involvement often exhibit seizure disorders. There is a large spectrum of seizure types that may be present ranging from petit mal to generalized tonic–clonic disorders. A preoperative history to determine the occurrence and frequency of seizures and the measurement of the serum levels of seizure medication should be performed. Dosage adjustment of medications may be necessary and consultation with the patient's neurologist, because some patients may require large doses of medication, resulting in supranormal serum levels which may be appropriate for that particular patient. Others may have adequate seizure suppression with lower serum levels.

Airway

The preoperative evaluation should include a survey for the presence of drooling, difficulty swallowing, choking on food or liquids, and regurgitation. Preoperative medications may need to include an anticholinergic, metaclopramide, and/or an H_2 blocker. Airway management during induction may require rapid sequence induction or awake extubation.

Pulmonary

Patients with cerebral palsy are frequently ex-preemies who have residual pulmonary disease from bronchopulmonary dysplasia or who have a history of regurgitation and aspiration of gastric contents. A preoperative assessment of pulmonary function by means of peripheral arterial saturation, chest x-ray, arterial blood gas, or pulmonary function tests (if possible and indicated) may be helpful in evaluation.

Nutrition

Many patients with cerebral palsy and difficulty in swallowing, choking on food, and regurgitation will be poorly nourished. These patients tend to be those most globally affected and are typically thin, pale, or sallow in appearance. These children are generally difficult to care for and frequently have severe spasticity. It is not uncommon for these patients to present for major pelvic and/or femoral osteotomies resulting from hip subluxation. Careful preoperative assessment with particular attention to their nutritional needs must be completed. Regurgitation and feeding difficulties could be made worse postoperatively as a result of the need for spica casts. The preoperative insertion of a feeding gastrostomy and/or a Nissen fundoplication may be indicated.

Spasticity

One of the most difficult management problems for the patient with cerebral palsy is the control of spasticity. Many patients are placed on muscle relaxants, and some have required rhizotomy. There are some patients on large doses of the γ-aminobutyric acid inhibitor baclofen who may be at risk for severe intraoperative hypotension and even cardiovascular collapse. The recommendation has been made to wean these elective patients from the drug if possible. This does present some problems in these patients with severe spasticity. Careful attention to possible drug synergy and intravascular volume status is necessary in those cases in whom withdrawal is impossible or not indicated.

Postoperative Pain Management

Spastic quadriplegic and diplegic patients are some of the most difficult to manage with regard to postoperative pain control. A single caudal injection using 0.25% bupivacaine with 1:200,000 epinephrine plus 30 μg/kg kilogram of preservative-free morphine in mildly spastic patients has proven to be very effective and carries less risk in these neurologically impaired patients than do systemic narcotics. A continuous caudal infusion via catheter of 0.125% bupivacaine with 1:200,000 epinephrine plus preservative-free fentanyl 2 μg/mL of mixture infused at a dose of 0.1 to 0.2 mL/kg/h is used in the most spastic patients. These patients are monitored in a special care unit designed to care for postoperative pain patients with special needs. Additional intravenous midazolam is often required during the postoperative period to treat excessive spasticity.

SPINE PROCEDURES

Scoliosis

Scoliosis or lateral deviation of the spine is classified as idiopathic, congenital, or neuromuscular. Disorders of the spine have the potential to affect other body systems significantly. The cardiovascular, pulmonary, and neuromuscular functions can be dramatically changed with progression of the disease. The psychosocial well-being of the individual also often suffers. In the United States, the regular performance of routine school screening has improved the ability of early diagnosis, leading to earlier treatment. Progressive scoliosis has the potential for serious cardiopulmonary compromise, while progressive kyphosis can result in spinal cord compromise.

Idiopathic

The most common type of lateral curve abnormality is idiopathic scoliosis. Approximately 85 to 95 percent of idiopathic curves diagnosed are found in the adolescent population. There is a female-to-male preponderance. A consistent physical finding is vertebral rotation with curve progression. The vertebral processes, ribs, and paraspinal musculature on the convex side of the curve are drawn posteriorly, and the ribs on the concave side are thrust anteriorly. A rib hump then is detected on the convex side. Most idiopathic curves are right sided. A left rib hump should lead to the search for other etiologies as the cause of the curvature, such as neurofibromatosis. Complications of curve progression are summarized in Table 22-4.

The surgical correction of scoliosis involves instrumentation of the deformity and spinal fusion with autogenous or allograft bone. The most common instrumentations employed are the Harrington distraction, the Luque segmental instrumentation, and the Cotrel method. A new methodology, the Modulock, is

Table 22-4 Cardiopulmonary Complications of Idiopathic Scoliosis

ALL CURVES > 60°	> 80°	> 100°
Decreased vital capacity	Pulmonary hypertension	Arterial hypoxemia
Atelectasis		
Altered regional lung perfusion		
Arteriovenous shunting		

currently being used in some centers in the United States. The potential for neurologic injury is greater with the Luque method because segmental wires must be passed beneath the lamina. However, the rigid fixation from the steel rods allows the patients to be mobilized more rapidly.

The quality of the bone fusion mass is of extreme importance in the correction of scoliosis. The bone graft is commonly obtained from the iliac crest, although some scoliosis surgeons utilize a rib graft, known as a thoracoplasty, as the preferred site. The rib graft has the cosmetic advantage of removing the rib hump. Pseudarthrosis, or local failure of complete fusion, is a complication of scoliosis surgery. It is usually manifested by pain and loss of correction and must be surgically repaired to prevent loss of further correction.

Congenital

Congenital curves are the result of defective vertebral formation and differ significantly from idiopathic curves in progression and surgical methods to achieve correction. Congenital spinal defects can be divided into three groups: (1) failure of vertebral formation, such as hemivertebrae and trapezoidal vertebrae, which can produce scoliosis or kyphosis; (2) segmentation errors, characterized by incomplete separation of vertebral bodies or posterior elements or ribs; and (3) mixed abnormalities. These spinal deformities are often evident in infancy and rapidly worsen with growth. If untreated, they can produce grotesque musculoskeletal malformation and severe cardiopulmonary disease and/or spinal cord compromise.

Congenital deformities of the spine are often associated with other congenital defects such as: renal agenesis, renal pelvis, horseshoe kidney, obstructive uropathy, genital hypoplasia, diastematomyelia, congenital hip dysplasia, congenital heart disease, hearing defects, Sprengel's deformity, KF deformity, and others. A child with congenital scoliosis should be carefully evaluated for the presence of other anomalies.

Surgical correction attempts to fuse the defect or, in the case of deformities leading to spinal cord compromise, inhibit the progression of the curve with rib or fibula strut grafts. Those patients with lateral curvature can be managed surgically via a costotransverse posterior approach with the goal of operating extrapleurally. However, those patients with kyphosis leading to potential cord damage likely will require a transthoracic approach to place rib or fibula graft.

Neuromuscular

Neuromuscular scoliosis or kyphoscoliosis is the term applied to patients who have a neuromuscular etiology for their scoliosis. Spina bifida, neurofibromatosis, cerebral palsy, spinal cord trauma, arthrogryposis, and the muscular dystrophies are but a few of the numerous causes of neuromuscular scoliosis.

Children with paralytic diseases, such as myelodysplasia (myelomeningocele) can have curves of large magnitude, leading to serious cardiopulmonary complications. Neuromuscular curves can progress after maturity. Often major double curves are present, and a combination of anterior and posterior procedures are necessary to achieve correction. Anterior procedures via thoracotomy may be necessary to release a rigidly fixed curve, thereby allowing maximal posterior surgical correction. The anterior–posterior procedures may be staged or performed during one anesthetic. These are extensive surgical procedures. Spinal correction often involves extension to the sacrum. The Luque technique provides a very rigid fixation that allows early mobilization. In the respiratory-compromised patient, this may be a key factor to timely extubation and postoperative recovery.

Kyphosis

A kyphotic curve is normal in the thoracic region, the normal being 20° to 40° in the adult. Abnormal kyphosis or round back may be idiopathic, congenital, or paralytic in etiology. Extreme kyphosis can result in spinal cord compromise and paraplegia. The more severe curves are seen in Scheuermann's disease in which there is anterior wedging of the vertebral bodies. Paralytic disorders can also produce extreme kyphosis.

The surgical treatment of kyphosis often involves both anterior and posterior procedures. Surgical correction is usually reserved for adolescents with a 70° or greater curve. Correction is difficult; instrumentation failure and pseudarthrosis occur more often than in scoliosis surgery.

Anesthetic Considerations

Preoperative Evaluation

Careful evaluation of the patient is necessary to ascertain the types of intraoperative monitoring needed, determine the requirements for postoperative ventilation, and plan for postoperative pain relief. The pediatric orthopedist should have performed the proper radiologic surveys to demonstrate the lesion and searched for associated congenital anomalies as appropriate. Consultations with medical and surgical specialists should have been completed before anesthesia and anticipated orthopedic procedures.

The anesthesiologist should perform a history and physical examination pertinent to the patient and procedures planned. The airway needs to be evaluated carefully, and cervical instability must be assessed. If postoperative ventilation is planned, nares patency is taken into consideration because nasal intubation is better tolerated in the pediatric population and is the preferred route in our institution. Thoughts about invasive line placement are important to review with the patient and family. Extensive procedures require arterial lines for continuous blood pressure and periodic arterial blood gas determination and are especially essential if induced hypotension and/or hemodilution are used. Central venous lines or Swan-Ganz catheters also may be indicated. Patients and families should be given explanations of these procedures.

Pulmonary function should be assessed. At a minimum, the vital capacity and forced expiratory volume are done to predict the outcome and as an adjunct for postoperative ventilatory parameters. The preoperative chest x-ray should be examined by the anesthesiologist to assess cardiopulmonary function and to plan for central venous access if indicated. Many patients will have deformed thoracic cages, and the introduction of central lines can be difficult because of rotation of the cervical and/or thoracic spine. Arterial blood gases on room air, a complete blood count with differential, complete chemistry panel, tests of coagulation and bleeding times, and urinalysis complete the laboratory evaluation.

Premedication

The patient should be adequately premedicated. Many of these children and adolescents are anxious, anticipate pain, and are aware of the potential complications. Our premedication regimen includes a H_2 blocker and oral meperidine and pentobarbital. Patients with congenital heart disease may require antibiotic prophylaxis preoperatively.

Intraoperative Anesthetic Management

Induction and Intubation

Anesthetic induction can be accomplished either by face mask or intravenously. The ability to manage the airway successfully is paramount. Some patients may have congenital craniofacial anomalies, cervical instability, or poor neck flexion or extension caused by a disease such as arthrogryposis. Mask fits may be poor, and intubations may be difficult and require fiberoptic management. If postoperative ventilation is planned, nasal intubation is preferred.

Double-lumen tubes are utilized for thoracotomies if the condition warrants and the age of the patient is appropriate. By allowing the surgeon unrestricted access to the thoracic spine, some trauma from packing the lung is avoided, and the procedures can be accomplished more expeditiously. Most patients tolerate one-lung ventilation well. It should be noted, however, that double-lumen tubes are difficult to position properly in the patient with scoliosis. The thoracic cage is shortened as a result of the vertebral rotation, and the usual bronchial angles also are distorted. Standard endobronchial tubes often have too much length between the distal tip and the endobronchial cuff to allow correct positioning in the bronchus intermedius while avoiding secondary bronchial obstruction. Fiberoptic and chest x-ray confirmation of position is advised.

Agents

Anesthetic agents are selected first on the basis of the patient's underlying medical and surgical diseases. Probably the most popular current techniques are a low-dose inhalation agent, usually isoflurane, and a continuous infusion of a narcotic, most commonly fentanyl. Muscle relaxants are not used, except for short-acting agents for intubation. Nitrous oxide is avoided in patients with a paralytic bowel, such as those with myelodys-plasia. At our institution, intrathecal preservative-free mor-phine may be injected early in the surgical procedure in those patients in whom postoperative ventilation is planned. We have found this to be an adjunctive anesthetic agent, allowing very low-dose inhalation administration.

Monitoring

Appropriate monitoring includes the usual Harvard standards plus arterial line monitoring for continuous blood pressure and intermittent arterial blood gas sampling. Posterior instrumen-tation cases with curves greater than 40° that require extensive dissection and decortication over several levels also are moni-tored with a central line. The addition of central venous pres-sure monitoring is an aid to volume replacement and may be used to aspirate air if an air embolus occurs. In patients with pulmonary hypertension, a conventional thermodilution Swan-Ganz catheter or oximetric thermodilution pulmonary artery catheter is placed in our institution.

Positioning

Positioning is crucial for a number of reasons. The head and neck must be carefully positioned. Some surgeons utilize tables such as the Hall frame, which have U-shaped "horseshoe" head rests. Others use various polyurethane face cushions to support the face and head. These are generally unsatisfactory because unnecessary pressure is placed on the face. Access to the face by the anesthesiologist is also limited. We have developed a procedure to immobilize the head using a Mayfield tong device to suspend the head and allow complete access to the face (Fig. 22-4).

Turning to the prone position can be problematic because hypotension can result; tubes and lines must be protected, and transducers must be rezeroed promptly.

Induced Hypotension

Induced hypotensive anesthesia to reduce the intraoperative orthopedic surgical blood loss has been a popular anesthetic technique for several decades. A variety of agents have been used for this purpose, and various authors have described their methods and agents. Usual recommendations include lowering the mean blood pressure to levels of 55 to 60 mmHg, using nitroprusside or nitroglycerin, with β-blockers to prevent the increased catecholamine release seen especially with sodium nitroprusside. An inhalation agent and narcotic infusion are used for maintenance of anesthesia. Intermittent bolus of a combination α-β-blocker as a substitute for continuous vasodilator infusion may also be used. Some orthopedic surgeons are con-

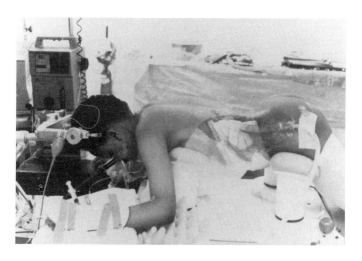

Figure 22-4 Spinal positioning on the CHOP (Children's Hospital of Philadelphia) frame with Mayfield tongs.

cerned about spinal cord blood flow and the levels of hypotension induced in their patients. We are now commonly keeping the mean blood pressure in the 60 to 65 mmHg range (systolic, 90 mmHg) for most procedures done at our institution. Monitoring must include Foley catheter and arterial and central venous lines as the minimum. Somatosensory cortical-evoked potentials can also be very helpful when induced hypotension or major manipulation of the spine is done.

Hemodilution

Deliberate normovolemic hemodilution can allow the patient to have normal intravascular filling pressures while losing blood which is relatively deficient in hemoglobin content. As long as the oxygen-carrying capacity is not seriously impaired, the patient's intravascular volume can be maintained with crystalloid and colloid. The hemoglobin-rich blood is then reinfused toward the conclusion of the procedure. Care must be taken to ensure that dilution of clotting factors does not become problematic. Hemodilution is often performed in conjunction with induced hypotension and hypothermia.

Blood Loss and Fluid Replacement

Extensive spinal surgery can be associated with the loss of 0.5 to 1.5 blood volumes. Careful estimates of ongoing losses are important. Sponges need to be weighed immediately, and an estimate of losses on the drapes and floor should be done. Hemodynamic monitoring is warranted. In large blood volume losses, metabolic acidosis may occur. Clotting abnormalities can develop from dilution of clotting factors. When using banked packed red blood cells, fibrinogen is usually depleted before platelets. Intraoperative measurement of prothrombin time, partial thromboplastin time, fibrinogen, and platelets should be performed when the blood loss exceeds 0.5 blood volume. Fresh-frozen plasma should be administered only if the clotting factors are abnormal and there is evidence of excessive bleeding in the surgical field. In pediatric patients, caution is suggested in the too rapid administration of fresh-frozen plasma or cryoprecipitate because the ionized fraction of Ca^{++} can decrease as a result of binding by the citrate used to preserve the fresh-frozen plasma. Cryoprecipitate is indicated if the measured fibrinogen decreases below 100 mg/dL and there is evidence of excessive bleeding in the wound. In our experience, it is exceedingly rare that thrombocytopenia is the cause of clotting abnormalities developing during spinal fusion.

Blood Salvage

Salvage techniques that may be utilized include autologous blood donation, cell-saving techniques, and autotransfusion methodologies. Some combination of blood salvaging should be employed in all cases in which significant blood loss is expected.

Hypothermia

The large exposure of the surgical wound creates problems in maintaining temperature homeostasis. All intravenous fluids should be warmed and inspired gases, heated and humidified. Even with all available precautions taken, hypothermia is virtually inevitable. Patients with significant hypothermia should be mechanically ventilated until temperature and acid base status is normalized (Table 22-5).

Neurologic Function Evaluation

Many surgeons are now performing spinal cord monitoring during spinal instrumentation. It should be noted, however, that such monitoring remains controversial in the orthopedic literature, and some surgeons are dubious of its value. If spinal cord monitoring is not performed, then after the surgical instrumentation is placed, a wake-up test or an evaluation of the ankle clonus test is performed to verify that no neurologic deficit is present. The anesthetic agents and adjuvants can have profound effects on these tests, and care should be taken in the choice of anesthetic. Appropriate communication with the surgeon and monitoring technicians is obviously important.

Air embolus has been reported as a complication of posterior spinal instrumentation, especially in association with the wake-up test. If a wake-up test is performed, continue to use positive

Table 22-5 Candidates for Postoperative Ventilation

Neurologic weakness

Acidosis, hypothermia

More than one blood volume loss, large volume replacement

Restrictive lung disease, pulmonary hypertension

Thoracoplasty, thoracotomy

Intrathecal morphine

pressure ventilation and avoid negative pressure ventilation in order to minimize the possibility of an air embolism.

Other Complications

Pneumothorax has been reported as a surgical complication of posterior spinal instrumentation. Other anesthetic complications that have been reported include cardiac dysrhythmias, hyperkalemia, myoglobinuria, and malignant hyperthermia.

Pain Management

Patients experience very significant postoperative pain after spinal instrumentations. Ideally, these patients should be managed by a group effort, which includes representatives from several major disciplines. Appropriate preoperative patient teaching should be done. Our regimen involves the administration of intrathecal preservative-free morphine to patients we intend to ventilate at least overnight (Table 22-5). An effective dose is 15 to 20 μg/kg administered as a single injection early in the procedure. The practice of early administration allows a decrease in the concentration of inhalation anesthetics, which is helpful in maintaining ankle clonus. Additionally, these patients are excellent candidates for patient-controlled analgesia use early in the postoperative phase.

Another alternative is epidural narcotic analgesia or caudal narcotic analgesia via indwelling catheters. Caution should be used in placing and maintaining catheters in the surgical wound. Our approach has been to tunnel the epidural catheter subcutaneously as one would for a Hickman or Broviac catheter. Biological filters should be inserted in line with the catheters, and injected drugs should be mixed under a pharmacy ventilated hood. We routinely remove such catheters after 48 h.

BIBLIOGRAPHY

Arthrogryposis

Baines DB, Douglas ID, Overton JH: Anaesthesia for patients with arthrogryposis multiplex congenita: What is the risk of malignant hyperthermia? *Anaesth Intensive Care* 1986; 14:370–372.

Hall JG: Arthrogryposis. *Am Fam Physician* 1989; 39:113–119.

Herring JA: Instructional case arthrogryposis. *J Pediatr Orthop* 1988; 8:353–355.

Laureano AN, Rybak LP: Severe otolaryngologic manifestations of arthrogryposis multiplex congenita. *Ann Otol Rhinol Laryngol* 1990; 99:94–97.

Klippel-Feil Syndrome

Bavinck JNB, Weaver DD: Subclavian artery supply disruption sequence: Hypothesis of a vascular etiology for Poland, Klippel-Feil, and Mobius anomalies. *Am J Med Genet* 1986; 23:903–918.

Daum REO, Jones DJ: Fiberoptic intubation in Klippel-Feil syndrome. *Anaesthesia* 1988; 43:18–21.

McBride WZ: Klippel-Feil syndrome. *Am Fam Physician* 1992; 45: 633–635.

Naguib M, Farag H, Ibrahim AEW: Anaesthetic considerations in Klippel-Feil syndrome. *Can J Anaesth* 1986; 33:66–70.

Winter RB, Moe JH, Lonstein JE: The incidence of Klippel-Feil syndrome in patients with congenital scoliosis and kyphosis. *Spine* 1984; 9:363–366.

Osteogenesis Imperfecta

Berkowitz ID, Raja SN, Bender KS, et al: Dwarfs: Pathophysiology and anesthetic implications. *Anesthesiology* 1990; 73:739–759.

Hortop JH, Tsipouras P, Hanley JA, et al: Cardiovascular involvement in osteogenesis imperfecta. *Circulation* 1986; 73:54–61.

Ryan CA, Al-Ghamdi A, Gayle M, et al: Osteogenesis imperfecta and hyperthermia. *Anesth Analg* 1989; 68:811–814.

Sillence DO, Senn A, Danks DM: Genetic heterogeneity in osteogenesis imperfecta. *J Med Genet* 1979; 16:101–116.

Cerebral Palsy

Eiben RM, Crocker AC: Cerebral palsy within the spectrum of developmental disabilities, in Thompson GH (ed): *Comprehensive Management of Cerebral Palsy.* New York, Grune and Stratton, 1982.

Paneth N: Birth and the origins of cerebral palsy. *N Engl J Med* 1986; 315:124.

Spine

Engler GI, et al. Somatosensory evoked potentials during Harrington instrumentation for scoliosis. *J Bone Joint Surg* 1978; 60A:529–532.

Kafer ER: Respiratory and cardiovascular functions in scoliosis and the principles of anesthetic management. *Anesthesiology* 1980; 52:339–351.

Weinstein SL: Idiopathic scoliosis: Natural history. *Spine* 1986; 11: 780–783.

Winter RB, Moe JH, Eilers VE: Congenital scoliosis: A study of 234 patients treated and untreated. *J Bone Joint Surg* 1968; 50A:15–47.

General Suggested Reading

Scoles PV (ed): *Pediatric Orthopedics in Clinical Practice.* Chicago, Year Book Medical Publishers, 1988.

Staheli LT (ed): *Fundamentals of Pediatric Orthopedics.* New York, Raven Press, 1992.

CHAPTER 23

Anesthesia for Pediatric Ear, Nose, and Throat Procedures

Susan H. Noorily
Allen D. Noorily

This chapter will describe the anesthetic management of commonly performed pediatric ear, nose, and throat procedures and the potential problems and complications that may be encountered. Pediatric airway emergencies (difficult intubations, foreign-body aspiration, epiglottis, and croup) have been discussed elsewhere in this handbook.

PEDIATRIC ENDOSCOPY AND LASER SURGERY

Endoscopy is performed on the pediatric patient for a variety of diagnostic and therapeutic reasons. It is used as an aid in diagnosing the presence of foreign bodies or other aspirated material, to evaluate the airways and esophagus after trauma, for investigating suspected pathologic or congenital abnormalities, and to obtain cultures. Endoscopy is also employed in the treatment of such problems as juvenile laryngeal papillomatosis, esophageal stenosis, and subglottic stenosis.

During such endoscopic procedures, there is an inherent conflict between the anesthesiologist's need to maintain a secure airway and the surgeon's need to visualize and obtain access to the operative site. Unfortunately, there are no ideal solutions. Various techniques have been developed, and these will be discussed. Overall, patient safety is the primary goal.

Operative Laryngoscopy, Esophagoscopy, and Bronchoscopy

Flexible and Rigid Bronchoscopes

There are two types of bronchoscopes in use for pediatric endoscopy. Flexible bronchoscopes are used primarily to diagnose airway pathologic conditions and as an aid to difficult intubations. The flexible bronchoscope provides access to distal airways that are not accessible to rigid bronchoscopes. The procedure can be performed in some children who are awake by using topical anesthesia. A major disadvantage of this type of bronchoscope is that it has a very small diameter. Instrumentation and suctioning are therefore difficult, and the fibers are easily damaged. In addition, the flexible bronchoscope is more difficult to sterilize.

Rigid bronchoscopes offer the advantage of a higher quality image and a large channel for instrumentation. This bronchoscope has two components (Fig. 23-1), a hollow metal tube, called a *sheath,* and a *telescope,* which houses a high-intensity halogen bulb that transmits light through tiny fibers, delivers

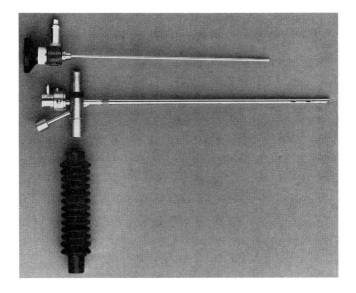

Figure 23-1 The bronchoscope has two components, the hollow metal tube, or sheath, and the telescope (top), which delivers high-intensity illumination and magnifies the operative site.

high-intensity illumination, and magnifies the operative site. The telescope fits within the sheath, and as a rule, visualization of the airway is performed with the telescope in place. Manipulation of the airway is performed with the telescope removed. There will be an air leak through the sheath if the telescope is not in place. Other methods of sealing this leak include the use of a sliding glass cover over the end of the bronchoscopic sheath and the application of the surgeon's thumb.

Pediatric sheaths are classified as infant or child size based on length. They are available in a range of diameters. The outer diameter (OD) of the bronchoscope corresponds to the OD of an endotracheal tube. Telescopes also come in varied sizes. This information is important to the anesthesiologist for several reasons.

The first is that a tight fit of the sheath within the patient's airway can result in mucosal ischemia and postoperative airway edema. Next, airflow through a small sheath becomes turbulent, such that resistance will increase as the flow rate is increased. Also, airflow through a small sheath can be inadequate for gas exchange. Recall that resistance is inversely proportional to the fourth power of the radius. High resistance impedes gas flow. Positive-pressure ventilation will be impaired and will require greater inspiratory pressures. In addition, the passive recoil of the infant lung and chest wall may be insufficient to allow adequate emptying, resulting in increased lung volume. Air trapping can occur with barotrauma and hemodynamic compromise, especially in paralyzed patients. Healthy infants can usually maintain adequate gas exchange for short periods of time while under general anesthesia. High resistance is more likely to be a hazard to sick infants.

The placement of the telescope will further impede air flow because it can occupy nearly the entire internal lumen of the small bronchoscopic sheaths. It is impossible to ventilate through a bronchoscope smaller than 3.0 mm when the telescope is in place.

To offset these potential dangers, it is best to allow spontaneous ventilation when feasible, use long expiratory times, periodically remove the telescope, and deliver low flows of O_2 (1 L/min) when the smallest sheaths are in use.

There are two types of rigid bronchoscopes. With the ventilating bronchoscope, instrumentation can be performed while positive-pressure ventilation is provided. This is accomplished with the two side ports within the bronchoscope sheath. When in use, both side ports must be past the glottis for adequate ventilation to occur. By contrast, an open bronchoscope allows simultaneous ventilation and instrumentation when a needle is attached to its proximal end (Fig. 23-2). The needle delivers in-

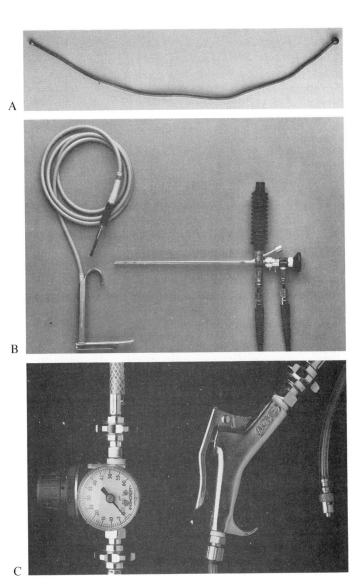

Figure 23-2 (A) Jet injector allows simultaneous ventilation and instrumentation using the Venturi effect. (B) The ventilating bronchoscope also allows ventilation during instrumentation, as long as both side ports are past the glottis. (C) Jet ventilation device-pressure output is controlled by adjusting the pressure valve on the handle. A good starting pressure in children is approximately 10 to 15 psi.

termittent bursts of oxygen at high pressure. This system is referred to as a jet injector (Sanders injector).

With the jet injector system, a Venturi effect is created, using room air. The patient receives less than 100% oxygen. Generally, good chest expansion can occur and will result in satisfactory ventilation at normal inflation pressures in adults and older children. In small children, the bronchoscopic lumen decreases in size and may fit tightly in the airway. A relatively strong jet may produce dangerously high inflation pressures. Expired gas may be unable to leak back around the bronchoscope through the glottis, and the lung will not completely empty. This can result in barotrauma and hemodynamic instability. Therefore, for safe ventilation in pediatric patients, a lower range of pressures should be used (10 to 20 psi for infants and 20 to 40 psi for older children).

Preoperative Evaluation

Most pediatric patients presenting for endoscopy have some degree of airway compromise. Many of these patients require multiple procedures. If an anesthesia record from a previous procedure is available, it can be extremely helpful. The old record will provide information regarding the ease of intubation, occurrence of airway obstruction, size of endotracheal tube and/or bronchoscope, anesthetic technique, and presence of postoperative stridor.

Some patients will have a history of prematurity or respiratory distress syndrome and abnormal pulmonary function. Some children will have a history of airway obstruction. The child may have a recent or current respiratory infection. All these factors play an important role in the anesthetic management.

The physical examination should focus on airway abnormalities and the cardiopulmonary system. Extensive laboratory tests are not necessary in most instances. A hemoglobin level may be useful because anemia can result in impaired tissue oxygenation. A chest x-ray should be taken if airway lesions or pulmonary impairment is suspected. This will also assess the efficacy of the bronchoscopy in patients requiring removal of a foreign body.

Anesthetic Management

Each patient and indication for endoscopy is different. Therefore, no best single anesthetic technique exists.

An older, cooperative child may tolerate being awake for endoscopy, especially when a flexible bronchoscope is used. Topical anesthesia alone is usually inadequate because the receptors for the gag reflex are deep to the surface mucosa. The gag reflex is mediated through cranial nerves IX and X. Cranial nerve IX can be blocked by injections into the palatoglossal arch bilaterally. Cranial nerve X can be blocked with topical anesthesia to the larynx, epiglottis, and pyriform sinus as a supplement to the injections. It is important to measure carefully the volume of local anesthetic used so that overdosage does not occur.

The majority of pediatric patients presenting for endoscopy will require general anesthesia. Premedication is not always necessary, but consideration should be given to the administration of drugs that block airway reflexes (e.g., anticholinergics or local anesthetics) and decrease gastric acidity and volume. Preoperative sedatives and narcotics should be avoided in the presence of any airway obstruction.

There are three methods of ventilation during bronchoscopy. One is an apneic technique. This is perhaps the least desirable method because the airway is not protected. The procedure time is limited for the surgeon. Hypoventilation can result in respiratory acidosis and dysrhythmias. The second, and most common, method is use of a ventilating bronchoscope through which inhalation anesthesia can be maintained. The risks include barotrauma and inadequate gas exchange, as previously discussed. The third method is jet ventilation. Its advantages include a better visual field for the surgeon and less interference with instrumentation. Anesthesia must be maintained with intravenous agents. Muscle relaxants are required. There are the risks of pneumothorax, inflation of the stomach, aspiration, and mucosal dehydration.

There are a few anesthetic goals that are shared independent of the technique used. The most important is preservation of adequate oxygenation and ventilation. Care must be taken during suctioning because this can remove oxygen from the airway and decrease the lung volume, promoting atelectasis. Some patients have pneumonia as a result of a foreign body. The foreign body must be removed before the resolution of the pneumonia. Maintaining adequate oxygenation in these patients can be challenging when the bronchoscope is in place because shunting occurs. In this case, the surgeon will have to pull the bronchoscope periodically back to ventilate the "good" lung to maintain a safe oxygen saturation. For all endoscopic procedures, the patient must remain still. Finally, every attempt should be made to achieve a rapid return of airway reflexes and consciousness at the end of the procedure.

Induction can be accomplished with an inhalational or intravenous technique. The choice will be based on airway anatomy and pathologic findings, the availability of intravenous access, and the patient's age. An endotracheal tube may be passed before the introduction of the bronchoscope, but this is not always necessary. Some surgeons prefer mask ventilation followed immediately by bronchoscopic intubation to minimize airway instrumentation.

At the end of the procedure, a child with an empty stomach and no airway compromise can be ventilated through a mask until awake. Otherwise, an endotracheal tube must be placed and not removed until the child is fully awake. Because stridor is common postoperatively, corticosteroids are often empirically administered before the procedure. In addition, racemic epinephrine (0.05 mL/kg) can be delivered by a nebulizer in the recovery room. A small percentage of patients will require reintubation as a result of upper airway edema. In this instance, an endotracheal tube smaller than the original one should be chosen.

Laryngeal Microsurgery with the Laser

Introduction to Laser Use

The word *laser* is an acronym for "light amplification by the stimulated emission of radiation." Several types of lasers are used in the various surgical subspecialties. The two types used for airway surgery are the CO_2 laser and the Nd:YAG laser. A laser acts as a very high-intensity beam light that is focused on a small spot causing precisely controlled incision, coagulation, or vaporization of tissue. The CO_2 laser emits infrared light, which is easily absorbed by the water contained in tissues. It is therefore used for excision of soft tissue. The Nd:YAG laser light is better absorbed by pigmented tissue. Laser light is potentially dangerous to anyone in the vicinity of its use if precautions are not taken. An accidentally misdirected or reflected beam of light can cause a burn.

Indications

The CO_2 laser is most frequently used in pediatric airway procedures to manage juvenile laryngeal papillomatosis. These are viral tumors that multiply and produce significant airway obstruction. Multiple laser procedures over several years are required to maintain a patent airway in these children because surgical destruction is only palliative. In most cases, these tumors regress spontaneously as the patient reaches puberty.

Anesthetic Management and Safety Precautions

Many of the principles that apply to pediatric bronchoscopy are important during laser surgery of the airway. In addition, laser surgery has some inherent hazards. The laser beam can ignite flammable materials, such as endotracheal tubes, breathing circuits, drapes, and lubricants. Smoke and products of combustion are generated. Human tissue can also be burned; the eyes are particularly vulnerable. Safety precautions can prevent most serious injuries. Eye protection is required for the patient and all operating room personnel because the CO_2 laser can cause corneal burns and retinal injury. Moistened eye patches and/or safety goggles will suffice. All metallic surfaces and exposed areas of the patient's skin must be covered with moist towels. Doorways should be labeled "laser in use." A final consideration is that special masks be worn by operating room personnel to prevent inhalation of smoke, which can contain viral particles if the laser surgery is being done for juvenile laryngeal papillomatosis.

Airway laser surgery is generally performed with the patient under general anesthesia. A patent airway and ventilation can be maintained either with or without an endotracheal tube in place. The advantages of using an endotracheal tube include assurance of a secure airway, protection of lower airways from tissue debris if a cuff is used, and avoidance of operating room pollution from anesthetic gases. However, there are also some disadvantages of placing an endotracheal tube. The endotracheal tube will obstruct the surgical site. Nonmetal tubes are combustible and can be ignited during laser surgery. The products of combustion can cause tracheobronchial or lung injury.

If an endotracheal tube is placed, there are a few options. Several varieties of metal tubes are available. The large sizes will have a cuff, which is inflated with saline solution so that if perforation occurs, any ignition site will be extinguished. The cuff should be protected with moistened gauze or cottonoids by the operating surgeon during laser use.

Another option is to protect a nonmetal tube. Most commonly, red rubber tubes are wrapped with metallic tape. The laser beam will be deflected off the metal tape. The surgeon should place moistened cottonoids around the endotracheal tube. The endotracheal tube cuff must be protected by a saline-soaked gauze cover. Saline must be used to fill the cuff instead of air. Wrapped tubes are not foolproof because burning material contacting the inner lumen can ignite the tube. Rough tape edges can injure tissues. The tape can detach and become a foreign body. Wrapping nonmetal endotracheal tubes with metallic tape does not offer protection from the Nd:YAG laser.

Although not recommended, unprotected tubes are sometimes used. Polyvinyl chloride, red rubber, and silicone can all be ignited by a focused CO_2 laser beam in the presence of 100% oxygen. If one of these tubes must be used, the oxygen concentration must be kept at or below 30%. Nitrous oxide will support combustion and should be avoided. Helium retards ignition better than air, but either can be used to reduce the oxygen concentration. The laser should be used at the minimum power setting, never more than 10 W, and the power burst should be limited to 10 s.

In a recent study, both stainless-steel tubes and copper or aluminum foil-wrapped red rubber tubes were not affected by the CO_2 laser, whereas plain red rubber endotracheal tubes and a specially manufactured tube of silicone and metal burned under laser fire.

Because of these risks, many anesthesiologists choose to do laser anesthetics without an endotracheal tube in place. One technique is pharyngeal insufflation by a nasopharyngeal catheter placed above the vocal cords. High-flow anesthetic gases are supplied, and the patient is allowed to breathe spontaneously. A suction catheter is placed near the patient's mouth to decrease "pollution." There are many disadvantages to this technique, including an unprotected airway, the risk of laryngospasm, stomach distention, catheter occlusion, hypoventilation, and operating room pollution.

Apneic techniques can also be employed. One method is to use controlled ventilation by mask or endotracheal tube with intermittent periods of apnea during laser use. The endotracheal tube would be removed before laser use and replaced at the first sign of decreasing oxygen saturation.

Jet ventilation, as described in the previous section, is a very effective method of ventilating patients during laser surgery. The jet injector cannot be composed of flammable material. Jet ventilation has been used in combination with endotracheal tube ventilation to provide the surgeon with access to supra- and subglottic areas of the vocal cords. Jet ventilation is contraindicated when major airway obstruction is present because of the increased risk of inadequate lung emptying and the resulting barotrauma.

Some patients requiring laser surgery of the airway will have a tracheotomy. Patients who are ventilated through a tracheotomy should never be anesthetized with a plastic tube during airway laser surgery. A metal tracheostomy tube should always be used. Metal tracheostomy tubes should not be fenestrated or the laser beam might travel down the trachea.

Before anesthetic induction, it is essential to have readily available emergency airway equipment. The surgeon must be present and prepared to secure the airway either endoscopically or surgically. Plans for the management of airway obstruction and fire should be discussed in advance.

It is preferable, but not necessary, to have intravenous access before induction. Preoperative atropine or glycopyrrolate administration should be considered to prevent excessive secretions and bradycardia. Inhalation induction with high oxygen concentrations is considered the safest method in children with airway pathologic disorders. Paralysis should be avoided until the airway is securely managed.

Anesthetic agents used during laser surgery will depend on the technique used. Volatile anesthetics are considered safe during laser procedures. The patient must not move during laser use, and muscle relaxants are usually administered. Dexamethasone (0.5 mg/kg) is given prophylactically for anticipated airway edema. Guidelines for emergence and extubation are the same as for bronchoscopy.

Management of Endotracheal Tube Fire

In the event of an endotracheal tube fire, the following steps should be taken:

1. Stop the gas flow.
2. Disconnect from the breathing system and extubate the patient.
3. Ventilate through the mask until reintubation is possible.
4. Reintubate.
5. Perform bronchoscopy immediately to assess the extent of the injury.
6. If the injury is severe, a tracheotomy should be performed.
7. Administer steroids (and antibiotics if indicated).
8. Admit to the intensive care unit.

The injury to the tracheobronchial tree occurs as a result of both the burn and toxicity from the products of combustion and smoke inhalation.

TONSILLECTOMY, ADENOIDECTOMY, AND OBSTRUCTIVE SLEEP APNEA

Tonsillectomy and Adenoidectomy

Background Information
Tonsillectomy and adenoidectomy are among the most commonly performed operations in the pediatric population. In the 1970s, it was estimated that approximately 750,000 children underwent one, or both, of these surgical procedures. More recently, this number has decreased because of the more specific indications for these operations and better antibiotic management of infections. The indications for adenotonsillectomy are varied and sometimes controversial. It is most often performed in children who have recurrent or chronic debilitating infections, acute peritonsillar abscess, or chronic upper airway ob-

struction from hyperplasia of the adenoids and tonsils (Fig. 23-3).

Adenotonsillectomy is usually performed as an outpatient procedure. In the past, this practice was considered controversial because of the shortened period of postoperative observation. Although the mortality rate from tonsillectomy is low, most deaths are associated with hypovolemia or airway compromise occurring as a result of postoperative bleeding. It is currently thought that outpatient adenotonsillectomy with a postoperative observation period of 3.5 to 6 h before discharge home is safe practice when the patient has good oral intake, a temperature of 38.5°C or less, no signs of airway distress, and no history of obstructive sleep apnea or other serious medical problems and lives a reasonable distance from the hospital.

Anesthetic Considerations

A careful medical history and physical examination should be performed. Inquire about any recent or current viral infections. It is important to consider the possibility of undiagnosed obstructive sleep apnea (OSA) in all children presenting for adenotonsillectomy, especially if there is a history of loud snoring. Therefore, a thorough cardiopulmonary history should be taken. (This will be discussed in greater detail in the section on OSA.) Parents should be questioned about recent aspirin ingestion because this can cause platelet dysfunction and lead to excessive perioperative bleeding.

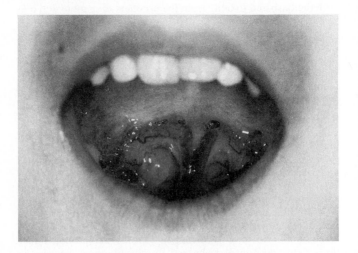

Figure 23-3 Hypertrophy of adenoids and tonsils.

Premedication is chosen on an individual basis. Antisialagogues and antiemetic medications can be useful. Atropine or glycopyrrolate is recommended to prevent vagal arrhythmias. Sedatives and hypnotics should be administered with extreme caution if airway obstruction is a significant factor because sedation and anesthesia can exacerbate OSA.

General anesthesia is the technique of choice in pediatric patients. In most cases, induction can take place either by inhalation or intravenous routes. Keep in mind that induction in a patient with OSA can provoke airway obstruction. This can usually be alleviated by jaw thrust or placement of an oral or nasopharyngeal airway, noting that a nasal airway might cause an adenoidal bleed. If the patient has normal airway anatomy and an uncomplicated intubation is anticipated, an intravenous induction is usually appropriate. It is essential to have equipment available for an unsuspected difficult intubation and emergency cricothyrotomy. If a difficult intubation is anticipated, an awake intubation should be performed when possible. However, in children, an inhalation induction with spontaneous ventilation is usually a more realistic alternative. Again, emergency airway equipment must be readily available.

An oral RAE (Ring-Adair-Elwyn, Glens Falls, NY) endotracheal tube is the preferred tube for this procedure. It is taped to the mandible, allowing for good surgical exposure. Before the incision, the surgeon will insert a mouth gag. It is important to check for breath sounds after gag placement because the endotracheal tube can be displaced or compressed by the gag.

Maintenance of anesthesia can be accomplished with either volatile gases as sole agents or in combination with other drugs. The patient must not move. Muscle relaxants are acceptable but need to be completely reversed at the end of the procedure before extubation. Steroids are sometimes administered to help reduce tissue edema. Postoperative pain can be significant, and a small dose of narcotic should be considered. Some surgeons infiltrate the operative field with a long-acting local anesthetic, which provides some postoperative pain relief. When local anesthetics are used, there may be complaints of difficulty swallowing because of inability to sense the action of the pharyngeal muscles. This may also produce drooling, although the airway is not compromised.

It is difficult to determine the exact blood loss that occurs during adenotonsillectomy, but on average, 5 to 10 percent of the patient's estimated blood volume is lost, depending on the technique employed. (If electrocautery is used as the sole surgical instrument for the procedure, then a blood loss of only 5 to 10 mL can be expected. If electrocautery is not used at all, the blood loss will be higher.) In addition to this, a significant amount enters the gastrointestinal tract. Therefore, an orogastric tube should be passed at the end of the procedure to empty the stomach with suction. Blood in the stomach is a potent stimulus for nausea. The nasopharynx also requires gentle suctioning. The mouth should be inspected for blood, blood clots, active bleeding, and other debris. Any throat packs, if used, must be removed. A potential complication of electrocautery use is thrombosis of the internal carotid artery. This can occur because the internal carotid artery is only a few millimeters from the operative site.

Deep versus awake extubation causes debate among some practitioners. Advocates of deep extubation claim that emergence is smoother, quicker, and accompanied by less coughing and blood pressure elevation. Although this may be true, an awake patient has protective airway reflexes intact and is better able to maintain airway patency. This may make awake extubation the safer alternative in certain patients, particularly those with OSA.

Patients are often transported to the recovery room in the lateral head-down or "tonsillar" position to prevent aspiration of blood and contact of secretions with the vocal cords, which could cause laryngospasm, especially in a patient who is not fully awake. In the recovery room, intravenous hydration should be continued because most children will be unable to take oral fluids for several hours.

Patients with OSA should be admitted to an intensive care area overnight. Relief of the obstruction does not always immediately relieve the apnea, and airway obstruction may persist postoperatively for a variable period of time.

Postoperative Bleeding

The most frequent complication associated with adenotonsillectomy is postoperative bleeding, possibly resulting in hypovolemia or airway obstruction. There are two vulnerable periods of potential rebleeding—up to 8 h after surgery and 1 week later. The majority of early postoperative bleeding occurs within the first 6 h. Most bleeding occurs as a slow oozing and manifests when the patient vomits a large volume of blood. When this happens, the patient needs to be rehydrated.

If the surgeon does not think that the bleeding can be controlled conservatively, the patient will be brought back to the operating room. Approximately 3 percent of patients who bleed postoperatively will return to the operating room. There are many potential dangers involved in reanesthetizing these patients. The patient can have respiratory obstruction from a blood clot, leading to hypoxia. The patient may be hypovolemic. The combination of hypoxia and hypovolemia can lead to cardiac arrest. The patient is considered to have a full stomach, making aspiration a hazard. The following are some suggestions to consider when faced with this emergency situation.

Preoperative

1. Draw blood for type and cross (if not already done) and hematocrit.
2. Ensure functioning intravenous line.
3. Restore the blood volume to normal.
4. Remove loose clots from the tonsillar beds and postnasal space with forceps.
5. Attempt to empty the stomach.

Induction

1. Have a large-bore suction readily available.
2. Emergency airway equipment and surgeons should be present.
3. Possible techniques:
    a. Intravenous rapid-sequence induction. Ketamine or etomidate may be the best choices for use as an induction agent when the intravascular volume status is uncertain.
    b. Inhalation induction with high oxygen concentrations and cricoid pressure is an alternative.
    c. Awake intubation would be ideal, but is difficult in children.

If bleeding is active, the head can be held in the lateral position during induction.

OSA

Background Information
As previously discussed, adenotonsillectomy is now a surgical procedure used to alleviate OSA. Hyperplastic tonsils and adenoids can cause very mild to very severe obstruction. In these patients, relaxation of the pharyngeal muscles during sleep produces airway obstruction when tonsillar and adenoidal tissues collapse into the airway. The diagnosis of OSA is made by a sleep study in which there are five episodes of apnea per hour, each lasting for at least 10 s, and a total of 35 episodes in a 7-h sleep period.

The patient with OSA may demonstrate signs of obstruction only during sleep. These signs include loud snoring, irregular respiratory patterns, breath pauses, and apnea. Respiration is usually noisy. Sleep disturbances are common. Chronic mouth

breathing, difficulty swallowing, and orthodontic malformations may be consequences of chronic obstruction.

Obesity is common among children with OSA. In addition to
enlarged tonsils and adenoids, a large uvula, long soft palate,
macroglossia, or retrognathia may cause OSA. Congenital
anomalies, such as Pierre Robin and Treacher-Collins syndromes, are associated with apnea. Children with neuromuscular disorders may obstruct from a lack of pharyngeal support.
Patients with Down's syndrome have frequent obstruction.
Children with pharyngeal flap corrections for cleft palate can
get OSA.

Cardiorespiratory Syndrome

Daytime somnolence and cor pulmonale are the most dramatic
effects of chronic obstruction from adenotonsillar hyperplasia.
This end-stage disease, sometimes referred to as cardiorespiratory syndrome, is uncommon. Treatment of such patients
may include medical therapy with digoxin, diuretics, steroids,
and supplemental oxygen. These patients may require airway
support with a nasopharyngeal airway or endotracheal tube.
Surgical procedures such as adenotonsillectomy, uvulopalato-
pharyngoplasty, and tracheostomy are often performed.

Management of OSA

In children, the tonsils and adenoids may be so hypertrophic
that they encroach on the airway, and in this case, adenotonsillectomy should be performed. However, there are no absolute
guidelines regarding the degree of obstruction that unequivo-
cally indicates the need for adenotonsillectomy.

A history and physical examination specifically directed at
the signs and symptoms of obstruction will usually be adequate
to diagnose airway obstruction from adenotonsillar hyperplasia. A description of the child's breathing during sleep is most
helpful. A cardiopulmonary history is essential to rule out right-
sided heart failure and pulmonary hypertension. An electrocardiogram should be obtained in the presence of an abnormal
chest x-ray, a history of exercise intolerance, or hepatic enlargement to look for right-axis deviation. On physical examination, an increased respiratory rate and loud P_2 would alert to
the possibility of more severe obstructive disease. If the history
and physical examination prove to be unhelpful when OSA is
suspected, a sleep study (polysomnograph) should be performed to help define the problem.

If surgical treatment of OSA is planned, the child must be
optimally managed medically before proceeding. Postoperative
intensive care should be anticipated and arranged for at least

24 h. A reversal of cardiopulmonary dysfunction by adenoton-sillectomy has been reported if an early diagnosis is made.

EAR SURGERY

Myringotomy and Tympanostomy Tube Insertion

The insertion of tympanostomy tubes is the most common operation performed in the United States (approximately 2 million per year) and is the most common procedure performed in pediatric outpatients.

The major indication for this procedure is chronic otitis media with effusion caused by poor eustachian tube function. Eustachian tube dysfunction may result from immaturity, respiratory tract infection, allergy, anatomic abnormality (cleft palate for example), excessive adenoidal tissue, abnormal ciliary function, compromised immunity, and nasopharyngeal tumors. This extensive list illustrates the wide spectrum of patients presenting for tympanostomy tubes, although most are healthy children. Otitis media is the most common disease of childhood, with the exception of viral upper respiratory tract infections. Tympanostomy tubes function by allowing sustained middle ear ventilation.

An experienced surgeon can usually perform this procedure in 10 min or less with the aid of an operating microscope. Therefore, in most cases, these children receive general anesthesia with an inhalation induction and maintenance by mask. Many anesthesiologists do not place intravenous catheters in healthy children because this can double the anesthesia time. Others place intravenous catheters in all patients, as a safety precaution. During the procedure, it is best to keep the patient stationary and move the operating microscope from one side of the table to the other. The surgeon may ask that the patient's head be turned slightly to allow better visualization of the tympanic membrane. The surgical incision of myringotomy is intensely painful, and therefore, the patient must be well anesthetized before the incision is made. However, children generally require little postoperative analgesia, allowing them to awaken easily and take fluids before discharge.

Nitrous Oxide Use

Nitrous oxide (N_2O) is 34 times more soluble than nitrogen. This can cause problems in a closed space because N_2O will enter the space faster than the nitrogen can escape. The volume of gas in the closed space will expand if the space is compliant. In a noncompliant space, the pressure will increase.

The middle ear is an air-filled, noncompliant space. Many studies have documented increases in middle ear pressure during N_2O use (Fig. 23-4). A patent eustachian tube will help to decompress the middle ear. If there is underlying ear disease, however, or edema from surgical trauma, this equalization of pressure may not occur. Tympanic membrane rupture and displacement of surgical grafts have been reported, although cases such as these are admittedly rare. Conversely, cessation of N_2O delivery might result in negative pressure.

Practically speaking, in middle ear operations, a closed space does not exist until the surgeon begins to close the middle ear. Each surgeon has their own individual bias regarding the use of N_2O during middle ear surgery. It is prudent to ask the surgeon about these concerns. If N_2O is believed to be an important addition to the anesthetic, it can be used if it is discontinued several (30 to 45) minutes before closing begins or at any time the surgeon appears to have difficulty with graft placement.

Induced Hypotension

A bloodless operative field is helpful to otologists performing microsurgery of the ear because a very small amount of blood can obscure their view. To achieve this goal, some anesthesiol-

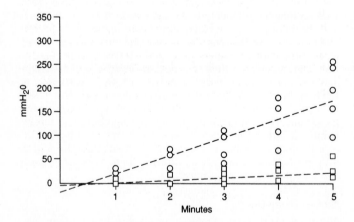

Figure 23-4 Middle ear pressure (vertical axis) versus time when exposed to nitrous oxide (upper curve ○) compared with control (□). (Reproduced with permission from Casey WF, Drake-Lee AB: Nitrous oxide and middle ear pressure: a study of induction methods in children. *Anaesthesia* 1982; 37:896–900.)

ogists have used induced hypotension; others have failed to find a correlation between the degree of hypotension and the surgeon's assessment of operating conditions. Young, healthy patients tolerate hypotension well, but compromised patients may be unable to perfuse vital organs sufficiently.

Other measures can be used to improve operating conditions. Many surgeons prefer to infiltrate the tissues with epinephrine to minimize blood loss. Traditionally, the maximal allowable dose of epinephrine without local anesthetic is 2 μg/kg when used with halothane and 3 to 5 μg/kg when used with isoflurane or enflurane. Elevation of the head of the operating table will promote venous drainage. However, this will also increase the risk of venous air embolism and may lower the blood pressure.

Use of Neuromuscular Blocking Agents

Facial nerve identification and preservation is an important part of otologic surgery. The use of neuromuscular blocking drugs during these procedures has been questioned. It is possible to provide skeletal muscle relaxation without complete paralysis. A surgeon, therefore, can elicit a response from direct nerve stimulation, even in the presence of small doses of these drugs. However, if the patient has any degree of facial nerve dysfunction preoperatively, neuromuscular blocking agents might interfere with nerve identification. In this case, such drugs, especially long-acting agents, are best avoided.

Both the surgeon and anesthesiologist agree that patient safety is of utmost importance. An immobile patient is essential during microsurgical procedures. Volatile anesthetic agents are ideal for microsurgery of the middle ear because N_2O and long-acting neuromuscular blocking drugs can be avoided, and a slightly lowered blood pressure, if desired, can be easily achieved.

Postoperative Care

Nausea and dizziness are common in patients who have had ear surgery. Therefore, consideration should be given intraoperatively to the avoidance of high-dose narcotics and administration of prophylactic antiemetic medication.

THE CHILD WITH UPPER RESPIRATORY SYMPTOMS

It is appreciated that many children with ear, nose, and throat complaints frequently have a runny nose. Is it safe to anesthetize a child who has a runny nose? The answer to this question is not clear-cut. Each patient is different, and the most important step in making a decision is to arrive at an appropriate diagnosis. Allergies and infections, which present with upper respiratory symptoms, are common medical problems in children—we must distinguish between these two processes.

Pediatric patients scheduled for ear, nose, and throat procedures often have infections within the tonsils, adenoids, or ears. These conditions often present with fevers and upper respiratory symptoms. At times, the prescribed surgical procedure is the only way to break the cycle of recurrent infections. Repeated postponement of the procedure does not help the situation. Each patient history must be carefully evaluated before administering an anesthetic in such cases because automatic cancellation of surgery creates a hardship for the child, family, and surgeon.

Noninfectious Causes of Upper Respiratory Symptoms

Vasomotor rhinitis and allergic rhinitis are causes of noninfectious upper respiratory symptoms. A crying child may develop a runny nose—a common scenario preoperatively. Children with allergies may also have a runny nose, and therefore, the parents must be carefully questioned about the precise symptoms. If they respond by saying that their child "is always like this," a noninfectious cause is probable. Children with noninfectious runny noses are candidates for elective surgery.

A major concern for the anesthesiologist is abundant secretions, which can lead to laryngospasm, coughing, apnea, and hypoxia. Also, allergic rhinitis can be a prodrome of asthma. Therefore, elective surgery is best scheduled in the allergic "off" season. These children will require supplemental oxygen and oxygen saturation monitoring during the postoperative recovery period.

Infectious Causes of Upper Respiratory Symptoms

Viral Respiratory Tract Infections

Certain viruses result in infections localized primarily in the upper airway, causing copious upper airway secretions and increased airway reactivity. Those viruses causing infections of the lower respiratory tract are more dangerous because their result can be increased reactivity, decreased compliance, and bronchospasm.

A child who has an upper respiratory infection will be sick for 2 or 3 days and return to normal activity within 3 or 4 days. A child with a lower respiratory infection will have the acute illness for 4 or 5 days and, although recovered within 1 or 2 weeks, will continue to have reactive airways.

The signs and symptoms occurring with respiratory infections can be similar to those occurring with noninfectious rhinitis. To complicate the diagnosis further, early in the presentation of respiratory infections, it may be impossible to differentiate between upper and lower respiratory infections. Both respiratory infections will increase the risk of the child developing perioperative complications. Fortunately, when a child has an infectious runny nose, the parents will usually state that their child is "coming down with something."

Sinusitis

Another common cause of a runny nose in children is sinusitis. Sinusitis usually presents with cough, purulent rhinorrhea, and possibly headaches. Antibiotics alone may not be effective in completely clearing the sinuses, and surgery is often required. A history of reactive airway disease is common in these patients, especially when nasal polyps are the cause of the sinusitis. A dry cough may be the only sign of reactive airway disease described by the parents.

Anesthetic Assessment

The history is the most important part of the evaluation. Most children with full-blown viral or bacterial infections will not come to the hospital for elective surgery. It is the children who present with a runny nose who are early in their symptoms that are difficult to assess.

The parents must be specifically questioned about the presence of fever, cough, wheezing, behavior and appetite changes, illness in close contacts of the child, and any recent respiratory infection. If a child with a runny nose is said to be in a normal state of health and has negative findings on physical examination, elective surgery can proceed. If the child has any of the signs or symptoms described, an infection is more likely.

In most cases, the physical examination of a child in the early stage of a viral illness is unhelpful because negative findings do not rule out an infectious process. However, a temperature of 38°C is suggestive of infection when accompanied by runny nose, cough, sneezing, or malaise. Laboratory tests (e.g., complete blood count) are not helpful early in the course of a viral infection. Any recent history of fever or cough is an indication for a chest x-ray. Routine chest x-rays are not advised. If, however, there is reason to suspect pneumonia, a chest film should be obtained to look for an infiltrate.

Anesthetic Management

Administration of anesthesia to a child with an upper respiratory infection is a controversial practice. Studies reveal conflicting information, but some conclusions can be drawn. Tait and Knight reported that children older than 1 year of age with an upper respiratory infection who underwent a short halothane anesthetic without endotracheal intubation for insertion of tympanostomy tubes demonstrated no increased incidence of respiratory complications. On the other hand, separate reports by Liu and associates, De Soto and co-workers, and Cohen and Knight, indicate that infants and children with such infections have an increased incidence of perioperative respiratory events, especially when intubated for the surgical procedure.

When a decision is made to proceed with surgery on a child with upper respiratory symptoms (infectious or noninfectious), the possible consequences of increased airway secretions and airway reactivity must be discussed with the parents.

Before induction, determine whether the patient will require intubation. For a short procedure, it may be safer to avoid intubation unless indicated for a specific reason. Anticholinergic drugs given preoperatively may help decrease airway reactivity.

The induction of anesthesia can be accomplished by an inhalation or intravenous technique. The inhalation induction should be conducted slowly because premature placement of an oral airway and high concentrations of anesthetic gas in the presence of increased secretions can lead to coughing, breath holding, or laryngospasm. An intravenous line should be started as soon as possible in these patients. Some anesthesiologists prefer to have intravenous access even when an inhalation induction is planned, especially if difficulty obtaining an intravenous line is anticipated.

Emergence can be associated with problems similar to that of induction in children with upper respiratory symptoms. The goal is a smooth return to an awake state. Airway stimulation must be avoided. Intravenous lidocaine may be helpful in accomplishing this goal. Of course, close observation will be required postoperatively.

If elective surgery is canceled because a child has a suspected respiratory infection, the procedure will need to be rescheduled. The child must be followed by the surgeon or pediatrician, but as a general guideline, a child with an upper respiratory infection can return for surgery 2 weeks after the cessation of symptoms. A child with a lower respiratory infection will require a period of 4 to 6 weeks after the cessation symptoms.

Summary

Administration of general anesthesia to children with upper respiratory symptoms is not benign. These children require special observation perioperatively. It is safest to avoid performing elective surgery on a child with a recent or active respiratory infection. Even children with noninfectious rhinitis are at an increased anesthetic risk, although these children are generally considered candidates for elective surgery. Endotracheal intubation is associated with an increase in perioperative complications in this group of patients.

BIBLIOGRAPHY

Berry FA: The child with a runny nose, in Berry FA (ed): *Anesthetic Management of Difficult and Routine Pediatric Patients.* 2nd ed. New York, Churchill Livingstone, 1990, pp 267–284.

Berry FA: Acute airway obstruction with special emphasis on epiglottitis and croup, in Barry FA (ed): *Anesthetic Management of Difficult and Routine Pediatric Patients.* 2nd ed. New York, Churchill Livingstone, 1990, pp 243–266.

Bluestone CD: Current indications for tonsillectomy and adenoidectomy. *Ann Otol Rhinol Laryngol* 1992; 101:58–64.

Brummitt WM, Fearon B: Anesthesia and pediatric endoscopy. *J Otolaryngol* 1981; 10:49–51.

Casey WF, Drake-Lee AB: Nitrous oxide and middle ear pressure: A study of induction methods in children. *Anaesthesia* 1982; 37: 896–900.

Chung F, Crago RR: Sleep apnoea syndrome and anaesthesia. *Can J Anaesth* 1982; 29:439–445.

Cohen MM, Cameron CB: Should you cancel the operation when a child has an upper respiratory tract infection? *Anesth Analg* 1991; 72:282–288.

Cohen SR, Geller KA: Anesthesia and pediatric endoscopy: The surgeon's view. *Otolaryngol Clin North Am* 1981; 14:705–713.

Crysdale WS, Russel D: Complications of tonsillectomy and adenoidectomy in 9409 children observed overnight. *Can Med Assoc J* 1986 135:1139–1142.

Davies DD: Re-anaesthetizing cases of tonsillectomy and adenoidectomy because of persistent postoperative haemorrhage. *Br J Anaesth* 1964; 36:244–250.

Davis RK, Simpson GT: Safety with the carbon dioxide laser. *Otolaryngol Clin North Am* 1983; 16:801–813.

DeSoto H, Patel RI, Soliman IE, et al: Changes in oxygen saturation following general anesthesia in children with upper respiratory infection signs and symptoms undergoing otolaryngological procedures. *Anesthesiology* 1988; 68:276–279.

Healy GB, Strong MS, Shapshay S, et al: Complications of CO_2 laser surgery of the aerodigestive tract: Experience of 4416 cases. *Otolaryngol Head Neck Surg* 1984; 92:13–18.

Hermens JM, Bennett MJ, Hirschman CA: Anesthesia for laser surgery. *Anesth Analg* 1983; 62:218–229.

Keon TP: Anesthetic considerations for laser surgery. *Int Anesthesiol Clin* 1988; 26:50–53.

Liu LMP, Ryan JF, Coté CJ, et al: Influence of upper respiratory infections on critical incidents in children during anesthesia. Presented at the 9th World Congress of Anesthesiology, Washington, DC, May 27–28, 1988.

Mangat D, Orr WC, Smith RO: Sleep apnea, hypersomnolence, and upper airway obstruction secondary to adenotonsillar enlargement. *Arch Otolaryngol Head Neck Surg* 1977; 103:383–386.

Markowitz-Spence L, Brodsky L, Syed N, et al: Anesthetic complications of tympanotomy tube placement in children. *Arch Otolaryngol Head Neck Surg* 1990; 116:809–812.

Ott NL, O'Connell EJ, Hoffman AD, et al: Childhood sinusitis. *Mayo Clin Proc* 1991; 66:1238–1247.

Pasternak LR: Anesthetic considerations in otolaryngological and ophthalmological outpatient surgery. *Int Anesthesiol Clin* 1990; 28:89–100.

Patel RI, Hannallah RS, Norden J, et al: Emergence airway complications in children: A comparison of tracheal extubation in awake and deeply anesthetized patients. *Anesth Analg* 1991; 73:266–270.

Potsic WP: Tonsillectomy and adenoidectomy. *Int Anesthesiol Clin* 1988; 26:58–60.

Reilly JS: Tonsillar and adenoid airway obstruction: Modes of treatment in children. *Int Anesthesiol Clin* 1988; 26:54–57.

Sanders RO: Two ventilating attachments for bronchoscopes. *Del Med J* 1967; 39:170.

Shott SR, Myer CM, Cotton RT: Efficacy of tonsillectomy and adenoidectomy as an outpatient procedure: A preliminary report. *Int J Pediatr Otorhinolaryngol* 1987; 13:157–163.

Sosi MB: Which is the safest endotracheal tube for use with the CO_2 laser? A comparative study. *J Clin Anesth* 1992; 4:217–219.

Spoerel WE, Grant PA: Ventilation during bronchoscopy. *Can J Anaesth* 1971; 18:178–188.

Tait AR, Knight PR: The effects of general anesthesia on upper respiratory tract infections in children. *Anesthesiology* 1987; 67:930–935.

Wald ER, Guerra N, Byers C: Upper respiratory tract infections in young children: Duration of and frequency of complications. *Pediatrics* 1991; 87:129.

Weinberg S, Kravath R, Phillips L, et al: Episodic complete airway obstruction in children with undiagnosed obstructive sleep apnea. *Anesthesiology* 1984; 60:356–358.

Weisberger EC, Miner JD: Apneic anesthesia for improved endoscopic removal of laryngeal papillomata. *Laryngoscope* 1988; 98:693–697.

Woods AM: Pediatric endoscopy, in Berry FA (ed): *Anesthetic Management of Difficult and Routine Pediatric Patients*. New York, Churchill Livingstone, 1990, pp 199–242.

Woods AM, Gal TJ: Decreasing airflow resistance during infant and pediatric bronchoscopy. *Anesth Analg* 1987; 66:457–459.

CHAPTER 24

Anesthesia for Pediatric Cardiac Surgery

Alan D. Zablocki

The approach to anesthetizing a child with congenital heart disease requires a multidisciplinary evaluation preoperatively. Knowledge about the type of defect, echocardiographic and sometimes cardiac catheterization data, and laboratory tests must be evaluated to formulate an anesthetic plan. This chapter will outline general preoperative anesthetic evaluation and intraoperative management of patients with congenital heart disease.

PREOPERATIVE EVALUATION

The medical and surgical history of the patient should include the following: the patient's age, the type of congenital heart disease, the clinical manifestations (e.g., symptoms of congestive heart failure [CHF], cyanosis, hypercyanotic spells, squatting, exercise intolerance, fatigue, failure to thrive, and growth retardation), the surgical repair or procedure planned, and the reason for the timing of the operation. Patients with congenital heart disease may have undergone multiple diagnostic studies, including cardiac catheterization. These findings should be summarized. Pertinent information from the most recent catheterization data should be outlined as follows: (1) characterization of the lesion (e.g., ostium primum atrial septal defect with cleft mitral valve), (2) pressures in the cardiac chambers (gradients across a stenotic valve or infundibulum should be noted), (3) O_2 saturations in the cardiac chambers (these help determine the location of the shunt), and (4) the degree of shunting. The location of both intracardiac and extracardiac shunts, if present, should be indicated with their direction and magnitude (e.g., Qp/Qs = 4.5/L where Qp = flow through the pulmonary circulation and Qs = systemic flow) and any unsuspected or concomitant lesions noted. It is very useful to draw a diagram of the defect and trace the path of blood through the heart—this maneuver helps us understand the pathophysiology (Fig. 24-1). It is also imperative to understand the surgical repair, what it will accomplish, and what the complications are. The history should obviously also include a routine pediatric preoperative evaluation, including other congenital anomalies, chromosomal aberrations, prematurity, overall health, medications, allergies, family history, recent upper respiratory infection symptoms, and previous surgery.

The physical examination and laboratory are also of importance in the evaluation process. Significant alterations in vital signs or hemodynamics; potential airway difficulties; and examination of the lungs for evidence of reactive airway disease, pulmonary edema, or infection should be noted (Table 24-1). Of particular importance is the presence or absence of cyanosis, which can serve to categorize the congenital lesion into one of two broad categories—too little pulmonary blood flow (cy-

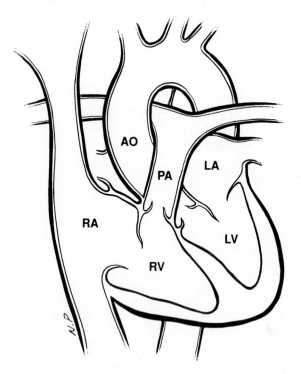

Figure 24-1 This sketch may be used as a basis for diagramming the cardiac defect and tracing the pathway of blood through the patient's heart.

Table 24-1   Physical Examination of the Child with Heart Disease

Vital signs	Heart rate, respiratory rate and pattern (e.g., tachypnea, grunting, flaring, and retractions), weight, and temperature
Cardiovascular system	Murmurs, extra heart sounds, signs of diminished peripheral perfusion, hepatomegaly
Pulmonary system	Rales, rhonchi, wheezing, cyanosis, clubbing
Airway	Congenital anomalies
Vascular access	Two peripheral intravenous cannulas, an arterial line, and a central venous line are usually needed. Anticipate potential difficulties. Arterial line may need to be placed in a specific site (e.g., previous Blalock Taussig shunt or coarctation).

anotic) or too much pulmonary blood flow (acyanotic). Our knowledge of which of these broad classifications by which the patient is best categorized may help anticipate other potential problems (e.g., the cyanotic lesions may be polycythemic, but acyanotic lesions may have electrolyte abnormalities caused by diuretic therapy and are more susceptible to recurrent pulmonary infections); (Table 24-2).

The American Society of Anesthesiologists (ASA) physical status of all pediatric cardiac surgical patients is at least ASA II, and some who arrive while receiving inotropic support and who are intubated may be classified as levels IV or V.

Table 24-2   Laboratory and Radiographic Studies

Laboratory	Hematocrit (polycythemia is a good indicator of the severity of systemic arterial hemoglobin desaturation), coagulation profile, electrolytes, glucose, calcium
Chest x-ray	Pulmonary vascular pattern, cardiomegaly, specific chamber enlargement, pneumonia
Electrocardiography	Hypertrophy, axis deviation, conduction defects

Of importance when talking to the parents and child in the preoperative visit is to inform them of the probability of needing postoperative ventilation and multiple lines and monitors. Older children may have specific questions that should be answered as honestly as possible. It has also proved very beneficial to involve the child in a preoperative teaching experience, which involves play therapy and a tour of the intensive care unit and operating room waiting areas. Meeting the nursing personnel that will be caring for the child postoperatively can be very reassuring for both the child and family.

Premedication is usually not necessary in children younger than 1 year of age, and even anticholinergics are best given in the operating room for antivagal effect. In older children, premedication is generally desirable, especially in certain circumstances, such as patients with tetralogy of Fallot who are at risk for development of hypercyanotic episodes caused by crying or agitation. Chronic medications should be given as usual.

PREOPERATIVE PREPARATION

Drugs

The key to successful intraoperative management is preoperative preparation and anticipation of potential problems. Drugs for pediatric open heart procedures should be drawn up beforehand and labeled with the drug name and concentration. A list of anesthetic drugs is contained in Table 24-3 and resuscitation drugs, in Table 24-4.

The precise dose of these drugs must be administered without an excessive volume. The correct dose of each drug should be calculated preoperatively and written down for quick reference. Almost all drugs can be administered undiluted if 1-mL syringes are used. The unit-dose system can be used, but reliance on this system can be detrimental in an emergency situa-

Table 24-3   Anesthetic Drugs

Atropine
Fentanyl or sufentanil (total dose, 50 to 100 µg/kg or 15 to 20 µg/kg, respectively)
Morphine
Thiopental
Muscle relaxants (e.g., succinylcholine, pancuronium, and vecuronium)
Volatile agents (e.g., halothane or isoflurane)
Reversal agents (e.g., neostigmine or atropine)

Table 24-4   Resuscitation Drugs—Bolus Injection

Calcium chloride	10%, may be diluted to 5% for neonates, 10 to 20 mg/kg
Bicarbonate	1 mEq/mL (0.5 mEq/mL for neonates), given according to base deficit
Epinephrine	1:10,000 (100 μg/mL) and a separate syringe with a concentration of 10 μg/mL → 1 to 10 μg/kg/dose
Phenylephrine	10 μg/mL → 1 to 5 μg/kg/dose
Isoproterenol	2 μg/mL. Add 0.1 mL from 200 μg/mL ampule (20 μg) to 10 mL of saline. Begin with 1 μg/kg/dose
Lidocaine	1% or 2%, 1 mg/kg
Atropine	0.5 mg/mL, 0.02 to 0.03 mg/kg

tion—it is preferable to know the correct dose of each agent and administer it from a 1-mL syringe.

Infusions of inotropes or vasodilators also must be administered in the correct dose without excessive volume. Several formulas are available for calculation of the appropriate concentration needed to achieve this as follows:

Dopamine	6 × body weight (in kilograms) equals the dose in milligrams to be added to 100 mL in a burette chamber. With this mixture, 1 mL/h = 1 μg/kg/min. As an alternative, 15 × weight (in kilograms) can be added to a 250-mL bag for the same concentration. For infants less than 10 kg, the dose may be doubled so that 1 mL/h = 2 μg/kg/min, and an infusion pump may be used, which allows the delivery of less than 1 mL/h. For children larger than 20 kg, the concentration may be reduced by a factor of 10 and the rate of infusion, increased by 10 because larger children can tolerate greater volumes.
Dobutamine	The preparation is identical to that for dopamine.
Nitroprusside, nitroglycerin	The preparation is identical to that for dopamine. If an infusion pump capable of de-

livering less than 1 mL/h is unavailable, the concentration may be reduced by one half, so that 1 mL/h = 0.5 μg/kg/min.

Epinephrine, isoproterenol

When 0.6 × body weight (in kilograms) is added to 100 mL, 1 mL/h = 0.1 μg/kg/min. In some cases, the concentration can be halved, so that 1 mL/h = 0.05 μg/kg/min.

It is helpful to have at least four infusion pumps available. At least one should be able to deliver less than 1 mL/h. It is not necessary to prepare all these infusions for all cases. If a repair of a complex anomaly in a small infant is planned, then all of them may be needed; conversely, an atrial septal defect repair in a healthy child may require none of them. All resuscitation drugs are given centrally into a central venous or right atrial line to achieve rapid results and to prevent tissue necrosis if a peripheral intravenous line infiltrates.

The equipment required for pediatric open heart procedures is identical to that required for routine pediatric cases with the addition of that needed for monitoring central venous and arterial blood pressure. A list of the equipment commonly used at our institution is shown in Tables 24-5 and 24-6.

In addition to monitors, two peripheral intravenous (IV) lines are ideal (with burette chambers or a pump, double stopcocks, and T-connectors). One line may be used for maintenance and one for volume replacement. The central line may be attached to pressure tubing by a T-connector and to a transducer for continuous monitoring of central pressures. If a

Table 24-5   Monitoring Equipment for Pediatric Open Heart Cases

Electrocardiography: one set of leads; V5 not needed
Precordial and esophageal stethoscopes
Pulse oximeter
Three transducers, with a male–male connector on one if postbypass left atrial monitoring is anticipated
Arterial line, 22 gauge (24 gauge for small infants < 5 kg)
Central venous pressure catheter, Cook catheter, 5-French double lumen, 5, 8, or 12 cm in length or Arrow 4-French double lumen, 5, 8, or 13 cm in length
Blood pressure cuff, appropriate size is width, at least 20 percent greater than the diameter of the extremity
Temperature probes, nasal and rectal
Capnography

Table 24-6   Miscellaneous Equipment for Pediatric Open Heart Cases

---

Airway equipment
Pediatric circle system with humidifier
Pediatric ventilator bellows—prolonged ventilation by hand is
   unsatisfactory for these procedures because both hands are
   needed for other tasks, such as administration of blood
   products
Atrioventricular sequential pacemaker
Defibrillator
Alternating-current fibrillator—used on brief procedures to
   produce ventricular fibrillation

---

double-lumen catheter is used, the other port may be used for infusions of inotropes or vasodilators when coming off cardiopulmonary bypass (CPB). Because it is difficult to reach the central line when the child is draped, heparin flush this port, then attach a carrier fluid (on a pump) and all necessary vasoactive drips with a bear claw or other multifusion device. Be sure all ports of the bear claw are flushed clear of air. Attaching the drips as close to the infant as possible eliminates dead space. Maintenance IV fluids should be a non-glucose containing isotonic crystalloid (except neonates, who may require dextrose 10% solution). Extra infusion pump sets and fluid bags should be available for additional drips if needed.

Fluids and blood products for infusion may be drawn into syringes and kept in a water bath (in a plastic bag, not in direct contact with water) for warming. A thermometer should be used to ensure that the temperature in the water bath does not exceed 41°C because hemolysis can occur when that temperature is exceeded.

Special Problems with IV Lines

Precautions to Prevent Fluid Overload
All fluids should be administered with an infusion pump in the neonate and small infant. If a fluid bolus is needed, it may be given with a syringe into a stopcock. Small bags of fluid—250 mL or less—should be used, and no more than 2-h of maintenance fluid should be in the burette chamber at any one time. Fluid totals should be tabulated and recorded frequently.

Precautions to Prevent Infusion of Air Bubbles
Most congenital cardiac defects involve a communication between the right and left sides of the circulation; therefore, it is

imperative that air bubbles be prevented from entering the circulation through lines. This requires meticulous preparation, including flushing of stopcock ports, filling drip chambers to the correct level, removing air from T-connectors by holding them upright and tapping them with fluid running, aspiration of air from injection ports on IV administration sets, and placing a drop in the end of each component when connecting parts of the line. Some recommend the use of bubble filters, but their use is not a substitute for meticulous technique. Sometimes, despite all efforts, a bubble will be observed in the tubing and must be removed before it reaches the patient. A convenient site is the T-connector—simply insert a 23-gauge needle into the T-port and let the IV fluid run wide open until the bubble is cleared. After the patient is prepared and draped, then access to the T-connector is difficult. If a bubble is observed past the most distal stopcock or connection, a simple way to remove it is to disconnect the tubing and insert a spinal needle down past the bubble and flush it back. Attempts to aspirate air back through a stopcock are usually ineffective and often counterproductive because they may allow more air into the system through a loose connection or around a line. Constant vigilance for air bubbles is mandatory throughout the procedure, especially during injection of drugs.

INTRAOPERATIVE MONITORING
AND INDUCTION OF ANESTHESIA

The operating room should be warm and all necessary drugs and equipment present in the room before bringing the patient in. The chart should be reviewed to update laboratory values, consults, and any other pertinent information.

Electrocardiographic leads, pulse oximeter probe, blood pressure cuff, and precordial stethoscope are placed on the patient before induction. Invasive monitoring is usually established after induction of anesthesia. Intravenous access may be established before or after induction, depending on the child's condition and the type of induction desired.

Induction Techniques

Several approaches are available for induction in a sick infant/child with CHF or cyanotic heart disease. Atropine is administered intravenously or intramuscularly. If an IV line is already in place, induction with high-dose narcotics (25 to 50 μg/kg of fentanyl or an equivalent dose of sufentanil) and pancuronium is the preferred approach. If there is no line intramuscular (IM) ketamine (4 to 6 mg/kg) is administered, followed by IM succinylcholine or, if a line can be quickly started, IV pancuronium.

In some instances, an inhalation technique can also be used—halothane is administered until loss of consciousness occurs, a line is inserted as soon as possible, and pancuronium is administered. The halothane is then discontinued, and narcotics are administered. If an IV line cannot be started quickly, IM succinylcholine is administered (4 mg/kg), and the airway is secured with an endotracheal tube. The halothane is then turned down to a low concentration until IV access is established. Avoid prolonged administration of a volatile agent in high concentration by mask while searching for IV access. Attention may be diverted during efforts at difficult access, and potentially dangerous myocardial depression and hypotension can ensue.

In the relatively healthy, older child, premedication is optional, and many different induction techniques may be chosen. Inhalation induction with halothane, rectal barbiturates, IV barbiturates, or IM ketamine are all acceptable alternatives.

Vascular Access

Two peripheral lines are recommended for vascular access. These should be as large as practical for the size of the patient because blood products are frequently required. Common sites include the dorsum of the hand or foot, external jugular, greater saphenous vein at the ankle, cephalic vein at the wrist, and the antecubital fossa. Surgical cut downs are needed on occasion. Once inserted, the line is taped in place, and the extremity is immobilized with an armboard.

Arterial lines are used on almost all cases. The site depends on the procedure and on any previous surgery (e.g., in a child with a previous right Blalock Taussig shunt, the left radial artery would be preferable). The technique of transfixing the artery has the highest success rate, especially in small infants. A T-connector is attached with a red label to avoid confusion with a peripheral IV line. As a general rule of thumb, a right radial arterial line is preferred in patients with coarctation of the aorta, interrupted aortic arch, and the presence of a left Blalock Taussig shunt. Otherwise, a left radial arterial line is preferred by a majority of practitioners because the placement of the aortic cannula in many small children may interfere with pressure readings in the right radial arterial line.

The central venous catheter serves two purposes: (1) monitoring of right-sided pressures (especially important postbypass) and (2) a direct central site for vasoactive drugs. A central line will be inserted in most cases, the exceptions being some extracardiac procedures (patent ductus arteriosus ligation) and some intracardiac procedures that are brief and unlikely to need resuscitation drugs (ostium secundum atrial septal defect re-

pair). The site of choice is the right internal jugular; alternate
sites include the left internal jugular, external jugular, femoral,
and basilic veins. Double-lumen catheters are preferred to single ones, when possible. For very small infants (up to 5 kg) the
catheter size is chosen according to weight: 2 kg, 2.5 French; 3
kg, 3 French (the 2.5 and 3 French are not available as double-
lumen catheters); 4 kg, 4 French; and 5 kg, 5 French.

If the catheter is too long, the surgeon can cut off the tip
once the right atrium is opened. If there is difficulty in line
placement, the surgeon can insert right atrial and left atrial lines
after the repair and before taking the patient off CPB.

The pulmonary artery (PA) catheter is seldom used prebypass because of the nature of most congenital defects. If it is
desired, a 6-French pediatric introducer can be inserted into the
internal jugular vein and the 5-French pediatric PA catheter inserted through it.

Alternatively, the PA catheter may be placed by the external
jugular or the greater saphenous vein or inserted directly into
the pulmonary artery or right ventricular outflow tract by the
surgeon. PA catheters are needed only in patients with severe,
reactive pulmonary hypertension.

Vigilance to monitoring devices is difficult during line insertion, but it must be maintained. After all lines are inserted, all
items must be securely taped, organized, and optimally positioned before preparing the patient and draping. After a small
patient is covered by a large drape, there is little access to the
IV sites.

MAINTENANCE OF ANESTHESIA

A high-dose narcotic technique is used for most procedures but
commits the patient to a period of postoperative ventilation. Inhalational agents may be used for brief procedures on relatively
healthy patients in whom extubation is planned. A moderate
dose of narcotics (35 to 40 μg/kg of fentanyl) may be used with
inhalational agents for patients in whom immediate extubation
is not planned, but overnight ventilation is not necessary either.
Nitrous oxide is best avoided on almost all cases because of its
effect on pulmonary vascular resistance and its ability to en-
large air bubbles.

After surgery has begun, a baseline activated coagulation
time (ACT) and arterial blood gases should be drawn. Heparin
may be given directly into the right atrium by the surgeon or
into a central line from which blood can be freely aspirated. An
ACT of greater than 400 s should be obtained before institution
of CPB. Cannulation can often be difficult in small patients, and
considerable blood loss may occur. The surgeon may request

hand ventilation during this time. Any obvious volume deficits should be replaced before cannulation. After the aortic cannula is in place, the patient may be transfused directly from the pump in increments of 5 to 10 mL/kg.

CPB

After cannulation, the surgeon will instruct the perfusionist to institute CPB. All palliative shunts are taken down and ligated before CPB to avoid flooding the lungs and distending the left ventricle during bypass. After stable bypass is initiated, the ventilator is turned off. All IV lines are turned off, and all drugs administered during CPB are given into the oxygenator. A bolus of narcotics and muscle relaxants is frequently given after CPB has begun. Volatile agents may be given during bypass by the pump.

Hypothermia

There is a wide spectrum of suggestions concerning myocardial preservation and hypothermia, depending on the age and size of the patient and the complexity of the intended repair. The extremes include (1) surgery done at normothermia with a fibrillating heart to (2) profound hypothermia with circulatory arrest. Most procedures are done using moderate hypothermia with cold, potassium-containing cardioplegia. Documentation on the anesthesia record should include bypass and cross-clamp times, cooling and rewarming, use of cardioplegia, and disappearance and return of cardiac electrical activity. Procedures done at normothermia with fibrillation are usually simple, such as atrial septal defect repair or pulmonary valvotomy. The surgeon will attach the leads for the alternating-current fibrillator and request the anesthesiologist turn it on. It should be left on until the surgeon requests it be turned off.

Procedures done with profound hypothermia and circulatory arrest are usually complex repairs in small infants. The purpose of circulatory arrest is to enhance exposure by removing cannulas from the field. Hypothermia may be achieved either by surface cooling with ice or by core cooling with CPB, the latter being more common. No effort to keep the patient warm is made before CPB in either case. Surface cooling involves placing ice bags over the head, right chest, abdomen, and proximal extremities. Care must be taken to avoid mechanical stimulation to the heart because ventricular fibrillation may occur. With either method, after 18° to 20°C is reached, the blood volume will be drained to the pump, the venous cannulas removed, and the pump turned off. Any intervention, such as administration of muscle relaxants, must be done before decannulation because there would be no way to do so afterward. After the repair is completed, the cannulas are reinserted, CPB reinstated, and rewarming begun.

Monitoring During CPB

The following parameters are monitored during CPB:

1. Electrocardiography. This monitors the electrical activity of the heart.
2. Mean arterial pressure. The lower limits of autoregulation of cerebral blood flow are not determined in pediatric patients, but they have been extrapolated from adult data. Mean pressures of 30 to 40 mmHg are common during CPB and appear to be without untoward sequelae. The range of acceptable mean pressures during CPB in pediatric patients is 20 to 60 mmHg.
3. Urine output. Diuresis usually occurs; although with moderate to profound hypothermia and low perfusion pressures, urine output often ceases. A reasonable goal is a urine output of 0.5 to 1 mL/kg/h. Mannitol (0.25 to 0.5 g/kg) and/or furosemide (0.5 to 1 mg/kg) may be needed if the urine output is less than this.
4. Central venous pressure. This should be measured above the superior vena caval cannula and should be near zero. High values may indicate obstruction of venous drainage, which may result in cerebral edema.
5. Temperature. The nasopharyngeal temperature is a good approximation of brain temperature. Rectal temperature is monitored as an index of less well-perfused tissues and is the usual end point of rewarming.
6. Muscle relaxation. Watch for diaphragmatic movement.
7. Pupils and sclera. The eyes may not be easily accessible but should be monitored intermittently for scleral edema and excessive pupillary dilation.
8. Laboratory data. With arterial blood gases showing metabolic acidosis with a base deficit greater than -5, treatment with bicarbonate is indicated. Cardioplegia is often removed by wall suction instead of cardiotomy suction to prevent excess K^+ loading. Hypokalemia may be treated by adding 0.5 to 1 mEq/kg of potassium to the pump. Hemodilution to a hematocrit of 25 percent is standard. Packed erythrocytes may be needed.
9. The surgical field. Try to see as much of the repair as possible.

REWARMING AND TERMINATION
OF CPB

Rewarming

The warming blanket is turned on and a vasodilator (nitroprusside or nitroglycerin) may be infused. Rewarming is considered adequate when a nasopharyngeal temperature of 37° to 38°C and a rectal temp of 35°C are reached. The rewarming period is a good time to prepare for the termination of CPB. Rezero and calibrate the monitors; obtain additional blood products from the blood bank; set up a heated humidifier, calculate the protamine dose, draw it up, and place it inside the cart; make sure the pacemaker is present and functional; start vasoactive infusions; review the doses of resuscitation drugs and be sure the drugs are available; draw up and warm blood products; and suction the endotracheal tube. Ventilate the patient before attempting to wean from CPB. Observe both lungs to ensure that neither extubation nor endobronchial intubation has occurred.

Blood Products

The following formulas can be used to calculate the amount of blood products needed:

$$\text{Milliliters of PRBCs needed} = EBV \times \frac{\text{Hct desired} - \text{Hct present}}{\text{Hct PRBCs}},$$

where PRBC = packed erythrocytes, EBV = estimated blood volume, Hct = hematocrit.

Fresh-frozen plasma = 15 to 20 mL/kg will raise the levels of all clotting factors into the range needed for adequate hemostasis.

Platelets = 0.2 units/kg will increase the platelet count by 100,000. If patient volume is overloaded, request platelet concentration into as small a volume of plasma as possible.

Termination of CPB

When warming is adequate, the surgeon will ask the perfusionist to decrease the venous return, which translocates volume from the pump to the patient. Mechanical ventilation of the lungs with 100% O_2 should begin at this time. The lungs may be observed on the field to ensure adequate inflation. The heart rate should be adequate before the patient comes off CPB because the cardiac output of infants is rate dependent. An increase in rate may be achieved by a bolus dose of atropine (0.02 mg/kg) or isoproterenol (0.02 to 0.05 µg/kg). Atrioventricular nodal conduction may be temporarily or permanently damaged by the surgical repair, and pacing may be required. If the patient has pulmonary hypertension or has undergone a complex or long repair, an infusion of an inotropic agent, such as dopamine or epinephrine, should be started several minutes before termination of CPB, in addition to a bolus dose of $CaCl_2$ (10 to 20 mg/kg). When venous return to the pump is terminated, the patient is off CPB. Under most circumstances, PA catheters are not used, so that thermodilution cardiac outputs are not available. Cardiac filling pressures should be optimized by transfusion from the pump in boluses of 5 to 10 mL/kg until right atrial pressures of 15 to 18 mmHg are reached. A qualitative estimate of myocardial contractility may be obtained by observation of the heart. If the patient is hypotensive and the heart appears hypocontractile or distended with high filling pressures, further inotropic support may be needed. In some patients, especially those with pulmonary hypertension, a vasodilator such as nitroprusside, nitroglycerin, or prostaglandin E_1 may be required for right ventricular afterload reduction.

After termination of CPB, the surgeon may need to measure pressures (Note: this may be done by using a male–male connector with stopcock on the arterial or central line transducer) in cardiac chambers to determine whether any residual gradient across a stenosis exists or O_2 saturations to detect residual shunts. The use of Doppler flow color mapping is a major technologic advance for this purpose and is used to assess the completeness of the repair. If the repair is incomplete, CPB may have to be reinstituted to complete the repair. Difficulty weaning from CPB is suggestive of an incomplete or inadequate repair. After the surgeon is satisfied, reversal of the heparin with protamine is done, with slow (1 mg/kg/min) administration of protamine. An ACT should be drawn 5 min after the protamine is injected to detect residual heparinization.

Volume requirements are often very large in the first few hours post-CPB. It is impractical and sometimes impossible to transfuse the entire volume of the oxygenator into a small patient, and this blood may be concentrated or discarded. After protamine reversal, blood products are given if needed. Citrate toxicity is not uncommon during this time period because large volumes of blood products relative to the patient's blood volume can be rapidly administered with a syringe. Any unexplained hypotension temporally related to blood product administration should be treated empirically with a calcium bolus. If the patient has needed inotropic support to wean from CPB, it is usually best maintained until arrival in the intensive care unit. The patient should be closely observed for hemodynamic deterioration during closure of the pericardium and the sternum. Hypokalemia is a common problem post-CPB and KCl may be administered at a rate of 0.5 to 1 mEq/kg/h with an infusion pump.

TRANSPORT AND RECOVERY

Organization is critical. The patient must be hemodynamically stable. Warming lights should be used after the drapes are removed, and efforts to prevent hypothermia during transport must be employed. All drug infusions are continued during transport. Transport monitoring includes: electrocardiography and blood pressure with the transport monitor, heart sounds and breath sounds with a precordial stethoscope, and oxygen saturation with the pulse oximeter. Some patients may be extubated in the operating room, but most will be left intubated and ventilated during transport. A Jackson-Rees system is used with a bag of the appropriate size. Generally, 100% oxygen is administered, regardless of whether the patient is extubated or intubated. Airway equipment, resuscitation drugs, blood products or volume expanders, and the pacemaker should accompany the patient to the unit.

Before leaving for the intensive care unit, call ahead to set ventilatory parameters. On arrival in the unit, continue to ventilate by hand until the ventilator is ready. Always assess breath sounds and chest excursion immediately after the child is connected to the ventilator. Either pressure- or volume-cycled ventilation may be used in infants and small children. An FiO_2 of 100% should be used until stable pulse oximetry readings or blood gas analysis are available. The anesthesiologist should remain present until the patient is hemodynamically stable and has adequate analgesia. Good communication with the pediatric intensive care unit team regarding the child's intraoperative course will facilitate optimal postoperative care.

BIBLIOGRAPHY

Hickey P, Wessel D: Anesthesia for congenital heart disease, in Gregory G (ed): *Pediatric Anesthesia.* New York, Churchill Livingstone, 1989, pp 833–892.

Hickey P, Wessel D: Anesthesia for treatment of congenital heart disease, in Kaplan J (ed): *Cardiac Anesthesia.* Orlando, FL, Grune & Stratton, 1987, pp 635–724.

Lake CL: *Pediatric Cardiac Anesthesia.* Norwalk, CT, Appleton and Lange, 1988.

Rothstein P: Anesthesia for children with congenital heart disease, in Thomas S (ed): *Manual of Cardiac Anesthesia.* New York, Churchill Livingstone, 1984, pp 259–292.

Stratford M, DiNardo J: Anesthesia for congenital heart disease, in DiNardo J, Schwartz M (eds): *Anesthesia for Cardiac Surgery.* Norwalk, CT, Appleton and Lange, 1990, pp 117–172.

CHAPTER 25

Acyanotic Congenital Heart Disease

Paul M. Seib
Deborah K. Rasch

Acyanotic congenital heart lesions account for the majority of congenital heart defects and often require surgical palliation or repair. They may present as isolated conditions or in association with other defects that require surgical intervention soon after birth, such as diaphragmatic hernia or esophageal atresia. Similarly, congenital heart disease (CHD) is commonly associated with chromosomal anomalies, such as Down's syndrome (40 percent of patients may have cardiac defects). The incidence of CHD is approximately 0.8 percent of live births, and as more persons with repaired CHD survive to have children, this incidence may be expected to increase. This chapter will review the most common shunts and obstructive lesions. A comprehensive review of these and less common lesions may be found in any of several excellent pediatric cardiology reference texts.

GENERAL DIAGNOSIS AND
MEDICAL MANAGEMENT

The approach to the diagnosis and treatment of CHD has changed rapidly in recent years, largely as a result of improvements in diagnostic imaging with echocardiography and magnetic resonance imaging; advances in cardiac Doppler technology, which allows the cardiologist to obtain hemodynamic information without cardiac catheterization; and new techniques for interventional cardiac catheterization, including balloon valvuloplasty and occlusion devices for the patent ductus arteriosus (PDA) and secundum atrial septal defect (ASD). Refinements in cardiac surgical techniques and in cardiopulmonary bypass have allowed complete repair of most lesions when significant symptoms occur, often in the first year of life, thus avoiding palliative procedures and the risk of multiple operations. Earlier complete repair helps avoid the detrimental effects of chronic congestive heart failure, such as myocardial fibrosis, failure to thrive, prolonged cyanosis, and developmental delay.

Goals for the care of infants and children with CHD should include:

1. *Early diagnosis,* including in utero diagnosis by fetal echocardiography or by postnatal echocardiography, which allows appropriate perinatal management. Cardiac catheterization may be necessary to clarify some aspects of the diagnosis or to perform palliative procedures, such as balloon atrial septostomy.

2. *Early intervention* to support cardiac output, oxygenation, and oxygen delivery. This may require the use of mechanical ventilation, inotropic agents, or vasodilators. Prostaglandin E_1 is used to maintain the patency of the ductus arteriosus in cases of ductal-dependent pulmonary blood flow (e.g., pulmonary valve atresia) or ductal-dependent systemic blood flow (e.g., coarctation of the aorta or critical aortic valve stenosis). The transition from fetal to neonatal circulation has a great effect on therapy and may necessitate that surgery be performed early or be delayed, depending on the perinatal changes in pulmonary vascular resistance (PVR). For instance, the arterial switch procedure for transposition of the great arteries with intact ventricular septum is ideally performed during the first 2 weeks of life while the left ventricle is still "prepared" to handle the elevated vascular resistance that it faced in utero. If surgery is delayed until after the PVR falls to its lowest point at 4 to 6 weeks of age, the left ventricle will thin, and it will be unable to handle the acute increase in afterload that occurs when the great arteries are surgically switched and it must pump against systemic (SVR) rather than PVR. Conversely, patients with complex single ventricle anatomy (e.g., tricuspid atresia) require initial palliative operations that restrict or augment pulmonary blood flow and allow the patients to have a more definitive repair when the pulmonary vascular resistance is low and the child has grown.

3. *Nutritional support* to allow adequate growth for the patient who may have chronic congestive heart failure (CHF) yet may still need to undergo surgical procedures for correction or palliation of the heart defect.

4. *Management of late complications,* such as arrhythmias, ventricular dysfunction, pulmonary vascular disease, or CHF. The realization that some of these late sequelae are difficult to manage has led to a more aggressive surgical approach emphasizing early complete

repair. For example, an arterial switch procedure is favored for repair of transposition of the great arteries because it avoids the extensive atrial suture lines required in the atrial baffle procedures (Mustard or Senning operation) formerly used to repair this defect. Such extensive atrial surgery predisposes the patient to sinus node dysfunction and atrial arrhythmias (atrial flutter and atrial fibrillation).

The discussion of CHD is conveniently divided into acyanotic and cyanotic lesions. The topic of this chapter, acyanotic heart disease, can be subdivided into (1) those lesions causing a left-to-right shunt and leading to excessive pulmonary blood flow and (2) obstructive lesions that limit cardiac output. Both types of lesions commonly result in what we see clinically as congestive heart failure. Occasionally, both types coexist and may exacerbate one another. In the neonate and infant, the age at presentation may be a hint as to the underlying pathophysiology because critical obstruction lesions are often present in the first week of life, while left-to-right shunt lesions present more commonly after the pulmonary vascular resistance reaches its nadir at 4 to 8 weeks of age.

LEFT-TO-RIGHT SHUNTS

Left-to-right shunts can occur at the level of the atria, the ventricles, or the great arteries, and shunts can occur at more than one level, making it difficult to decide which shunt is clinically most important. Some examples of left-to-right shunts, along with their hemodynamic and clinical effects, are discussed in this section.

Atrial Level Shunts

There are four types of ASD which result in atrial level left-to-right shunts (Fig. 25-1).

1. *Ostium secundum defects* are the most common and are located in the middle of the atrial septum in the region of the fossa ovalis. These defects are associated with normal atrioventricular valves and a small percentage are associated with anomalous pulmonary venous drainage.
2. *Ostium primum defects* occur in the lower end of the atrial septum and result from a failure of the endocardial cushions to close this area. A cleft in the anterior leaflet of the mitral valve is almost always present and occasionally results in significant mitral insufficiency.

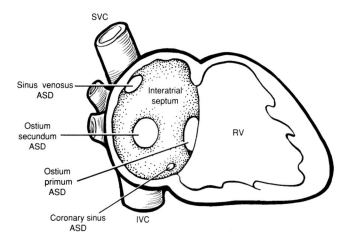

Figure 25-1   The types of atrial septal defects (ASD) based on their location within the atrial septum (see text for description of each type). SVC = superior vena cava; IVC = inferior vena cava; RV = right ventricle.

3. *Sinus venosus defects* occur in the area where the superior vena cava (SVC), and rarely the inferior vena cava enter the right atrium (RA). These defects are usually associated with partial anomalous pulmonary venous drainage; most commonly of the right upper lobe pulmonary veins to the SVC–RA junction.
4. *Coronary sinus defects* are rare and are located immediately next to the coronary sinus.

Despite the different names for these defects, the physiology is the same. Large defects product significant volume overload of the right heart but rarely result in overt CHF. The amount of the left-to-right shunt is determined by the size of the defect and the relative compliances of the two ventricles. At birth, the ventricles are of about equal thickness and compliance. The pulmonary vascular resistance falls normally and the pulmonary artery pressure remains normal; therefore, the right ventricle becomes thin and more compliant. With both atrioventricular valves open in diastole, blood flows preferentially left to right toward the more compliant right ventricle. These patients are rarely symptomatic but may have a slim build. The left precordium may bulge and be hyperdynamic as a result of the underlying, volume-overloaded right ventricle. Auscultation reveals a systolic ejection murmur at the upper left sternal border, a widely split second heart sound, which may be "fixed" and not vary with respiration, and a "scratchy" diastolic murmur at the lower left sternal border in the presence of a large left-to-right shunt. The chest x-ray shows prominence of the right atrium and cardiomegaly with mildly increased pulmonary vascular markings. The electrocardiogram typically demonstrates sinus rhythm, right atrial enlargement, and right ventricular hypertrophy reflected as an rSR′ pattern in lead V1 indicative of right ventricular volume overload. Left axis deviation of the frontal plane QRS axis should suggest a primum ASD. Echocardiography can adequately define the anatomy of most ASD, and cardiac catheterization is usually not necessary. Surgical repair involves direct suture closure of many secundum defects or patch closure. Baffling of anomalous pulmonary veins to the left atrium or repair of a cleft mitral valve may also be required. Late sequelae of unrepaired ASD include CHF (often precipitated by atrial arrhythmias), pulmonary hypertension, and paradoxic embolus resulting in stroke.

It is of note that isolated partial anomalous pulmonary venous return can be clinically indistinguishable from an ASD and should be suspected when there is right ventricular volume overload without an ASD.

Patients with complete atrioventricular canal defects (CAVC) have both a primum ASD and a large ventricular septal defect (VSD) in the inlet portion of the ventricular septum. These result from failure of fusion of the endocardial cushions that normally close the lower atrial septum and the inlet ventricular septum (Fig. 25-2). The atrioventricular valves (AV valves) have abnormalities ranging from a simple cleft mitral valve to a common AV valve with only an anterior and posterior leaflet and no chordal attachments to the ventricles. Such valves may be mildly to severely insufficient. These defects have a wide spectrum of anatomic variations that affect the clinical presentation and course. For instance, some CAVC defects have a large atrial defect, a cleft mitral valve with mild regurgitation, and only a small VSD. They behave clinically like a large ASD. More typical of CAVC defects are large atrial and ventricular defects, a common AV valve, and moderate AV valve insufficiency. They are especially common in patients with Down's syndrome. These patients almost always have the onset of severe CHF in infancy associated with failure to thrive. Physical examination findings are similar to those in patients with a large VSD with the additional findings of the murmur of AV valve insufficiency. They are frequently refractory to medical therapy and require surgical repair in infancy. Initial complete repair is preferable, in which the ventricular and atrial defects are closed with a patch of pericardium or Dacron and the AV valves are

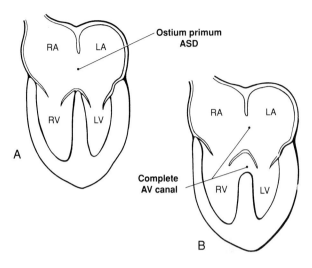

Figure 25-2 (A) Ostium primum atrial septal defect (ASD), usually associated with a cleft in the anterior leaflet of the mitral valve. RA = right atrium; LA = left atrium; RV = right ventricle; LV = left ventricle. (B) Complete atrioventricular (AV) canal defect with large atrial and ventricular components and a common AV valve.

suspended and attached to the patch such that two AV valve orifices are created. Potential complications include residual leaks around the atrial or ventricular patches, complete AV block, residual AV valve insufficiency or stenosis, ventricular dysfunction, and pulmonary hypertensive crisis. This latter problem can be catastrophic and occurs because many patients with CAVC have elevated pulmonary vascular resistance and muscular hypertrophy of the pulmonary arterioles, making them prone to hypoxic pulmonary vasoconstriction. Postoperatively, agitation or suctioning of the endotracheal tube may result in pulmonary hypertensive crisis and rapid deterioration. Such patients may require sedation and mechanical ventilation for several days postoperatively until the pulmonary vascular bed becomes less sensitive. Palliative procedures, such as a pulmonary artery band, are usually reserved for complex cases of CAVC in which there is straddling (chordal attachments in both ventricles) or overriding (shift of the anulus) of the AV valves. An aortopulmonary shunt may be performed in cases of CAVC with tetralogy of Fallot. In general, the cumulative morbidity and mortality of palliative procedures followed by complete repair is higher than that of initial complete repair.

Anesthetic Management

Except for cases of ostium primum ASD associated with endocardial cushion defect, these children are quite active and do not have evidence of heart failure. Therefore, anesthetic induction may be accomplished using either an intravenous technique or inhalational induction. Narcotics are given judiciously to provide postoperative analgesia but to also allow for early postoperative extubation. Cardiopulmonary bypass times are usually very short, and myocardial preservation may be accomplished using cold cardioplegic solution with aortic cross clamping or induced fibrillation without cross clamping. Low-dose inotropic support with dopamine or dobutamine is usually instituted for weaning from cardiopulmonary bypass.

Postoperative complications, although rare, include atelectasis as a result of incisional pain and arrhythmias related to atriotomy (premature atrial contractions, supraventricular tachycardia, or low atrial pacemaker). The long-term results of the operation are uniformly good with mortality rates of close to zero.

For infants with complete AV canal defects, anesthetic management is more difficult. These infants present with severe CHF and often fail to thrive despite medical management. Therefore, these infants do not tolerate the myocardial depressant activity of inhalational agents, and ketamine may increase left-to-right shunts as a result of increases in SVR. High-dose narcotic anesthesia using fentanyl (30 to 50 μg/kg) will provide hemodynamic stability, with the least alteration in shunts. Care must be taken to maintain normocarbia and, if tolerated, to lower FiO_2 after the child is intubated because lowering of PVR that accompanies hyperoxia will increase both atrial and ventricular level left-to-right shunts and decrease systemic cardiac output.

The surgical approach is via a right atriotomy, and in small infants, deep hypothermia and circulatory arrest may be necessary. Valvular defects are repaired by suturing the clefted areas, and the ASD and VSD are repaired using a pericardial patch. The valve leaflets must also be suspended from the patch. The ease of weaning from cardiopulmonary bypass depends on left ventricular chamber size, the presence and degree of mitral valve regurgitation, and the degree of preexisting pulmonary hypertension. Most of these infants are transported to the intensive care unit while paralyzed and sedated to be weaned very cautiously from the ventilator because postoperative pulmonary hypertensive crisis may occur. Significant inotropic support may be necessary in these patients as a result of low cardiac output syndrome. If significant AV valve regurgitation is present, the infant may have to go back on bypass to attempt surgical revision. Amrinone may be useful in cases where pulmonary artery hypertension and/or left ventricular failure exist.

Ventricular Level Shunts

There are four types of VSD, based on their location within the interventricular septum. The terminology used to describe these defects has varied over the years as more has been learned about the embryology and surgical anatomy of these lesions. Soto and colleagues recently proposed a classification based on the surgical point of view. Van Praagh and associates have also proposed a classification system for these defects based on their location relative to the four main anatomic and developmental components of the interventricular septum. Ventricular septal defects may lie within one region only or extend into adjacent regions of the septum. The older terminology is listed below along with that used by Van Praagh and associates (in parentheses) (Fig. 25-3).

1. Perimembranous (conoventricular)
2. Trabecular (muscular)
3. Inlet (AV canal type)
4. Supracristal (conal septal)

The most common cardiac defect (28 percent of all lesions), VSD may occur alone or may frequently be associated with other defects. Although these different types of defects vary with regard to their location, their clinical effects depend on whether they are small, medium, or large. Most large defects and some moderate-sized defects require surgical intervention; small defects rarely do.

Large VSDs usually result in CHF with an onset at 4 to 8 weeks of age, coincident with the nadir in the pulmonary vascular resistance. The large left-to-right shunt and the complex physiologic responses that occur result in the clinical picture we recognize as CHF (Fig. 25-4). How large is a large defect? When a VSD diameter is equal to or greater than the aortic anular diameter, it is large. The degree of left-to-right shunt is determined by the balance between the PVR and the SVR. The pressures in the right and left ventricles are equal, and the systolic pulmonary artery pressure is also equal to the systemic pressure unless there is pulmonary stenosis. Thus, the term "pulmonary hypertension" is misleading in this setting because it is obligatory when there is a large defect. It does not mean that PVR is irreversibly elevated. Prolonged exposure to high pulmonary blood flow at high pressure, especially when there

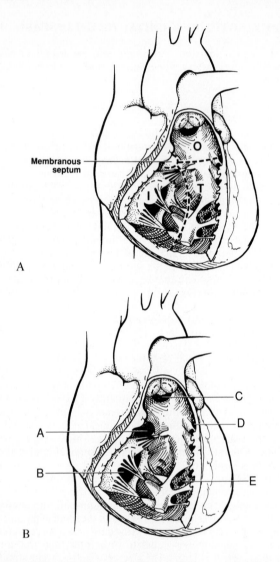

Figure 25-3 (A) Four components of the ventricular septum as viewed from the right ventricular side. I, inlet septum (or septum of the atrioventricular canal) lies between the tricuspid anulus and the chordal attachments of the tricuspid valve. T, trabecular septum is bordered by the inlet septum and the apex inferiorly and extends superiorly to the supraventricular crest, which separates it from the smooth-walled outlet septum, O. The trabecular septum may be considered to have a sinus septum component bordering the inlet septum and a

is cyanosis, leads to the development of pulmonary vascular obstructive disease (PVOD) and the irreversible elevation of PVR seen clinically in the Eisenmenger syndrome.

Moderate-sized VSDs are "restrictive," meaning that they are smaller than the size of the aortic anulus such that the size of the defect restricts flow from the left to right ventricles. The balance between the PVR and SVR still plays a role when the defect is larger, but this balance becomes less important as the defect becomes smaller. The right ventricular and pulmonary arterial pressures are less than the left ventricular pressure, and the risk of developing PVOD is greatly reduced, although a fairly large left-to-right shunt may still exist.

Moderate-sized defects may spontaneously become smaller or close completely when surrounding tissue grows over the defect. Small VSDs pose a risk for endocarditis but seldom require closure, except in the case where they are located immediately under the aortic valve (supracristal or conal septal defects) and cause aortic valve insufficiency.

Physical examination findings depend on the size of the defect. Large defects are associated with tachypnea, tachycardia, an increased anteroposterior diameter of the chest, hyperdynamic precordium, no thrill, a loud holosystolic murmur, a gallop rhythm, and a diastolic flow rumble at the apex because of excessive pulmonary blood flow returning across the mitral valve. Hepatomegaly is also present, but peripheral edema and pulmonary rales are rare findings in children. Moderate defects with a large shunt may have findings similar to these, but the murmur is usually louder, and a precordial thrill is present, caused by the jet of blood through the restrictive defect directed anteriorly into the right ventricle. Thus, VSD murmurs frequently get louder as the defect gets smaller, and the diastolic rumble disappears as the left-to-right shunt becomes smaller. Small defects have a higher pitched murmur, and as the VSD gets very small, the thrill disappears, and the murmur becomes progressively shorter. The chest x-ray shows cardiomegaly, in-

---

Figure 25-3 (*continued*)   smooth septal band component extending up to the outlet septum. The outlet septum is also called the distal conal septum. (B) Ventricular septal defects based on their anatomic location (see text). A = perimembranous or conoventricular defects; B = inlet defect or ventricular septal defect of the atrioventricular canal type; C = supracristal or conal septal defects; D and E = muscular defects in the septal band (D) and apical portion of the trabecular septum (E). (Adapted with permission from Adams FH, Emmanoulides GC, Riemenschneider TA: *Moss' Heart Disease in Infants, Children, and Adolescents*, ed 4. Baltimore, Williams and Wilkins, 1989, p 191.)

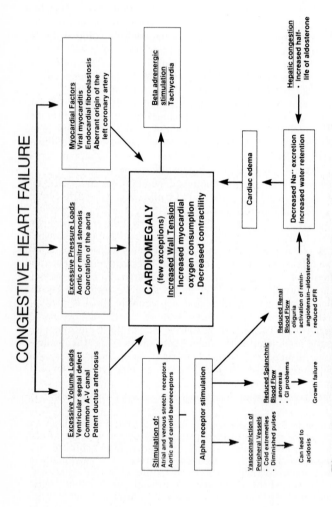

Figure 25-4 Congestive heart failure. A-V = atrioventricular; GI = gastrointestinal; GFR = glomerular filtration rate.

creased pulmonary vascular markings, and left atrial enlargement in large and moderate-sized defects with large shunts (Fig.
25-5). Electrocardiography shows left atrial enlargement, left
ventricular hypertrophy, and may show biventricular hypertrophy. Both test results are normal in a small VSD.

Surgical repair in infancy is undertaken for severe CHF, usually associated with failure to thrive. If medical therapy is successful in controlling these symptoms, elective repair of large
defects is performed at 6 months to 2 years of age to avoid the
development of PVOD. The defect is usually closed with a
patch of synthetic material (e.g., Dacron) through a right ventriculotomy or, preferably, through the tricuspid valve. Potential complications include residual leak around the patch,
damage to the tricuspid valve, ventricular arrhythmias, and
complete heart block as a result of injury to the conduction system that runs along the posterior rim of the defect. Pulmonary

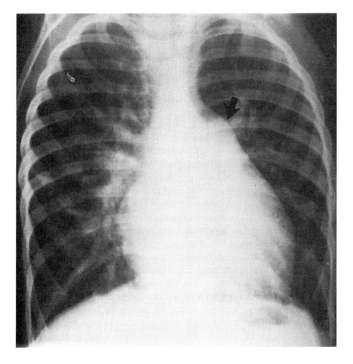

Figure 25-5   Chest x-ray of a 6-month-old infant with a ventricular septal defect. Note increased pulmonary vascular
markings and prominent pulmonary component to cardiac silhouette (arrow).

artery banding to restrict pulmonary blood flow is usually reserved for patients with multiple muscular VSDs, small infants
(< 2 kg), or patients with complex single ventricle anatomy who
require palliation until they are large enough to undergo more
definitive surgery, such as a Fontan operation. Its potential
complications of distortion of the branch pulmonary arteries,
inadequate or excessive restriction, and the need for reoperation to remove the band have made this technique less preferable than complete repair.

Anesthetic Management

Anesthetic management of children with VSDs depends on the
size of the shunt, the age of the patient, and clinical symptoms.
For children 1 year of age or older with small to moderate-sized
shunts, oral premedication with 0.3 to 0.5 mg/kg of midazolam
provides for a smoother transition from the parents to the operating room. Younger, sicker infants require no premedication.

Anesthetic induction for children with small to moderate-
sized defects may be accomplished using either an intravenous
route or with inhalational agents. Because of the left-to-right
shunt, induction times will be shortened when inhalational
agents, such as halothane, are used because shunted blood re-
circulating through the lungs will be partially saturated, thus
changing the alveolar concentration less and speeding the induction.

Intravenous agents, on the other hand, are likely to have a
slower onset because of the same recirculation phenomenon.
For infants with larger shunts who present with pulmonary hypertension and right heart failure, intravenous induction with
fentanyl 10 to 20 μg/kg is preferred because greater hemodynamic stability is afforded. Maintenance of anesthesia may be
accomplished with narcotics, inhalational agents, or as in most
cases, a combination of the two. Older children with lesser-
sized defects can often be weaned from the ventilator early in
the postoperative period so that a lower total narcotic dose
might be preferable. Sicker, younger infants should remain intubated postoperatively because they may not tolerate the normal fluid shifts encountered postcardiopulmonary bypass. Infants who present with CHF preoperatively may also benefit
from continuous monitoring of left atrial pressure by a left atrial
catheter inserted during the operation. Inotropic support will
likely be necessary in these patients for hours to days postoperatively, and they should be weaned very slowly because small
changes sometimes result in significant decreases in cardiac
output. Vasodilator infusions, such as nitroglycerin or amrinone, may be helpful in cases of right ventricular failure and
pulmonary hypertension.

Great Artery Level Shunts

PDA and aortopulmonary window (AP window) are the two
great artery level shunts (Fig. 25-6). Although they have different origins, they have almost identical physiologic effects resulting from a large communication between the great arteries.
A left-to-right shunt results, which as in the case with a large
VSD, is determined by the balance between the PVR and the
SVR. The AP window is almost always large, but a PDA frequently constricts enough to result in only a moderate or small
shunt, and many patients are asymptomatic. A PDA is frequently associated with other congenital cardiac lesions; an AP
window usually occurs alone.

A PDA results from persistent patency of the fetal ductus
arteriosus, which functions in utero to shunt almost all the right
ventricular output from the pulmonary arteries to the descending aorta where it returns to the placenta. Postnatally, especially in the setting of a premature infant, a large left-to-right
shunt may result and complicate hyaline membrane disease.
Occasionally, maintaining patency of the ductus is desirable, as
with cyanotic lesions with very limited pulmonary blood flow
(e.g., pulmonary valve atresia) or to provide systemic blood
flow (e.g., hypoplastic left heart syndrome, coarctation of the
aorta, or critical aortic valve stenosis).

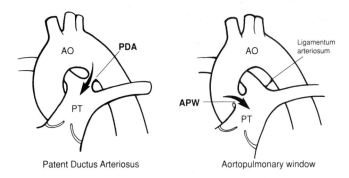

Patent Ductus Arteriosus   Aortopulmonary window

Figure 25-6 (A) Patent ductus arteriosis (PDA) arising from
the anterior surface of the descending aorta and entering the
left pulmonary just distal to the bifurcation of the main pulmonary artery (MPA). AO = aortic arch; PT = pulmonary
trunk. (B) Aortopulmonary window (APW) between the adjacent portions of the ascending aorta and MPA has virtually no
length and is usually a large communication. (Adapted with
permission from Perloff JK: *The Clinical Recognition of Congenital Heart Disease,* ed 3. Philadelphia, WB Saunders, 1987,
p 467.)

The classic physical examination findings of a loud, continuous, "machinery" murmur, bounding pulses, and CHF may be seen in many patients, but in the neonate or in the presence of elevated PVR, the murmur may be short and systolic only, and the pulses may be normal. Chest x-ray shows cardiomegaly and increased vascularity, and the electrocardiogram demonstrates left ventricular hypertrophy in the presence of a large shunt. Both may be normal with a small PDA. Echocardiography identifies a PDA between the descending aorta and left pulmonary artery and differentiates it from an AP window, which connects the ascending aorta and main pulmonary artery. Associated lesions can be evaluated and cardiac function assessed. Referral for surgical closure of an isolated PDA is usually made on the basis of echocardiographic findings alone, without cardiac catheterization.

Indomethacin causes ductal constriction and is frequently used to achieve nonsurgical closure of the PDA, but when unsuccessful or contraindicated (e.g., renal dysfunction or active bleeding), surgical ligation is performed. In the premature infant, this is usually accomplished by placing a clip on the ductus. In the older child, double ligation and division of the PDA is preferred. The surgical approach is through a left thoracotomy. A PDA occlusion device has been developed that can be positioned across the PDA through a catheter during cardiac catheterization. The device has "feet" attached to patch material at each end, which are positioned at the aortic and pulmonary ends of the ductus, respectively. When open, they occlude the ductus. This device is still undergoing final approval by the Food and Drug Administration, although well over 200 successful human implantations have been performed.

An AP window consists of a round, window-like communication between the walls of the ascending aorta and the main pulmonary artery. It is usually a large, nonrestrictive communication that is associated with a large left-to-right shunt and severe CHF. Surgical repair is performed through a median sternotomy, and the defect is closed with a patch while, at the same time, separating the great arteries.

Anesthetic Management
Preterm infants requiring PDA ligation often have other medical problems and a compromised cardiopulmonary status. Therefore, these infants most often require operation in the neonatal intensive care unit to reduce transport risks, such as hypothermia and accidental extubation. Anesthetic induction with fentanyl 5 to 10 µg/kg and pancuronium 0.1 to 0.2 mg/kg is the preferred method because inhalational agents are not well tolerated in this group of patients. The infant is then positioned in

the lateral decubitus position, and a left thoracotomy incision is made. Umbilical artery catheters, if present, are useful for both monitoring devices and vascular access. However, if an arterial line is not already in place, it is usually unnecessary to insert one solely for use during the procedure. When the vascular clips are placed, an increase in systemic diastolic blood pressure supports adequate ductal closure. Blood products should be available, and warmed syringes of albumin or other volume expander are essential in case rapid resuscitation should be needed; however, blood loss is usually minimal. Vagal reflexes caused by traction on the recurrent laryngeal nerve may occur; pretreatment with atropine 0.02 mg/kg (minimum 0.1 mg) is recommended. These infants generally require ventilatory support postoperatively because of preexisting pulmonary disease.

Older infants and children undergoing PDA ligation may be induced with a variety of intravenous agents or an inhalational induction, preferably with halothane. These children can be safely maintained on inhalational agents, and the procedures are generally short. Judicious use of narcotics to provide postoperative pain relief but still allow for extubation at the end of the procedure is desirable. Intermediate-acting muscle relaxants are also preferable because of the short length of the case. Some centers also consider epidural analgesia postoperatively to reduce splinting and improve pulmonary mechanics.

Most pediatric patients who present with AP window will be infants who are very ill as a result of severe CHF and pulmonary hypertension. Therefore, an intravenous narcotic–relaxant technique is best suited for anesthetic induction and maintenance.

Although the repair is entirely extracardiac, cardiopulmonary bypass is necessary. For patients who require operation during the newborn period, weaning from bypass might be expected to be more complicated because of the severity of preexisting heart failure. However, most of these infants recover and have an excellent prognosis. On the other hand, the infant that presents later in life for repair who has developed PVOD is much more difficult to manage during the postoperative period as a result of reactive airway disease and intermittent episodes of severe pulmonary hypertensive crisis.

OBSTRUCTIVE LESIONS

Obstructive CHD may occur within the heart or great arteries, and it is the most common cause of CHF in the first week of life. Occasionally, obstruction may occur at more than one site (e.g., aortic valve stenosis with coarctation of the aorta) or may exacerbate an associated left-to-right shunt lesion (coarctation of the aorta with VSD). Lesions such as critical aortic valve stenosis may result in severe left ventricular dysfunction, which is present in utero but well compensated for by the fetal circulation. Postnatal closure of the ductus arteriosus results in acute, severe decompensation of a left ventricle now faced with providing systemic blood flow that had been provided largely by the right ventricle before closure of the ductus.

Left Heart Obstructive Lesions

Intracardiac obstruction to blood flow in the left heart may occur at almost any point in the path of blood flow between the pulmonary veins and the aorta. The most common lesions would include aortic valve stenosis, subaortic stenosis, coarctation of the aorta, interrupted aortic arch, and mitral stenosis.

Aortic valve stenosis occurs most commonly in association with a bicuspid aortic valve, in which case, it is usually mild. More extreme aortic valve deformities may result in severe aortic valve stenosis (gradient > 75 mmHg) or a "critical" aortic valve stenosis, in which there is severe left ventricular dysfunction and inadequate cardiac output. As noted previously, infants may acutely develop shock when the ductus arteriosus closes; older children may have the more typical symptoms of CHF, dyspnea, chest pain, or syncope. Physical examination findings depend on the severity of the stenosis and the cardiac function. A hyperdynamic apical impulse is usually present, and a thrill is often felt in the suprasternal notch. A systolic ejection click is heard at the sternal border or apex, followed by a systolic ejection murmur at the midleft and right upper sternal borders, which radiates to the neck. The murmur becomes longer as the stenosis increases. If cardiac function is poor and the patient in shock, the murmur may be barely audible, and pulses may be absent. The decrescendo diastolic murmur of aortic insufficiency often coexists. Chest x-ray shows a prominent ascending aorta and frequently a normal heart size with straightening of the left heart border ("left ventricular contour"). Cardiomegaly occurs with reduced left ventricular function or in the presence of aortic insufficiency. The electrocardiogram may show left ventricular hypertrophy but is not very sensitive to mild or moderate hypertrophy. Echocardiography provides information about the valve anatomy (e.g., bicuspid or dysplastic), left ventricular function, and Doppler estimation of the valve gradient and degree of aortic insufficiency.

Many valves are amenable to balloon valvuloplasty, which can lower the gradient without causing or significantly worsening the aortic insufficiency, thus delaying the need for surgery. Although many patients will eventually require aortic valve replacement, delaying this procedure until the child is larger allows the use of an adult-size valve, avoids the need for anticoagulation in an active child, and potentially reduces the number of valve replacements over the child's lifetime. Surgical results for aortic valve stenosis in infants have improved greatly in recent years, and the decision whether to perform surgical or balloon valvuloplasty as the initial procedure for aortic valve stenosis varies from institution to institution.

Subaortic stenosis is usually caused by a fibrous or fibromuscular ridge of tissue arising from the ventricular septum and protruding into the left ventricular outflow tract. It is frequently associated with other lesions, such as VSD, coarctation of the aorta, mitral stenosis, or double-outlet right ventricle. When present, such lesions tend to progress over time and can also recur after surgical resection. The hemodynamic effects are very similar to aortic valve stenosis, but the jet of blood directed against the usually normal aortic valve may induce aortic valve insufficiency. The physical examination, chest x-ray, and electrocardiographic findings are similar to those in aortic valve stenosis, although there is usually no ejection click, and the murmur may be slightly lower on the chest. Surgical resection is indicated when the stenosis is severe (gradient > 75 mmHg) or when there is progressive aortic insufficiency. It is usually performed through the aortic valve. Potential complications include damage to the aortic valve, complete AV block, and iatrogenic VSD caused by excessive resection.

Coarctation of the aorta and interrupted aortic arch may be considered together because their pathophysiology and presentation are almost identical. Coarctation of the aorta usually occurs as a discrete narrowing of the aorta immediately distal to the origin of the left subclavian artery, which consists of a thickened ridge of media and intima of the aortic wall. Sometimes the origin of the left subclavian artery is also stenotic. Traditionally described as "preductal" lesions that present in infancy or "postductal" types, which supposedly present in adulthood, most coarctations are located immediately opposite the insertion of the ductus arteriosus and are best termed "juxtaductal." Additionally, there may be hypoplasia of the aorta proximal to the coarctation that may involve the "isthmus" between the left subclavian artery and the aortic end of the ductus arteriosus or even extend into the transverse aortic arch. Such hypoplasia is frequently associated with intracardiac lesions, such as a VSD. The association of coarctation of the aorta with a bicuspid aortic valve is as high as 85 percent; few adults identified with bicuspid valve have coarctation of the aorta. Interrupted aortic arch exists when there is complete discontinuity between the ascending and descending aorta and is classified based on the site of interruption (Fig. 25-7). Type A interruption occurs dis-

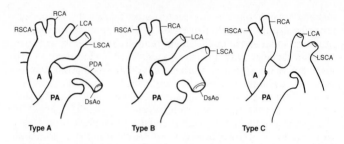

Figure 25-7 Classification of interrupted left aortic arch: Type A, distal to the left subclavian artery (LSCA); Type B, between the LSCA and the left carotid artery (LCA); and Type C, between the LCA and the right carotid artery (RCA) as it arises from the innominate artery. The patent ductus arteriosus (PDA) supplies blood flow distal to the interruption in all cases. RSCA = right subclavian artery; A = aorta; PA = pulmonary artery; DsAo = descending aorta.

tal to the left subclavian artery; Type B is proximal to the left subclavian artery and distal to the left carotid artery and is the most common form of interruption; and Type C is between the innominate artery and the left carotid artery and is the least common form. All these types have a PDA supplying blood to the distal aorta, and a VSD is almost always present. Interrupted aortic arch also has a greater association with great artery abnormalities, such as truncus arteriosus and double-outlet right ventricle with subpulmonary VSD (Taussig-Bing anomaly). Type B interruption is especially prone to be associated with the DiGeorge syndrome of thymic aplasia, immune deficiency, and hypocalcemia because of absence of the parathyroid glands.

Coarctation of the aorta tends to present either with CHF in infancy or with hypertension in childhood or young adult life. Patients with interrupted aortic arch almost always present in infancy with CHF.

The infant with one of these two defects usually becomes symptomatic in the first week of life with symptoms of CHF or shock. The development of symptoms is usually coincident with closure of the ductus arteriosus and the acute afterload imposed on the left ventricle. Even after the pulmonary end of the ductus closes, the aortic end may remain patent, and this area immediately across from the coarctation ridge may provide a path for blood flow to the descending aorta, thus delaying the development of symptoms. Over several weeks, closure of the aortic end of the ductus occurs, and ductal tissue in the wall of the adjacent aorta may constrict, resulting in significant obstruction. Patients with less severe coarctation or those with many collateral vessels may not develop symptoms in infancy and, thus, may not have their condition diagnosed until they are recognized to have hypertension later in life. These patients are usually asymptomatic and are only detected if blood pressure measurement is made a part of routine well-child care. Potential complications of untreated coarctation of the aorta include left ventricular hypertrophy or dysfunction, endocarditis, or intracranial hemorrhage caused by rupture of cerebral aneurysms that occur with increased frequency in patients with coarctation. If repair is delayed into the second or third decade of life, the associated hypertension may fail to resolve despite adequate relief of the obstruction.

Physical examination findings depend on the age of the patient, the severity of the coarctation, the collateral flow, and the presence of associated lesions. Infants with "critical" coarctation or interrupted aortic arch have overt CHF with tachypnea, grunting respirations, normal or low blood pressure, poor perfusion, and absent femoral pulses after closure of the ductus arteriosus. They may develop severe acidosis and oliguria. Before the development of prostaglandin E_1 to restore or maintain ductal patency, these patients were the highest anesthetic and surgical risk. Patients with less severe coarctation, more developed collaterals, and good left ventricular function may be asymptomatic or have more subtle CHF, weak femoral pulses, and upper extremity hypertension. Careful measurement of blood pressure in the upper and lower extremities and simultaneous palpation of upper and lower extremity pulses to detect delayed or diminished pulses is imperative to diagnose coarctation. A precordial systolic murmur is usually present but is nonspecific for coarctation although the murmur may be continuous in the presence of severe obstruction with well-developed collaterals. When a VSD is present, the murmur is the same as that in isolated VSD. Differential cyanosis (pink upper extremities and cyanotic lower extremities) may occur when lower body blood flow is provided by right-to-left flow at a PDA. Chest x-ray usually shows a normal or only mildly enlarged heart size with a left ventricular contour unless there is critical coarctation or an associated intracardiac left-to-right shunt. Rib notching as a result of enlarged intercostal collateral arteries is rarely seen before 5 years of age. The anteroposterior view may show pre- and poststenotic dilatation to the descending aorta along the left edge of the spine, referred to as a "3 sign." The electrocardiogram in infancy shows right ventricular hypertrophy because the right ventricle supports systemic blood flow by the PDA. Beyond infancy, the electrocardiogram may be normal or eventually show left ventricular hypertrophy with more severe or long-standing coarctation. The echocardiogram can identify the location and severity of aortic obstruction in these conditions, evaluate associated defects, and assess ventricular function. The collateral circulation is not seen well by echocardiography. Frequently, the initial aortic arch repair is carried out on the basis of echocardiographic information alone, and cardiac catheterization is performed after the initial arch repair to assess associated defects.

Surgical repair of coarctation of the aorta is performed by resection with end-to-end anastomosis, left subclavian flap angioplasty, (Fig. 25-8) patch enlargement, or conduit placement. Repair of interrupted aortic arch involves reestablishing continuity of the aorta by anastomosis of the subclavian or carotid artery to the distal aorta, by tube graft interposition, or preferably, by direct anastomosis of the proximal and distal aorta. Banding of the pulmonary artery may be performed for control of the shunt because of the VSD, but most surgeons prefer to close the VSD at the time of the initial arch repair by doing both procedures through a median sternotomy.

Mitral stenosis in children is usually congenital and caused by deformities of the mitral valve, such as parachute mitral valve, mitral arcade, or commissural fusion. A supravalvular mitral ring may also occur and result in an identical clinical picture. Rheumatic mitral stenosis is much less common in the United States but remains the leading cause of mitral stenosis in children in Latin America and the Middle East. Infants with significant mitral stenosis are usually symptomatic with dyspnea, poor feeding, cough, orthopnea, sweating, and failure to thrive. They are usually fussy, tachypneic, and tachycardiac. They have an increased anteroposterior chest diameter, retractions, a hyperdynamic precordium, a gallop rhythm, and a crescendo diastolic murmur at the apex, which may be hard to hear because of the tachycardia. A high-pitched decrescendo systolic murmur of mitral regurgitation frequently coexists. The pulses are low volume and perfusion poor. Chest x-ray shows cardiomegaly, left atrial enlargement, and increased pulmonary vascular markings with pulmonary edema. Electrocardiography demonstrates left atrial enlargement and right ventricular hypertrophy if there is pulmonary hypertension. Echocardiography can delineate the valve anatomy better than angiography, while also assessing the valve gradient, ventricular function, and associated defects. Transesophageal echocardiography is especially helpful in larger children, both preoperatively and in the operating room at the time of valve repair. Cardiac catheterization of such patients may be undertaken to delineate further the hemodynamics, to evaluate associated lesions, or to perform balloon valvuloplasty of the mitral valve. Surgical intervention is performed for CHF and failure to thrive refractory

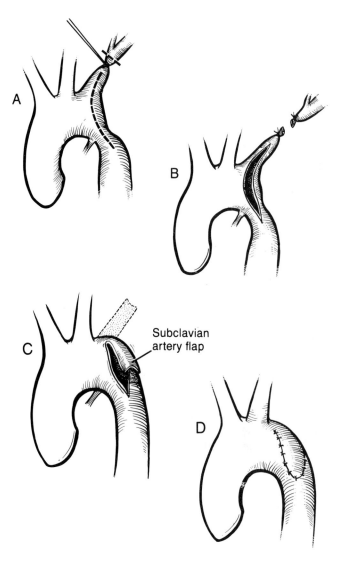

Subclavian
artery flap

Figure 25-8 Subclavian flap angioplasty.

to medical management. The goal of surgery, especially in small children, is valvuloplasty to relieve stenosis and avoid or delay the need for valve replacement.

Anesthetic Management
Most left heart obstructive lesions, with the exception of post-ductal coarctation of the aorta, present in the newborn period and may develop severe CHF or shock. Many of these lesions are ductus dependent and require prostaglandin infusion to maintain ductal patency to preserve systemic flow. The left heart is hypertrophied and at risk for myocardial ischemia. Bradycardia is very poorly tolerated in this group of patients because of a fixed stroke volume limited by the obstruction. The SVR, heart rate, and diastolic pressure should be maintained at near preinduction levels to prevent myocardial ischemia. In older children with aortic stenosis, adequate premedication is essential. However, most infants presenting for this type of surgery will be quite ill, and no premedication is necessary.

Anesthetic induction is best accomplished with fentanyl 10 to 20 μg/kg and pancuronium 0.1 to 0.2 mg/kg, and the patient is maintained on the narcotic/air/oxygen. In cases of aortic stenosis, injury to the conduction system or iatrogenic creation of a VSD may occur, especially during resection of subvalvar aortic stenosis, which may result in postoperative CHF. Both continued inotropic support for several days and temporary pacing may be necessary in these patients.

Interrupted aortic arch complex may require cardiopulmonary bypass if a VSD exists in association or a very hypoplastic aortic isthmus is present. Occasionally, two aortic cannulas may be necessary to provide flow to the arch vessels and the lower extremities during bypass. Profound hypothermia and circulatory arrest are often necessary. As in critical aortic stenosis, these infants are quite unstable and are prone to myocardial ischemia and arrhythmias. Fentanyl anesthesia is preferred. These infants often require prolonged mechanical ventilation and continued inotropic support. Perioperative mortality rates remain high.

Right Heart Obstructive Lesions

Many lesions that cause obstruction to blood on the right side of the heart result in cyanosis (e.g., tricuspid atresia, tetralogy of Fallot, or pulmonary valve atresia) and are discussed elsewhere. Pulmonary valve stenosis is the most common right heart obstructive lesion and rarely causes detectable cyanosis.

Pulmonary valve stenosis (PVS) usually occurs as an isolated defect caused by fusion of the valve commissures or a bicuspid pulmonary valve. Occasionally, the valve is severely dysplastic, as in patients with Noonan's syndrome. Although rare now, congenital rubella infection is associated with severe stenosis of the pulmonary valve and the main and branch pulmonary arteries.

Most patients with pulmonary valve stenosis are asymptomatic, even in the presence of severe obstruction. Neonates with severe PVS and suprasystemic right ventricular pressure may present with cyanosis and right ventricular failure, but most patients' conditions are diagnosed after evaluation of the murmur. Physical examination reveals a well-developed child, who is often described as "cherubic" because of their chubby, round faces. Cyanosis is typically absent, although some patients with more severe obstruction may become cyanotic with crying as a result of right-to-left shunting at a patent foramen ovale. A precordial thrill is present at the left upper sternal border in the presence of moderate-to-severe obstruction. A harsh systolic ejection murmur at the left upper sternal border is frequently preceded by an ejection click. The murmur radiates to the back and also to the axillae in the presence of pulmonary artery branch stenosis. Hepatomegaly and a murmur of tricuspid regurgitation occur with right ventricular failure but are rare. The electrocardiogram is sensitive for right ventricular hypertrophy and may show asymmetric T wave inversion in the anterior chest leads with severe obstruction. Chest x-ray usually shows a normal heart size with dilatation of the main pulmonary artery. Pulmonary vascular markings are diminished only with severe stenosis.

Echocardiography identifies the anatomy of the pulmonary valve and whether it is dysplastic. It also provides information on right ventricular function and associated lesions. Doppler echocardiography is used to estimate the pulmonary valve gradient and correlates well with gradients measured at the time of cardiac catheterization.

Intervention to relieve pulmonary stenosis is undertaken for Doppler-estimated valve gradients in excess of 40 mmHg. The current treatment of choice for isolated valvar pulmonary stenosis is balloon pulmonary valvuloplasty at the time of cardiac catheterization. This technique is highly effective and safe; it provides long-lasting relief of obstruction. Patients with dysplastic valves have less favorable results and frequently require surgical valvotomy. When there are other associated lesions or multiple levels of pulmonary stenosis in the main or branch arteries, surgical valvotomy is usually performed at the time that the other lesions are repaired.

Anesthetic Management

Because most patients with pulmonary valve stenosis are asymptomatic, either an intravenous induction with fentanyl 10 to 20 µg/kg or inhalational induction with halothane is acceptable. Premedication in the older infant or child will ease the stressful transition from the parents to the operating room. In cases of severe pulmonary stenosis, tachycardia may increase the gradient across the pulmonary valve and reduce the cardiac output by shortening the diastolic filling time.

Therefore, avoidance of agents that produce tachycardia in these patients is desirable. Most of these children have a relatively uncomplicated course and may be extubated within a few hours postoperatively; therefore, narcotics should be titrated to provide postoperative pain relief, yet allow removal of the ventilatory support.

The neonate who presents with critical pulmonary stenosis and intact ventricular septum is quite different and is often hemodynamically unstable. These patients continue to have a high perioperative mortality rate. Prostaglandin infusions and inotropic support are often in use before arrival in the operating room. Anesthetic induction is best accomplished with fentanyl 5 to 10 µg/kg/dose and titrated carefully to prevent hypotension. The right ventricle is hypertrophied and noncompliant, leaving it vulnerable to ischemia. Dysrhythmias are common during cannulation and are often poorly tolerated. Pulmonary valvotomy is often combined with a systemic-to-pulmonary shunt, particularly if the pulmonary valve orifice is small. These infants often have a prolonged recovery phase and require inotropic and ventilatory support for several days to weeks postoperatively.

BIBLIOGRAPHY

Artman M, Graham T: Congestive heart failure in infancy: Recognition and management. *Am Heart J* 1982; 103:1040–1055.

Coles JG, Williams WG, et al: Surgical experience with reparative techniques in patients with congenital mitral valve anomalies. *Circulation* 1987; 76(suppl III):III-117–III-122.

Hoffman JIE: Congenital heart disease: Incidence and inheritance. *Pediatr Clin North Am* 1990; 37:25–43.

Kirklin JW, Colvin EV, McConnell ME, et al: Complete transposition of the great arteries: Treatment in the current era. *Pediatr Clin North Am* 1990; 37:171–177.

Mas MS, Bricker JR: Clinical physiology of left to right shunts, in Garson A, Bricker JT, McNamara DG (eds): *The Science and Practice of Pediatric Cardiology*. Philadelphia, Lea & Febiger, 1990, p 999.

Morriss MJ, McNamara DG: Coarctation of the aorta and interrupted aortic arch, in Garson A, Bricker JT, McNamara DG (eds): *The*

Science and Practice of Pediatric Cardiology. Philadelphia, Lea & Febiger, 1990, p 1353.

Mullins CE: Pediatric and congenital therapeutic cardiac catheterization. *Circulation* 1989; 79:1153–1159.

Soto B, Ceballos R, Kirklin JW: Ventricular septal defects: A surgical viewpoint. *J Am Coll Cardiol* 1989; 14:1291–1297.

Van Praagh R, Geva T, Kreutzer J. Editorial comment: Ventricular septal defects: How shall we describe, name, and classify them? *J Am Coll Cardiol* 1989; 14:1298–1299.

SUGGESTED READINGS

Adams FH, Emmanouilides GC, Riemenschneider TA: *Moss' Heart Disease in Infants, Children, and Adolescents,* ed 4. Baltimore, Williams and Wilkins, 1989.

Aiemer G, Jonas RA, Perry SB, et al: Surgery for coarctation of the aorta in the neonate. *Circulation* 1986; 74(suppl 1):1-25–1-31.

Bernhard WF, Keane JF, Fellows KE, et al: Progress and problems in the surgical management of congenital aortic stenosis. *J Thorac Cardiovasc Surg* 1973; 60:404–419.

Braulin EA, Lock JE, Foker JE: Repair of type B interruption of the aortic arch. *J Thorac Cardiovasc Surg* 1983; 86:920–925.

Campbell J, Delorenzi R, Brown J, et al: Improved results in newborns and undergoing coarctation repair. *Ann Thorac Surg* 1980; 20:273–280.

Castaneda A, Mayer JE, Jonas RA: Repair of complete atrioventricular canal in infancy. *World J Surg* 1985; 9:590–597.

Doty DB, Lamberth WC: Repair of ventricular septal defects. *World J Surg* 1985; 9:516–521.

Edmunds LH, Wagner HR, Heymann MA: Aortic valvotomy in neonates. *Circulation* 1980; 61:421–427.

Eggert LD, Jung AL, McGough EC, et al: Surgical treatment of patent ductus arteriosus in preterm infants: Four year experience with ligation in the newborn intensive care unit. *Pediatr Cardiol* 1982; 2:15–18.

Freedom RF, Benson LN, Smallhorn JR: *Neonatal Heart Disease,* ed 1. London, Springer-Verlag, 1992.

Friesen RH, Lichtor L: Cardiovascular effects of inhalation induction with isoflurane in infants. *Anesth Analg* 1983; 62:411–414.

Garson A, Bricker JT, McNamara DG: *The Science and Practice of Pediatric Cardiology,* ed 1. Philadelphia, Lea and Febiger, 1990.

Neuman GG, Hansen DD: The anesthetic management of preterm infants undergoing ligation of patent ductus arteriosus. *Can J Anesth* 1980; 27:248–253.

Perloff JK: *The Clinical Recognition of Congenital Heart Disease,* ed 3. Philadelphia, WB Saunders, 1987.

Rizzoli G, Blackstone EH, Kirklin JW, et al: Incremental risk factors in hospital mortality after repair of ventricular septal defect. *J Thorac Cardiovasc Surg* 1980;80:494–505.

Robinson S, Gregory GA: Fentanyl-air-oxygen anesthesia for ligation of patent ductus arteriosus in preterm infants. *Anesth Analg* 1981; 60:331–334.

Tabak C, Moskowitz W, Wagner H, et al: Aortopulmonary window and aortic isthmic hypoplasia. *J Thorac Cardiovasc Surg* 1983; 86:273–279.

Vincent RN, Lang P, Chipman CW, et al: Assessment of hemodynamic status in the intensive care unit immediately after closure of ventricular septal defect. *Am J Cardiol* 1985; 55:526–529.

CHAPTER 26

Cyanotic Congenital Heart Disease

Mary Dale Peterson
Deborah K. Rasch

The majority of deaths from congenital heart disease in the first year of life are caused by cyanotic lesions. The primary pathophysiologic state is hypoxemia, which leads to other compensatory mechanisms to increase available oxygen. Polycythemia increases blood viscosity, which increases vascular resistance and sludging and may produce renal, pulmonary, and cerebral thromboses. Secondary complications include brain infarct in children younger than 2 years of age and abscess in children older than 2 years of age. Fortunately, with advances in cardiac surgery and myocardial preservation, these complications are rarely seen because corrective surgery or palliation is done much earlier, even during the newborn period.

Cyanosis occurs usually in lesions in which:

1. Pulmonary blood flow is decreased (e.g., tetralogy of Fallot [TOF]).
2. Mixing of systemic and pulmonary venous return occurs (e.g., transposition of the great arteries).

This chapter will discuss the major cyanotic congenital heart lesions and the anesthetic implications of the individual conditions.

TRANSITIONAL CIRCULATION

Many infants who present with cyanotic heart disease have so-called ductal-dependent lesions: tricuspid atresia, pulmonary atresia, critical pulmonic stenosis, in which pulmonary blood flow (which cannot go right ventricle [RV] to pulmonary artery [PA]) goes right atrium (RA), left atrium (LA), left ventricle (LV), aorta (AO), patent ductus arteriosus (PDA), to PA (this is left-to-right flow through the PDA).

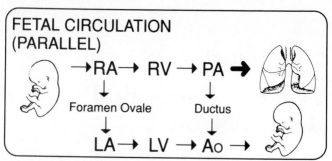

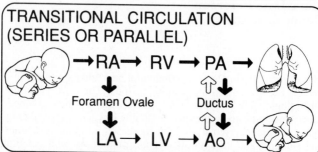

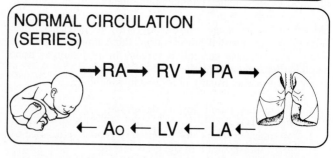

Figure 26-1 Transitional circulation. Schematic representation of the course of circulation during transition from a fetal-type circulatory pattern to an adult-type circulatory pattern. RA = right atrium; RV = right ventricle; PA = pulmonary artery; Ao = aorta; LV = left ventricle; LA = left atrium. (Reproduced with permission from Ryan JF, Todres ID, Coté CJ, et al: *A Practice of Anesthesia for Infants and Children.* Orlando, FL, Grune and Stratton, 1986, p 176.)

Prostaglandin E_1 is infused initially at a dose of 0.05 to 0.1 μg/kg/min to maintain ductal patency until palliative or definitive repair occurs (Fig. 26-1).

SHUNTING

The majority of shunts in congenital heart disease involve communications of various sizes across normally intact structures at the level of the atrium, ventricle, and/or great vessels. Major determinants of flow across the shunts are:

1. Shunt orifice size.
2. Outflow resistance (i.e., systemic vascular resistance [SVR] or pulmonary vascular resistance [PVR] or both).

In simple shunts (shunt without obstructive lesion), with a small orifice, the amount of flow is determined by the difference in pressures between chambers. As the orifice size increases, the flow becomes more dependent on outflow resistance (i.e., SVR or PVR, Table 26-1).[1]

In complex shunts (shunt with obstructive lesion), the shunt flow magnitude and direction is largely fixed by the obstruction size and not related to the outflow resistance. Therefore, PA pressures or PVR manipulation is of virtually no importance in managing TOF (Table 26-2).

Anesthetic factors to be managed in the operating room include pressure differentials within the chambers on either side of a shunt, such as RA and RV pressures, which can be managed with manipulation of preload by volume infusion, choice of inhalation and intravenous agents, or the use of venoconstrictors. Outflow resistance (SVR, PVR, or both) can also be managed. The SVR is manipulated with α-agonists. The classic example is using phenylephrine injection to raise SVR in TOF (Table 26-3).

For practical purposes, acute increases in left-to-right shunts are usually well tolerated, except for a few situations, such as pulmonary atresia in which increasing flow through the PDA may result in systemic hypotension and metabolic acidosis secondary to low tissue oxygen delivery. Acute increases in right-to-left shunts, which is a far more frequent problem during anesthesia, often results in life-threatening hypoxemia or acidemia.

[1]Laura McDaniel, M.D., lecture series, University of Texas Medical Branch at Galveston, 6/19/92 (communication).

Table 26-1   Simple Shunts: No Obstructive Lesions

RESTRICTIVE SHUNTS (SMALL COMMUNICATIONS)	NONRESTRICTVE SHUNTS (LARGE COMMUNICATIONS)	COMMON CHAMBERS (COMPLETE MIXING)
Large pressure gradient	Small pressure gradient	No pressure gradient
Direction and magnitude more independent on PVR/SVR	Direction and magnitude more dependent on PVR/SVR	Bidirectional shunting
Less subject to control	More subject to control	Net Qp/Qs totally depends on PVR/SVR
Examples: small VSD, small PDA Blalock shunts, and small ASD	Examples: large VSD, large PDA, and large Waterston shunts	Examples: single ventricle, truncus arteriosus, and single atrium

PVR = pulmonary vascular resistance; SVR = systemic vascular resistance; VSD = ventricular septal defect; PDA = patent ductus arteriosus; ASD = atrial septal defect.

Reproduced with permission from Hickey P, Wessel D: Anesthesia for treatment of congenital heart disease, in Kaplan J (ed): *Cardiac Anesthesia*, ed 2. Philadelphia, WB Saunders, 1987, p 647.

Table 26-2   Complex Shunts (Shunt and Obstructive Lesion)

PARTIAL OUTFLOW OBSTRUCTION	TOTAL OUTFLOW OBSTRUCTION
Shunt magnitude and direction largely fixed by obstruction	Shunt magnitude and direction totally fixed
Shunt depends less on PVR/SVR	All flow goes through shunt
Orifice and obstruction determine pressure gradient	Pressure gradient depends on orifice
Examples: tetralogy of Fallot, VSD and pulmonic stenosis, and VSD with coarctation	Examples: Tricuspid atresia, mitral atresia, pulmonary atresia, and aortic atresia

VSD = ventricular septal defect.

Reproduced with permission from Hickey P, Wessel D: Anesthesia for treatment of congenital heart disease, in Kaplan J (ed): *Cardiac Anesthesia,* ed 2. Philadelphia, WB Saunders, 1987, p 648.

Table 26-3   Techniques to Manipulate Vascular Resistances

VASCULAR RESISTANCE	INCREASES	DECREASES
Pulmonary	Acidosis and high $PaCO_2$	Alkalosis (pH 7.6) and low $PaCO_2$
	Atelectasis	Normal functional residual capacity (appropriate lung volumes)
	Hypoxia	Oxygen (high fraction of inspired oxygen is a poor vasodilator compared with pH, and toxic for prolonged periods)
	Sympathetic stimulation	Block sympathetic stimulation (anesthesia)
	Direct manipulation	
Systemic	Vasoconstrictors	Potent inhalation agent
	Direct manipulation	Vasodilators

SPECIAL PREOPERATIVE CONSIDERATIONS

Children with cyanotic heart disease and elevated hematocrits (> 45 percent) do not tolerate long periods of fasting. Therefore, intravenous fluids may be necessary preoperatively.

All children with congenital heart disease need to receive appropriate bacterial endocarditis prophylaxis if the surgical procedure has a risk for bacteremia. For "clean" cardiovascular surgery, cefazolin or other first-generation cephalosporin at a dose of 25 mg/kg should be given intravenously or intramuscularly within 2 h of the incision and continued every 6 h for 24 to 48 h. Vancomycin 10 mg/kg may be substituted in hospitals with resistant staphylococcal organisms.

As in all patients who have the potential for right-to-left shunting, all lines should be free of air bubbles, and careful injection techniques (do not inject to the end of a syringe) should be used.

Numerous preoperative sedation regimens can be used successfully in these children. In children prone to hypercyanotic episodes (tetralogy of Fallot [TET] spells), the oral route may be preferable. If heavy parenteral sedation is chosen in cyanotic children, these children should be monitored and given supplemental oxygen if needed.

It is important to note previous surgical interventions. Blood pressure measurements should not be made in an arm that is on the side of a Blalock-Taussig shunt or a subclavian flap coarctation of the aorta repair. The cardiac catheterization data can also be helpful in assessing potential vascular access problems (e.g., absent or thrombosed inferior vena cava (IVC) or bilateral superior vena cavae).

CHOICE OF ANESTHETIC TECHNIQUE

The condition of the patient and the proposed surgery are major considerations for choosing anesthetic agents. Greeley and colleagues have compared the effects of halothane and ketamine on arterial oxygen saturation in children with cyanotic heart disease. Patients induced with halothane, nitrous oxide (70%), and oxygen (30%) had significant increases in oxygen saturation despite a reduction in the mean arterial pressure (80 to 60 mmHg). This is thought to be the result of: (1) decreased systemic oxygen utilization and (2) a decrease in dynamic infundibular pulmonary stenosis in those patients with TOF caused by the negative inotropic effect of halothane. Ketamine 6 mg/kg IM also had a beneficial effect on oxygen saturations and may be a preferred induction technique in children with poor venous access. Nitrous oxide has a mild depressant effect on systemic hemodynamics, but no changes occur in PA pressure in infants with elevated PVR. It can be useful in speeding induction but should probably be avoided in patients with severely depressed cardiac function. Nitrous oxide also has the potential for expanding microbubbles.

High-dose narcotics with fentanyl or sufentanil have been successfully used in infants with severe complex cyanotic congenital heart diseases. This technique is well tolerated hemodynamically and decreased the stress response in infants undergoing heart surgery compared with conventional halothane anesthesia. The use of pancuronium with high-dose fentanyl is recommended to offset the vagotonic effect of fentanyl. This technique is most suitable for sick infants and children who will be ventilated in the postoperative period.

SPECIFIC LESIONS

The major congenital heart lesions causing cyanosis are best remembered by the rule of five T's because the names of these lesions begin with the letter "T" (Table 26-4). The following is a discussion of the pathophysiology of the cyanotic lesions and the specific anesthetic implications of the individual forms of cyanotic heart disease in infants and children.

TOF

TOF (Fig. 26-2) is the most frequently occurring congenital heart lesion that is responsible for cyanosis caused by too little pulmonary blood flow. It consists of (1) RV outflow obstruction (both infundibular and valvular stenosis occur in 74 percent of cases, and there may be additional areas of stenosis in the main PA or its branches), (2) ventricular septal defect (VSD, classically subaortic and very large), (3) overriding aorta, and (4) RV hypertrophy (RVH). The clinical status of newborns with TOF varies with the degree of RV outflow obstruction. If obstruction is minimal, pulmonary flow may be actually increased—this constitutes the "pink TET." At the other end of the spectrum,

Table 26-4   The Most Common Forms of Cyanotic Heart Disease in Infants

Tetralogy of Fallot

Transposition of the great vessels

Tricuspid atresia

Total anomalous pulmonary venous return

Truncus arteriosus

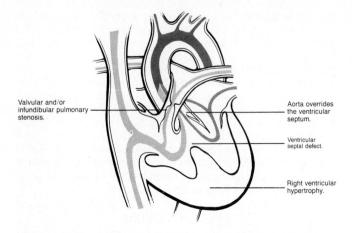

Valvular and/or infundibular pulmonary stenosis.

Aorta overrides the ventricular septum.

Ventricular septal defect.

Right ventricular hypertrophy.

Figure 26-2 Tetralogy of Fallot consists of right ventricular outflow obstruction, ventricular septal defect, overriding aorta, and right ventricular hypertrophy.

complete atresia of the pulmonary valve may result in severe cyanosis immediately after birth. In addition to the baseline cyanosis present at all times, hypercyanotic episodes (TET spells) may occur frequently in these infants. These are thought to be the result of a sudden additional decrease in pulmonary flow secondary to spasm of the pulmonary outflow tract. Squatting may help those hypoxemic spells by increasing SVR and augmenting venous return. PVR is usually normal because the pulmonic stenosis protects the lungs from excessive blood flow through the VSD. The presence of significantly frequent or severe TET spells is an indication for earlier operation. Occasionally, propranolol may be used to temporize until the surgery can be done.

Physical examination reveals a systolic ejection murmur with or without a click. Peripheral oxygen saturation, growth parameters, and hematocrit are useful to determine the degree of hypoxemia. Chest x-ray shows evidence of RVH, with an upturned apex (boot shape) and decreased pulmonary vascular markings (Fig. 26-3). Electrocardiography shows RVH and right-axis deviation.

In the severely cyanotic newborn, a systemic artery to PA shunt may be established in selected cases to provide palliative relief from the effects of too little pulmonary blood flow. Providing the size of the anastomotic opening is not restrictive, the diameter and length of the shunt govern the amount of pulmonary flow. The most common shunt performed is the subclavian

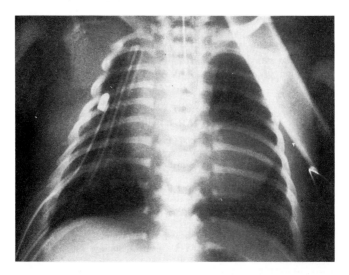

Figure 26-3 Tetralogy of Fallot. The pulmonary vascular markings are decreased, the cardiac apex is upturned, and there is an absence of the main pulmonary artery shadow as a component of the cardiac silhouette. The result is a "boot-shaped" heart.

to PA (Blalock-Taussig) shunt because the relative size of the subclavian artery appears best suited to give adequate flow without producing pulmonary edema.

Anesthesia is a challenge for these small, cyanotic infants, who come for urgent shunts to improve pulmonary blood flow. Induction of these patients requires an anesthetic technique that attempts to avoid right-to-left shunting. Ketamine 1 to 2 mg/kg IV or 6 mg/kg IM can be used for induction with maintenance anesthesia provided by narcotics. Depending on the stability of the infant, halothane may also be used in judicious concentrations. If the infant has had a recent heart catheterization, special attention to the patient's starting hematocrit is essential because these infants do not tolerate anemia well. For infants with cyanotic heart disease, we recommend transfusion of packed red blood cells if the hematocrit falls below 40 percent, especially if the infant is having TET spells. This can greatly improve the stability of these infants. Should the patient develop a TET spell under anesthesia, the following may be tried to ameliorate the degree of infundibular spasm and promote pulmonary blood flow:

1. Hyperventilate with 100% oxygen.
2. Maintain high preload (volume, leg raising, and aortic compression).
3. Increase SVR by giving phenylephrine 1 μg/kg IV.
4. Increase the depth of anesthesia if the blood pressure is stable.

Traditionally, when the palliated child approaches 2 years of age, the repair of the defects included in the TOF complex can be accomplished. More recently, however, infants are being repaired much earlier during infancy. Instead of doing a shunting procedure, patients with favorable anatomy are being corrected as soon as they begin to show signs of worsening cyanosis or an increased frequency of hypercyanotic episodes. Milder forms of tetralogy require only resection of the obstructing musculature with or without pulmonary valvotomy and closure of the VSD. More hypoplastic forms of RV outflow require a pericardial patch over the RV outflow tract.

The operative mortality rate from the palliative procedures in uncomplicated TOF is only one to two percent and total correction, one to five percent. Weaning from cardiopulmonary bypass (CPB) may be difficult if residual obstruction is present in the RV outflow tract or the main PA. Residual VSD will be tolerated better by the patient than residual obstruction during weaning from CPB, but if large, it may cause congestive heart failure in the postoperative period. PA saturations greater than 80 percent during ventilation with a FiO_2 less than 50% indicate a significant left to right shunt. Most patients with TOF will have some degree of RV dysfunction from CPB, right ventriculotomy, and pulmonary insufficiency. A right bundle branch block pattern on electrocardiography is common. If residual pulmonic obstruction or significant shunt are also present, the patient may need significant inotropic support during the postoperative period.

Transposition of the Great Vessels (TGV)

Cyanosis occurs in patients with TGV because there is no exchange of blood between the systemic and pulmonary circulations (Fig. 26-4). Mixing of the two circulations must occur through a PDA, patent foramen ovale, or coexisting anomalous intracardiac defect, such as VSD, for the infant to survive. The clinical picture of transposition of the great arteries depends on the amount of mixing and the site of mixing between the two circulations.

Chest x-ray initially shows a normal-sized heart with a narrow upper segment and rather egg-shaped lower portion of the cardiac silhouette (Fig. 26-5). As failure develops because of a

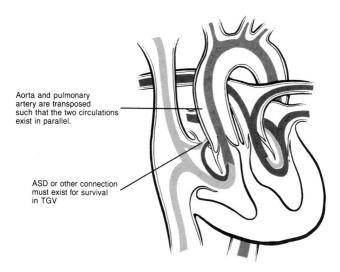

Aorta and pulmonary
artery are transposed
such that the two circulations
exist in parallel.

ASD or other connection
must exist for survival
in TGV

Figure 26-4 Transposition of the great vessels (TGV). Mixing of the systemic and pulmonary circulations through a ductus arteriosus, patent foramen ovale, or coexisting anomalous intracardiac defect, such as atrial septal defect (ASD), is necessary for survival.

fall in PVR, cardiomegaly occurs especially if a VSD is present. Whether or not a murmur is present depends on the presence or absence of a VSD or PDA. As with other cyanotic defects, if the PDA is large or a VSD is present, cyanosis will be minimal in the newborn period. If no murmur is heard, these babies may be missed on a normal newborn examination until the PDA begins to close and they become acutely cyanotic.

The observation that infants with TGV and a large atrial septal defect (ASD) survived without serious complications early in life led to the development of a palliative procedure known as interatrial septectomy—the Blalock-Hanlon procedure. However, the operative mortality rate was approximately 50 percent because these infants were critical hemodynamically and did not tolerate anesthesia and surgery well. Then, in the early 1960s, William Rashkind introduced the balloon atrial septostomy, in which an enlarged intraatrial communication is created during cardiac catheterization. Balloon septostomy has very low morbidity and mortality rates and often produces adequate mixing to stabilize these infants until a definitive procedure can be done early in the newborn period or to allow growth of these

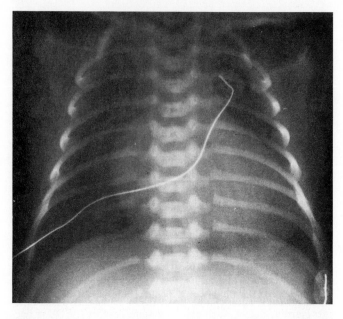

Figure 26-5 Transposition of the great vessels. Note the large oval heart and the narrow mediastinum, resulting in the "egg-on-a-string" cardiac silhouette. In this early film, pulmonary vascular congestion has not yet occurred.

infants when their defect is more complex or when they have a poorly developed LV.

If this procedure fails to produce satisfactory results or the infants present at an age older than 2 to 3 months, when septostomy has a higher incidence of tearing the septum or rupture, then an atrial baffling procedure (Mustard or Senning) or arterial switch operation may be done. All children with TGV require hemodynamic correction because, despite good intraatrial mixing, many of these children die before the age of 3 years from complications of polycythemia, thromboemboli, and hypoxemic cardiomyopathy when uncorrected. The Senning procedure is done for infants (> 3 months of age) and involves the use of the infant's own interatrial septum instead of synthetic material to create an intraatrial baffle. The advantage of this procedure in smaller infants is that this tissue, unlike synthetic material, continues to grow with the baby and there is less need for reoperation. Intraatrial baffle repairs (Mustard or Senning) are done with a hospital mortality rate less than five percent, but late sequelae, including right ventricular failure, atrial dysrhythmias, tricuspid regurgitation, pulmonary venous obstruction, or superior vena cava obstruction have prompted surgeons to use the arterial switch (Jatene) operation (Fig. 26-6). The arterial switch operation is a newer procedure that has the advantage of preserving the natural relationships between the great vessels and their respective ventricles. The coronary arteries must be transplanted, making this a more technically difficult operation. Although this repair was initially done in infants with a large VSD, so that the LV was prepared to accept systemic afterload, the repair has been extended to infants, within the first 2 weeks of life before a drop in PVR, with TGV and an intact septum. Even infants who present later may undergo an arterial switch operation if their LV is "prepared" with a PA banding procedure.

Complications from anatomic repair include supravalvular aortic and pulmonary anastomotic stenoses. LV dysfunction is common in the initial postoperative period. Although postoperative myocardial infarction has been reported, the infant's myocardium can recover, and few ventricular wall motion abnormalities are present in long-term follow-up.

In our institution, most infants undergo an arterial switch operation if anatomically feasible. For those infants with unfavorable coronary anatomy (e.g., single coronary artery) or a double-outlet RV (when the two great arteries are in a side-by-

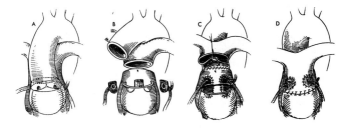

Figure 26-6 Arterial switch repair (Jatene operation). A. The aorta and main pulmonary artery are divided. B. The coronary arteries are excised with the ostea intact in a flap of tissue from the native aortic root. C. The coronary arteries are sutured to the neo-aorta (previously the pulmonary trunk), and the ascending aorta is reattached using one end to end anastomosis. D. The pulmonary arteries are then reattached to the old aortic root, which now becomes pulmonary outflow tract. [Reproduced with permission from Trusler G, Freedom R, Arciniegas E (eds): *Pediatric Cardiac Surgery*. Chicago, Mosby Year Book, 1985.]

side relationship), the Damus-Kaye-Stansel operation is an alternative to arterial switch (Fig. 26-7). In this operation, the coronary arteries are not transferred. Instead, flow from the LV to the aorta is established by anastomosing the proximal cut end of the PA to the side of the aorta. The right ventricle is joined

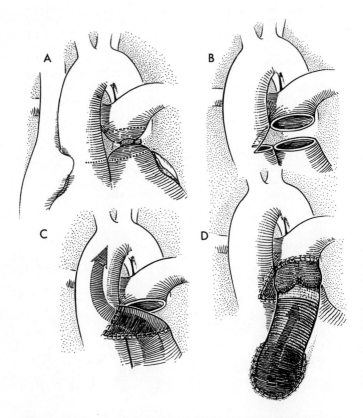

Figure 26-7 The Damus-Kaye-Stansel operation. A. The pulmonary trunk is isolated and divided from the pulmonary valve and right ventricle. B. An incision is made into the side wall of the ascending aorta. C. Pericardium or homograft material is then used to anastomose the pulmonary trunk to the side of the aorta. This allows systemic flow to be ejected via the native pulmonary valve which acts as the neo-aorta. D. The pulmonary outflow tract is recreated from the wall of the right ventricle usually by means of a homograft to the bifurcation of the main pulmonary artery. [Reproduced with permission from Trusler G, Freedom R, Arciniegas E (eds): *Pediatric Cardiac Surgery.* Chicago, Mosby Year Book, 1985.]

to the distal PA with a valved conduit. The aortic valve is kept closed by aortic pressure, which is greater than RV pressure (Fig. 26-7).

These operations are usually carried out under hypothermic total circulatory arrest. Nondepressant anesthetic techniques, such as high-dose narcotics, are used in these infants. Because of the circumferential aortic, pulmonic, and coronary artery suture lines of the arterial switch procedure, major bleeding can be a problem postbypass. We insist on the availability of fresh whole blood (< 24 h old) and fresh components before operating on these infants.

Ventricular dysfunction occurs frequently and must be aggressively treated with inotropes and occasionally coronary vasodilators. If severe, the surgeon may have to free up a coronary artery if it is kinked.

Tricuspid Atresia

This complex is the third most common cause of cyanotic heart disease and is one of the more severe and life-threatening forms of cyanotic heart disease. As would be expected by its name, no valvular orifice is present in the area of the tricuspid valve in these patients and no communication exists between the RA and RV. Classification of the forms of tricuspid atresia depends on the arrangement of the great vessels and presence or absence of a VSD (Table 26-5).

In the absence of a VSD and the presence of either critical pulmonary stenosis (PS) or pulmonary atresia, there is severe underdevelopment of the RV because it receives no flow in utero. Most of these patients will be deeply cyanotic, with the exception of those with a large VSD without PS. In most cases, auscultation of the chest reveals no murmur and a single second heart sound (there is no pulmonary component). Chest x-ray shows decreased pulmonary vascular markings, and electrocar-

Table 26-5   Classification of Tricuspid Atresia

Type I:	Normal Position of the Great Vessels
	No VSD and pulmonary atresia
	Small VSD and pulmonary stenosis
	Large VSD with pulmonary stenosis
Type II:	Transposition of the Great Vessels
	VSD and pulmonary atresia
	VSD and pulmonary stenosis
	VSD without pulmonary stenosis

VSD = ventricular septal defect.

diography shows left axis deviation and pure left ventricular hypertrophy. Prostaglandin infusion is necessary to maintain the PDA until a systemic to PA shunt can be performed for palliation. If there is a small or absent communication between the RA and LA, then balloon septostomy is usually performed to improve mixing and decompress the RA.

When the child outgrows the systemic to PA shunt, venous shunting procedures connecting the systemic venous return to the PAs can be done. This establishes a series circuit, which improves systemic oxygenation and reduces the volume load on the ventricle, which will lead to ventricular dysfunction. There have been many modifications to the original Fontan procedure initially described in 1971. The optimal age for the Fontan procedure is controversial. In our institution, if a child needs improved oxygenation before 2 years of age or if there are other risk factors for a Fontan (pulmonary hypertension, atrioventricular valve regurgitation, ventricular dysfunction, or small and/or stenotic PAs), the operation performed is a bidirectional cavopulmonary (Glenn) anastomosis as a step to an eventual Fontan. In this operation, the superior vena cava is transsected and the distal end anastomosed to the right PA in such a way as to provide bidirectional flow to the right and left PAs (Fig. 26-8). In the Fontan procedure and its modifications, the systemic

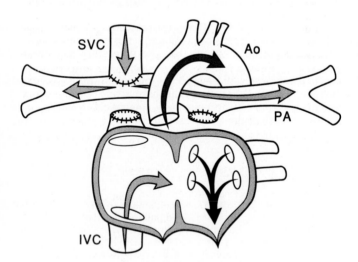

Figure 26-8 The bidirectional Glenn shunt. SVC = superior vena cava; Ao = aorta; PA = pulmonary artery; IVC = inferior vena cava.

venous blood from the superior and inferior vena cava is directed into the PAs.

Anesthesia can be induced with moderate doses of narcotics if an IV line is in place, or halothane 1 to 1.5% may be used. Central venous catheters (preferably internal jugular) should be shorter than usual so as not to interfere with the anastomosis and to be proximal to the cannulation sites. This catheter will reflect the PA pressure after repair, provided there is no anastomotic obstruction. The arterial line should not be placed in the extremity with a previous shunt. Blood must be readily available because many of these cyanotic children have excessive collateral vessels that may be encountered before bypass. Previous aortopulmonary shunts must be sought before CPB and ligated as bypass is initiated.

Children who have had a Fontan operation are very sensitive to changes in PVR. Because of the Fontan series circuit, increases in PVR will reduce cardiac output from limited return to the ventricle. Factors that increase PVR, as previously described, should be avoided. Fenestration of the atrial baffle or an adjustable ASD may allow blood to "pop off" into the left side while PVR is transiently high post-CPB. The oxygen saturations will be decreased, but cardiac output and overall oxygen delivery is improved with markedly diminished mortality. The fenestration may be closed in some catheterization laboratories, or the adjustable ASD may be closed with a simple subcutaneous operation.

Besides PVR, the other important factor post-CPB in these patients is ventricular function. Because children with parallel circulation and previous shunts have volume overload to the ventricle, the ventricle may have poor relaxation properties (diastolic dysfunction). This results in a lowered preload accepted by the ventricle and low cardiac output. Pulmonary blood flow will also decrease. This is more common in children with small, hypertrophied ventricles. After this dysfunction is noted, it can be difficult to treat because most inotropic support used to treat low cardiac output syndromes may worsen diastolic relaxation. Likewise, vasodilators may lower ventricular volume and worsen the diastolic dysfunction. Maintenance of adequate circulating blood volume is critical.

Agents that promote ventricular relaxation are theoretical but as yet unproved therapy. Amrinone may be beneficial in this circumstance. Ventricular-assist devices when pharmacologic management has failed have also been used in children.

In the hemodynamically stable postoperative Fontan patient, attempts are made to wean from the ventilator in an expeditious fashion because this may improve pulmonary blood flow. Chylothoraces and pericardial effusions are common after

Fontan operations and can be problematic, requiring long hospitalizations.

Total Anomalous Pulmonary Venous Return (TAPVR)

TAPVR may produce congestive heart failure in infancy as a
result of the combined mechanisms of pulmonary venous
congestion and pulmonary volume overload without mixing between the two circulations. Because of the anomalous connection, pulmonary venous blood drains either directly into the RA
or systemic veins into the right side of the heart. Obviously, for
systemic arterial flow to be adequate, an intracardiac communication or a PDA must coexist. TAPVR of four types may be
seen (Fig. 26-9): (1) supracardiac forms drain into the azygos
vein or superior vena cava, (2) cardiac types drain into the RA,
(3) infracardiac types drain into the ductus venous or inferior
vena cava, or (4) a mixture of these may occur. Obstruction to
pulmonary venous drainage almost always occurs with infradia-
phragmatic forms, is frequently associated with cardiac and supracardiac forms, and is only occasionally associated with
mixed forms. The presentation of the patient depends on
whether or not there is obstruction to pulmonary venous drain-

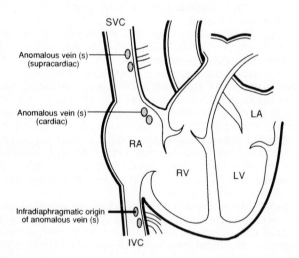

Figure 26-9 Types of total anomalous pulmonary venous return—the classification depends on the location of the anomalous drainage to the right heart. SVC = superior vena cava;
RA = right atrium; RV = right ventricle; IVC = inferior vena
cava; LV = left ventricle; LA = left atrium.

age, leading to pulmonary edema, and the type and degree of intracardiac communication that determine their degree of cyanosis. In most cases, the infant is cyanotic, and no murmur is heard. The cardiac silhouette is often normal in size, but there is a haziness extending from around the cardiac border in the shape of a "snowman" in those with supracardiac drainage from an anomalous vertical vein. Pulmonary congestion is always present, but it is exaggerated with obstruction of the anomalous channel (Fig. 26-10). The electrocardiogram usually shows RVH.

No satisfactory palliative procedures exist for TAPVR. Open intracardiac surgery must be performed in early infancy to establish an unobstructed communication between the pulmonary veins and the LA. If not, these infants go on to develop severe irreversible pulmonary hypertension and are no longer operative candidates. The operative mortality in this group is still higher than in other forms of cyanotic congenital heart disease (incidence rates, 10 to 20 percent). However, with the use of profound hypothermia and circulatory arrest, these numbers are improving. In the cardiac and supracardiac forms, balloon septostomy can be helpful as a preoperative means of improving mixing. This is usually unsatisfactory for long-term results.

Two basic surgical procedures are used. In the infracardiac and supracardiac types, anastomosis of the anomalous veins to the posterior wall of the LA is done, and the anomalous vein(s) is ligated near its insertion into the right-sided venous structures to prevent oxygenated blood from returning to the RA. In the cardiac form, an intraatrial baffle is created to shunt oxygenated blood to the left side. The operative morbidity and mortality is dependent largely on the size of the LV chamber and the presence of hypoplasia of the aortic valve.

These infants are usually very ill if the pulmonary veins are obstructed and require emergency surgery for repair. A high-dose narcotic technique is usually employed. These infants will usually require inotropic support in the immediate postoperative period. Pulmonary hypertension can be severe and must be aggressively prevented and treated. We usually continue anesthesia with fentanyl and vecuronium for 24 to 48 h in an attempt to lessen the pulmonary hypertensive crises that these patients may have. Low doses of dopamine (2 to 3 $\mu g/kg/min$) may be useful in improving renal dysfunction.

Truncus Arteriosus

Truncus arteriosus results from abnormal or incomplete development of the truncoconal ridges, which grow caudad in a spiral fashion during the 3rd to 4th weeks of gestation to separate the truncus arteriosus of the fetus into the aorta and PA. This pro-

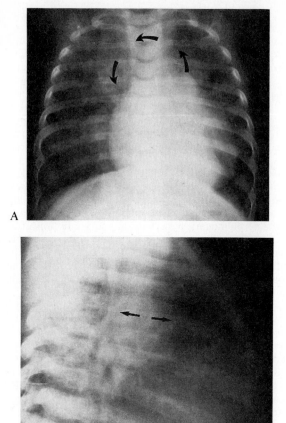

Figure 26-10 (A and B) Total anomalous pulmonary venous return, Type I. The pulmonary vascularity is increased. The superior mediastinal widening is the result of the enlarged anomalous inverted U-shaped vein (arrows), which drains the lungs into the superior vena cava. The result is the characteristic "snowman" cardiomediastinal configuration.

duces incomplete separation of the aorta and PA and a VSD. Four types of truncus occur (Fig. 26-11). Regardless of the anatomic variety, the patient with truncus has a common outlet for both RV and LV output. Pulmonary blood flow varies depending on the size and takeoff of the pulmonary circuit, but some degree of cyanosis is usually present. For those patients with Types I to III truncus arteriosus, congestive heart failure may develop from increased pulmonary blood flow. Chest x-ray shows concavity of the PA component to the cardiac silhouette (Fig. 26-12).

Almost 50 percent will die in the 1st month of life if untreated. Operative repair is difficult, and the exact approach depends on the anatomic defect. Previously, the basic principle of the operation was to create a division within the truncus using Teflon grafting material. Thus, two separate channels for blood flow to exit the heart were created, and the VSD was patched closed. More recently, the common trunk is used to create the neoaorta, and homograft material is used to create a new outflow tract from the RV to the main PA. This group of patients continues to have a higher perioperative mortality rate, approximately 20 percent.

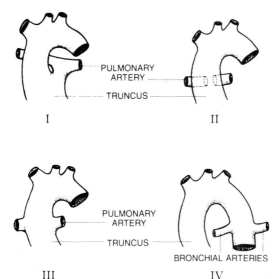

Figure 26-11 Types of truncus arteriosus—the classification depends on the point of insertion of the pulmonary artery into the truncus.

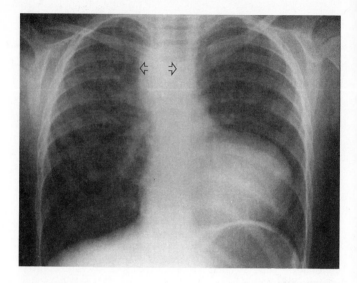

Figure 26-12   Truncus arteriosus. The main pulmonary artery is concave, and the apex of the heart points laterally. Pulmonary vascular congestion is variable in this condition. There is often a right aortic arch (arrows).

The anesthetic considerations are similar to those in other infants presenting with congestive heart failure and increased pulmonary blood flow. Usually, a high-dose narcotic anesthetic is used in these sick infants. Poor myocardial function and persistent pulmonary hypertension are common in the postoperative period. Anesthesia with fentanyl and vecuronium is usually maintained for 24 to 48 h if there is pulmonary vascular instability. Truncal valve insufficiency can also be a problem and should be treated with vasodilator therapy.

BIBLIOGRAPHY

Anderson RG, Obata W, Lillehei CW: Truncus arteriosus: Clinical study of 14 cases. *Circulation* 1957; 16:586–590.

Arciniegas E: Tetralogy of Fallot, in Arciniegas E (ed): *Pediatric Cardiac Surgery*. Chicago, Mosby-Yearbook, 1985.

Baffles TG, Johnson FR, Potts WT, et al: Anatomic variations in tetralogy of Fallot. *Am Heart J* 1953; 46:657–662.

Fink BS: *Congenital Heart Disease: A Deductive Approach to its Diagnosis*. Chicago, Year Book Medical Publishers, 1975.

Greeley WJ, Bushman GA, Davis DP, et al: Comparative effects of halothane and ketamine on systemic arterial oxygen saturation in children with cyanotic heart disease. *Anesthesiology* 1986; 65: 666–668.

Hess JH: Congenital atresia of the right auriculo-ventricular orifice with complete absence of the tricuspid valve. *Am J Dis Child* 1917; 13:167.

Hickey PR, Hansen DD: Fentanyl- and sufentanil-oxygen-pancuronium anesthesia for cardiac surgery in infants. *Anesth Analg* 1984; 63:117–124.

Hickey PR, Hansen DD, Strafford M, et al: Pulmonary and systemic hemodynamic effects of nitrous oxide in infants with normal and elevated pulmonary vascular resistance. *Anesthesiology* 1986; 65:374–378.

Jatene AD, Fontes VF, Souza LCB, et al: Anatomic correction of transposition of the great arteries. *J Thorac Cardiovasc Surg* 1982; 83:20–26.

Keith JD, Rowe RD, Vlad P: *Heart Disease in Infancy and Childhood.* ed 3. New York, Macmillan, 1978.

Kirklin JW, Barratt-Boyes, BG: *Cardiac Surgery.* New York, Wiley, 1986.

McGoon DG, Wallace RB, Danielson GK: The Rastelli operation: Its indications and results. *J Thorac Cardiovasc Surg* 1973; 65: 865–870.

Murphy ME, Aglira BA, Chin AJ, et al: Two-dimensional and Doppler echocardiographic assessment of transposition of the great arteries following neonatal anatomic correction (Jatene operation). *Circulation* 1985; 72:111–345.

Ryan JF, Todres ID, Coté CJ, et al: *A Practice of Anesthesia for Infants and Children.* Orlando, FL, Grune and Stratton, 1986.

Stark J, de Leval M: *Surgical Techniques for Congenital Heart Defects.* London, Grune and Stratton, 1983.

CHAPTER 27

Pediatric Cardiac Surgery: Postoperative Care

Deborah K. Rasch
Joseph J. Naples
Frederick L. Grover
John H. Calhoon

Postoperative management of the pediatric cardiac surgical patient requires a comprehensive understanding of many variables. Knowledge of the infant's cardiac disease for which the surgery is required, the duration of cardiopulmonary bypass, and any difficulties encountered during the surgical repair are essential for anticipating the occurrence of postoperative problems. An understanding of physiologic responses of the cardiovascular system to alteration of ventilation is the foundation for manipulation of hemodynamic variables to improve cardiac dynamics (e,.g., infants with complete atrioventricular canal often have pulmonary hypertension which may improve with mild hyperventilation). Electrolytes should be monitored at intervals, and abnormalities must be promptly managed because there is an increased risk of dysrhythmias in the hypokalemic patient after cardiopulmonary bypass, especially if the patient received digoxin preoperatively.

Many specific aspects of patient care after cardiac surgery may be guided by management protocols, such as those included in this chapter; however, each patient must also be evaluated individually. Communication between the surgeon and the anesthesiologist or intensivist is mandatory, and all physicians responsible for the patient's postoperative care must be kept informed of interventions initiated or planned for the patient. Figure 27-1 is an example of the general postoperative orders used at our institution. General considerations for postoperative management of these children will be discussed with coverage of specific postoperative syndromes.

POSTOPERATIVE MECHANICAL VENTILATION

Adequate ventilation and oxygenation for the pediatric patient after cardiac surgery are essential for optimal hemodynamics. The fraction of inspired oxygen (FiO_2) is initially set at 1.0 until pulse oximetry or blood gas data are available. Then, provided hemodynamics are stable, the FiO_2 can be lowered in a stepwise fashion. Care should be taken when adjusting ventilation because lung function is often abnormal in these patients and hypoxemia will not be well tolerated, especially in unstable patients. Cardiopulmonary bypass (CPB) decreases lung function, the extent of which is directly related to the duration of the bypass. A significant increase in pulmonary morbidity occurs when CPB lasts longer than 120 to 150 min. Hypothermic circulatory arrest has not been shown to increase postoperative pulmonary complications. Some authors would even suggest that pulmonary function may be improved because of a reduction in the time spent on CPB. Preexisting lung disease, pulmonary congestion, and pain in the postoperative period all further impair pulmonary mechanics. Therefore, ventilator changes are usually made in one category at a time (i.e., FiO_2, peak pressure, tidal volume, positive end-expiratory pressure, or rate). We prefer a volume ventilator for these patients because, by setting the tidal volume instead of a peak pressure, the ventilator will allow for changes in lung compliance resulting from postoperative fluid shifts.

As mentioned, ventilation often has a significant impact on hemodynamics during the postoperative period. Chronic increases in pulmonary blood flow (ventricular septal defect, A-V canal) may produce pulmonary vascular changes, which result in pulmonary hypertension. These elevated pulmonary pressures may not subside immediately postoperatively, and increased right ventricular afterload may lead to right ventricular failure. Similarly, patients undergoing right ventriculotomy as a part of the surgical repair (i.e., an outflow tract patch in tetralogy of Fallot) will be at risk for right ventricular dysfunction. For these patients, mild hyperventilation (PCO_2 of 28 to 32 mmHg and pH of 7.45 to 7.5) is desirable because alkalosis can reduce pulmonary artery pressures and improve hemodynamics. On the other hand, in the newborn with hypoplastic left heart syndrome or another lesion that is amenable to palliation rather than total repair, pulmonary congestion may continue to be a problem in the postoperative period. Air trapping, interstitial edema, and variable areas of atelectasis resulting from continued pulmonary overcirculation are often difficult to manage. These patients benefit from normocarbia and may require vigorous pulmonary toilet and prolonged mechanical ventilation.

PEDIATRIC CARDIAC SURGERY POSTOPERATIVE ORDER

Procedure:
Allergies:
Weight: Body surface area:

1. Vital signs every 20 min until stable, then ICU routine.

2. NPO. NG tube to low wall suction.

3. Chest tubes to –10 cm H_2O pressure.

4. Foley catheter to gravity drainage.

5. Record intake and output every hour.

6. Chest x-ray (to evaluate lung fields, cardiac size, endotracheal tube position, and the position of intracardiac lines and chest tubes) and ECG (to look for evidence of conduction and abnormalities, arrhythmia, or ischemia) now and the following morning.

7. Complete blood count, platelet count, serum electrolytes, glucose, serum Ca^{++}, and arterial gases (ABGs) approximately 20 min after arrival in the ICU.

8. ABG, K^+, hematocrit every 4 to 8 h. For infants < 1 year, measure ionized Ca^{++} and glucose.

9. Ventilator: FiO₂ _____,   Rate_____/min
                TV_____, mL   PEEP_____cmH₂O

10. Intracardiac or CVP lines: D5½ NS with 1 unit heparin/mL of fluid at 2 mL/h.

11. Arterial line: 0.9 NS with 1 unit heparin/mL of fluid at 2 mL/h.

12. IV fluids: D5½ NS (infants < 6 mo, D10½ NS) with 10 mEq KCl/500 mL. Total fluids per 24 h_____mL (this value is usually ½ maintenance

13. Medications:

    Cefazolin, 25 mg/kg/dose, given every 8 h _____mg.
    Morphine sulfate IV bolus, 0.05 to 0.1 mg/kg/dose, every hour prn _____mg.

                          OR

    IV drip, 15 mg/30 mL saline, beginning at 0.1 mg/kg/h and titrated to effect.

Figure 27-1 Pediatric cardiac surgery postoperative order form.

Fentanyl IV drip, 1000 μg/50 mL saline beginning at 2 μg/kg/h and titrated to effect.

Diazepam 0.1 to 0.3 mg/kg/dose _____mg IV every 3 to 4 h prn (can be synergistic with narcotics to decrease narcotic requirements; however, benzodiazepines may cause cardiac depression).

Acetaminophen suppositories, 10 mg/kg _____mg prn T ≥ 38.5° C.

14. Inotropes:

Dopamine
Dobutamine } 50 mg/50 mL, titrate to effect; usual
Amrinone   starting dose = 5 μg/kg/min

Epinephrine
Isoproterenol } 1 mg/50 mL, titrate to effect;
Phenylephrine   usual starting dose =
Norepinephrine   0.05 μg/kg/min

15. Dilators:

Sodium nitroprusside } 50 mg/50 mL, titrate to
Nitroglycerin   effect; usual starting
                       dose = 0.5 μg/kg/min

_____
Physician's Signature

Figure 27-1 (*Continued*)

Weaning from ventilatory support and extubation may be possible in the simple case (atrial septal defect, patent ductus arteriosus [PDA], or coarctation) at the end of the procedure. However, the smaller infant and the infant undergoing more complex repair will often benefit from mechanical ventilation for 12 to 24 h postoperatively, or longer, depending on the patient's clinical condition. Vigorous pulmonary toilet and bronchodilator aerosol treatments (albuterol, 0.1 mg/kg/dose) can be very beneficial in the child with preexisting lung disease or preoperative increased pulmonary blood flow.

The criteria for extubation include a variety of clinical and laboratory data, the least important of which are arterial blood

Table 27-1   Criteria for Extubation

Adequate arterial blood gases.

Spontaneous ventilation on continuous positive airway pressure 2 to 4 cmH$_2$O or low rate (4 to 6/min).

Absence of significant tachypnea. Acceptable respiratory rates depend on the age of the child as follows: birth to 6 mo, 60 breaths/min; 6 mo to 2 yrs, 40 to 50 breaths/min; $\geq$ 2 yrs, 30 breaths/min.

Minimal secretions.

Fraction of inspired oxygen 40% or less.

Vital capacity is less useful in younger children who may not be able to cooperate with the test.

Negative inspiratory pressure of -30 to -40 cmH$_2$O correlates better with successful extubation.

---

gases. Although blood gas values should be in the normal range, the other parameters listed in Table 27-1 are more important determinants of successful extubation. In addition to adequate pulmonary function for extubation, stable hemodynamics must be present (i.e., normal blood pressure, adequate cardiac output as evidenced by urine output of 1 mL/kg/h, warm extremities with good pulses and no acidosis, and no significant arrhythmias). Adequate surgical hemostasis with minimal chest tube drainage, normothermia, and stable serum electrolytes are also important. The patient must be awake and able to cough and clear secretions. Residual anesthetic and/or analgesic drugs and muscle relaxants must be adequately cleared from the body or reversed. Routine preparation for extubation should be carried out according to the steps in Table 27-2. Persons experienced

Table 27-2   Preparations for Extubation

Empty stomach; suction nasogastric tube.

Clear airway, mouth, and nasopharynx of secretions.

Have humidified oxygen ready: hood, mask, or nasal prongs.

Bag and mask for ventilation, laryngoscope, and appropriate endotracheal tubes in the event that reintubation is required.

Remove endotracheal tube while applying positive pressure.

Place in a fraction of inspired oxygen at least 10% higher than before extubation.

Determine arterial blood gases 5 min postextubation.

Table 27-3 Other Pulmonary Therapies After Extubation

Continue chest percussion and postural drainage.

In older children, incentive spirometry can be helpful.

Suction pharynx carefully (vigorous suctioning causes edema and agitation).

Supplemental oxygen as indicated per arterial blood gases measurements or pulse oximetry and physical signs.

Repeat daily chest x-ray until monitoring lines are removed.

in pediatric endotracheal intubation should be available for at least 30 min to 1 h after extubation to evaluate the child's respiratory status and to reintubate the patient if necessary. Other interventions that are helpful after extubation to encourage better pulmonary mechanics are shown in Table 27-3. These are equally as important as airway maintenance before the endotracheal tube is removed.

Respiratory failure may result from any of a number of factors in the pediatric patient after cardiac surgery. Difficulties may be encountered in three major areas: (1) upper airway, (2) pulmonary system, and (3) central nervous system. The abnormalities that can occur and their causes are listed in Table 27-4 with recommendations for treatment. Although an exact cause may be unclear at the time the respiratory failure occurs, a systematic approach to diagnosis and treatment is necessary. Of primary importance, however, are establishment of a clear, secure airway and improvement in oxygenation and ventilation. These are essential because even a short period of hypoxemia is poorly tolerated by the cardiovascular system that has recently undergone surgery.

SPECIFIC POSTOPERATIVE PROBLEMS

Serum Potassium

Most often after CPB, the patient will be hypokalemic as a result of hemodilution, glycosuria, and diuretics administered while on CPB; however, if cardiac output is low or acidosis is present, hyperkalemia may occasionally be encountered.

It the serum potassium level is less than 3.5 mEq/L:

1. Give 0.5 to 1 mEq/kg over 1 h by a syringe pump to a maximum dose of 20 mEq.
2. Repeat the serum potassium measurement 1 h after treatment in Step 1.

Table 27-4 Causes of Respiratory Failure in Postoperative Patients

AREA	CAUSE	ETIOLOGY/SYMPTOMS	TREATMENT
Upper airway	Postintubation croup	Most common postoperative upper airway problem. Stridor and/or "barking" cough. Risk factors: 1. Age 1 to 4 yrs 2. Tight-fitting endotracheal tube (air leak > 25 cmH$_2$O) 3. Prolonged intubation.	Cool mist. Racemic epinephrine 0.05 mL/kg in 2 to 3 mL saline to maximum dose of 1 mL of epinephrine. Controversial: Dexamethasone 0.2 to 0.5 mg/kg IV initial dose followed by 1 mg/kg/day. Reintubate with a smaller tube if hypercarbia, hypoxia, or increased work of breathing occur.
	Unrecognized vascular ring	Stridor, usually present both pre- and postoperatively. May be more noticeable because of edema from airway manipulation perioperatively.	Airway maintenance; division of vascular ring.
	Vocal cord paralysis	Rare cause of airway obstruction, results from inadvertent trauma to recurrent laryngeal nerve in thorax. Hoarseness and stridor are present.	Observe for respiratory distress; usually no intervention necessary.

Pulmonary system	Atelectasis	Most common intrapulmonary problem; result of lung changes from CPB, secretions, and immobility. Hypoxemia, hypercarbia, and fever may result.	Chest physiotherapy and endotracheal tube suctioning or encouragement of cough. Adequate pain control. bronchodilators (albuterol 0.1 mg/kg), flexible bronchoscopy in severe cases.
	Pulmonary edema	Etiology includes low cardiac output or fluid shifts postoperatively, persistent left-to-right shunts, and left heart obstructive lesions.	Mechanical ventilation to treat hypoxemia and hypercarbia then treat cause: 1. Inotropes or vasodilators to improve cardiac output 2. Diuretics (furosemide) to treat intravascular volume overload 3. Evaluate for residual shunts.
	Pleural effusion	Serous effusions are associated with low cardiac output, particularly after ventriculotomy; chylothorax may result from inadvertent damage to thoracic duct (PDA ligation, coarctation, Blalock-Taussig shunt).	Treat with thoracentesis or thoracostomy tube to improve symptoms; then evaluate and treat cause when possible.

(Continued)

475

Table 27-4 (*Continued*)

AREA	CAUSE	ETIOLOGY/SYMPTOMS	TREATMENT
	Diaphragm paralysis	Acute respiratory distress occurring after extubation in an infant who has done well on minimal ventilator settings; usually caused by topical hypothermia (ice slush placed in chest for myocardial preservation, which injures phrenic nerve). Asymmetric chest movement; affected hemidiaphragm will be elevated on chest x-ray.	Reintubation may be necessary; usually return of function occurs within 2 to 4 weeks for transient injuries. Vigorous pulmonary toilet.
Central nervous system	Residual anesthetic or analgesic	Infant may be agitated while the endotracheal tube is in place with adequate ABG. Once extubated, respirations slow down and patient may be unarousable.	Stimulation to breathe. If residual narcotic effect, a small dose of naloxone, 3 to 5 µg/kg may be helpful. If no improvement in neurologic status, may need to reintubate.

476

Residual muscle relaxant	Comfortable on minimal settings. Fatigue and respiratory distress ocurs on extubation because of muscle weakness, jerky movements, and anxious expression.	Reverse muscle relaxant with atropine, 0.02 mg/kg, neostigmine, 0.06 mg/kg. Support ventilation until reversal is adequate.
Seizures	Common after circulatory arrest. Usually on postoperative day 2 or 3. Occasionally, may be the result of emboli (air or clot) and result in symptoms of stroke. Metabolic problems (hypoglycemia or hypocalcemia). Cerebral edema as result of cerebral ischemia should be ruled out.	Protect the airway and ventilate with 100% oxygen. Treat seizure with IV phenobarbital, 10 to 15 mg/kg; lorazepam, 0.1 mg/kg IV; or diazepam, 0.3 mg/kg IV. CT scan to look for structural defect, i.e., intracranial bleeding. Use phenytoin cautiously in cardiac patients because conduction abnormalities may occur.

IV = intravenous; CPB = cardiopulmonary bypass; PDA = patent ductus arteriosus; ABG = arterial blood gases.

477

3. If the serum potassium level is still less than 3.2, repeat Steps 1 and 2.

   Note: These high concentrations should be administered through a central venous route when possible.

If the serum potassium level is 3.5 to 4.0 mEq/L, a slightly lower dose, 0.2 to 0.4 mEq/kg, may be given over a 1-h time period. In all cases of hypokalemia, the total daily dose of potassium being administered in the intravenous (IV) fluid should be increased, especially if diuretics are being used.

If the serum potassium is more than 5.0 mEq/L, remove potassium from all IV fluids and recheck in 1 h and thereafter when indicated. Be sure, however, that the specimen was not hemolyzed and that the value is accurate to prevent withholding of potassium in a patient who may actually be hypokalemic. (Note: If the patient is oliguric or has any significant renal dysfunction, do not "treat" hypokalemia. Until adequate urine output is achieved [0.5 to 1.0 mL/kg/h], potassium is withheld from IV fluids.)

These IV therapy guidelines apply only during the first 24 to 48 h after the operation. Thereafter, oral potassium supplementation is usually the method of choice (3 to 4 mEq/kg/day in three divided doses).

Hypocalcemia

Hypocalcemia may occur postoperatively in newborns and sick infants because of their reduced ability to mobilize calcium from bone. Citrate in blood products administered during the postbypass phase and dilution of serum ionized Ca^{++} by CPB add to the problems with calcium homeostasis. A low ionized Ca^{++} fraction can significantly reduce cardiac performance in the postoperative period and should be treated promptly. Calcium chloride therapy is preferred because a more ionized fraction is available than with calcium gluconate preparations. The dose is 10 to 20 mg/kg IV infused slowly over 1 to 2 min; then repeat the serum Ca^{++} value. If additional citrated blood products are given, repeat doses of CaCl may be indicated.

Postoperative Hypertension

Hypertension in the immediate postoperative period is quite common after coarctation repair and other surgical procedures involving the aortic arch and valve. Elevated blood pressure should be controlled because of its adverse effects on the performance of the cardiovascular system and the increased risk of bleeding as a result of severe hypertension. During the immediate postoperative period (approximately the first 24 h), sodium nitroprusside therapy is most commonly used although nitroglycerin and trimethaphan camsylate (in coarctation) may be used.

Criteria for Treatment

The criteria for treatment of elevated blood pressure will vary from patient to patient; however, if the patient's systolic arterial pressure is 30 mmHg higher than the preoperative level or the diastolic pressure is 15 mmHg higher, treatment is usually indicated. In selected cases, a lower systolic or mean arterial pressure limit will be selected to improve the hemodynamic state or because of an increased risk of bleeding.

Treatment

Treatment during the first 24 h postoperatively is aimed at pain control and/or vasodilator therapy. Morphine 0.05 to 0.1 mg/kg IV may be given to aid in control of hypertension and may be especially helpful at the onset of treatment. If pain control is assessed to be adequate, then nitroprusside at a dose of 0.5 to 8 μg/kg/min titrated for a mean arterial pressure at or slightly above preoperative levels is usually begun. The maximum permissible dose is 10 μg/kg/min because prolonged administration of nitroprusside or infusion of higher doses for a short period of time may lead to cyanide toxicity. Metabolic acidosis and tachyphylaxis are indications to discontinue the infusion. Nitroprusside is always infused into a right atrial catheter or a central venous pressure line that is attached directly to the nitroprusside line without any other free flush lines connected to it to prevent inadvertent bolus of the medication and resultant hypotension. When discontinuing nitroprusside, we should also be careful not to flush the line to prevent an inadvertent bolus injection.

If the patient remains hypertensive during the first postoperative day or continues to require large doses of vasodilator to control blood pressure, other antihypertensive medications may be considered. The vasodilator should be tapered off within 12 h unless continued strict antihypertensive management is specifically indicated. (Note: Because of the effect of nitroprusside on preload [increased venous capacitance], left-sided and right-sided filling pressures are usually lowered by this intervention. This requires reevaluation of the desirable left atrial or central venous pressure when nitroprusside is used for hypertension. Usually a lower filling pressure is acceptable.)

Volume and Hemoglobin Status

The following management protocol is a guide to routine adjustments of volume and hemoglobin in patients without excessive bleeding. For each patient, a desirable level of filling pressure, central venous or left atrial pressure is chosen on the basis of the individual patient's overall cardiac performance. In general, the desirable range of right-sided filling pressure will be between 6 and 14 mmHg mean pressure after ventriculotomy. The occasional patient, however, will require higher filling pressure for optimal hemodynamics. The optimal filling pressure will therefore be specified in the early postoperative evaluation and should be maintained with an appropriate infusion of volume, either packed cells, 5% albumin, or fresh-frozen plasma, depending on the patient's hemoglobin concentration and coagulation status. Changes in the hemodynamic state at any time during the postoperative course may necessitate a change in the desirable filling pressure. If it is necessary to infuse more than 20 to 30 mL/kg of volume to maintain favorable hemodynamics over a 1- to 2-h period, the patient should be carefully evaluated for excessive blood or fluid loss and the surgeon notified.

If volume infusion is indicated (and filling pressure confirmed as accurate with recalibration and rezero of the transducer if necessary), the guidelines listed in Table 27-5 may be helpful.

Most postoperative cardiac surgical patients who have undergone CPB will be overweight and exhibit peripheral edema the first 24 to 48 h after surgery. Often the central venous or left atrial pressure will be relatively low and the intravascular volume, down. After translocation of fluids ceases in the postoperative period, mobilization of excess fluids begins to occur, which may compromise cardiopulmonary function. If urine output is low and blood pressure is normal with elevated filling pressures, a diuretic may be indicated.

Furosemide, 0.5 to 1.0 mg/kg/dose, is very useful to encourage diuresis. The daily measurement of the hematocrit and total serum protein (TSP) may guide therapy. A drop in hematocrit and TSP without evidence of abnormal blood loss (i.e., chest tube output or excessive blood drawing) suggests intravascular volume overload. The normal TSP equals 4.5 to 6.5 mg/dL. If

Table 27-5 Guidelines for Volume Infusion

In older children if hemoglobin is less than 10.0 mg/dL (hematocrit, less than 30 percent), packed cells should be infused.

If the hemoglobin is above 10.0 mg/dL, a colloid solution can be infused.

For newborns, a hematocrit of 40 to 45 percent should be maintained; for small infants (2 to 6 mo), 35 to 40.

the TSP is low and the renal response to furosemide is poor (i.e., less than 2 mL/kg/h urine output for 2 h after furosemide administration), the patient may benefit from furosemide 1 mg/kg IV followed by albumin 1 g/kg IV over 3 to 6 h, and then furosemide 1 mg/kg IV at the end of albumin infusion.

Chest Drainage

If the patient's chest tube drainage is excessive, this should be taken into account in planning volume replacement and managed so that clinically apparent hypovolemia does not occur. If early postoperative bleeding is excessive, a choice from among the following interventions is to be considered:

1. Obtain an activated clotting time and, if abnormal, administer additional protamine (1 mg/kg to a maximum of 50 mg slowly IV).
2. Administer fresh-frozen plasma 10 to 20 mL/kg empirically or on the basis of an abnormal prothrombin time.
3. If a reason exists to suspect inadequate platelet function or an inadequate platelet count, consider platelet transfusion. However, the need for this intervention is rare, except in repair of cyanotic conditions or in the newborn as a result of dilutional thrombocytopenia.

We should always maintain a high level of suspicion of cardiac tamponade during the early postoperative period but, particularly, when any of the following occurs.

1. Excessive bleeding that stops over a short period of time.
2. Continued moderate bleeding.
3. Mediastinal widening on chest x-ray.
4. Unexpected or unexplained deterioration of hemodynamics.
5. Gradual increase in both right- and left-sided filling pressures with tendency for equalization of right- and left-sided pressures.

Arrhythmias

The patient's hemodynamics, oxygenation, ventilator function, acid–base status, and serum K^+ should be evaluated whenever significant arrhythmias occur. The doses of agents, such as theophylline preparations, catecholamine infusions, digoxin, and antiarrhythmics, should also be reevaluated. Premature atrial contractions are fairly common after cardiac surgery and are probably the result of the atriotomy for cannulation for bypass or edema of the atrial wall caused by perioperative fluid shifts. These dysrhythmias are most often benign and do not require specific treatment.

Ventricular electrical instability and ventricular tachycardia (e.g., premature ventricular contractions [PVCs]) do warrant investigation and usually require treatment. If the PVCs are greater than 6/min, there is coupling or multifocal PVCs, runs of ventricular tachycardia, or PVCs that interrupt the T wave of the preceding beat.

1. Immediately give lidocaine 1 mg/kg intravenously. If PVCs return, the dose may be repeated to a total dose of 3 mg/kg IV over a period of approximately 20 to 30 min while an infusion is being prepared.
2. Check for hypoglycemia, hypoxemia, and hypercarbia. Correct serum potassium as in the previous protocol.
3. Check intracardiac and percutaneous line placement to be sure they have not migrated into the ventricle.
4. If the ventricular dysrhythmias respond to lidocaine initially but return, begin an infusion of 20 to 50 μg/kg/min of lidocaine.
5. Failure to control the arrhythmia with lidocaine would warrant the use of bretylium 5-mg/kg bolus, followed by an infusion.

Supraventricular tachycardia is common after procedures involving the atria (e.g., Mustard or Senning procedure for transposition of the great vessels). These rhythms may be difficult to distinguish from sinus tachycardia in the infant whose sinus rate may increase to 200 to 220 beats/min. If the rate is 240/min or more, the diagnosis of supraventricular tachycardia (SVT) is more obvious. Another characteristic is that the SVT is usually sudden in onset and does not respond to volume infusion. Sinus tachycardia is most often caused by volume depletion or sympathetic stimulation, and the rate will decrease with volume administration or analgesic administration. The treatment of SVT is as follows:

1. Initial treatment consists of vagal maneuvers, the most effective of which in an infant is an ice bag placed over the bridge of the nose and supraorbital region.
2. If this is ineffective, digoxin is the drug of choice in most instances, unless the hemodynamics are unstable. In this case, synchronized cardioversion with 0.5 to 1 joul/kg is performed. The digoxin dose is one half the total digitalizing dose, or 10 to 15 μg/kg IV. After 30 min to 1 h, an additional dose of 5 to 7.5 μg/kg may be administered

if the tachycardia has not resolved. Another 5 to 7.5 μg/kg may be administered after 8 h, followed by maintenance therapy at 6 to 10 μg/kg/day.

3. More recently, adenosine 0.1 mg/kg has been used successfully to convert pediatric patients in SVT. It must be administered by a "shotgun" method because of its very short half-life (6 to 10 s). The adenosine dose and a flush syringe are placed on a stopcock so that the adenosine may be given followed by the flush to ensure the achievement of an adequate serum level. Cessation of the SVT is often followed by a sinus pause of 2 to 3 s before a normal sinus rhythm returns. If the initial dose fails to convert the dysrhythmia, then it may be doubled to a maximum of 12 mg IV.

4. Another drug that may be used is verapamil, 0.1 to 0.15 mg/kg/dose, repeated every 5 to 10 min for three doses. This drug may cause hypotension, especially if administered rapidly, which can compromise already unstable hemodynamics. Newborn and small infants are particularly sensitive to the cardiac depressant effects of these drugs, and therefore, verapamil is contraindicated in the newborn and young infant. Other drugs (digoxin and β-blockers) should be tried first.

5. If atrial wires are in place, overdrive pacing will occasionally work. Connect the pacemaker to wires and increase the rate output to 10 to 15 percent faster than the patient's intrinsic rate. When capture occurs, as evidenced by an increase in heart rate, slowly dial down the rate to the desired range and turn the pacemaker off. (Note: A special pacemaker unit will be required as the standard unit will only achieve a rate of 180 bpm.)

Hypoglycemia

Low peripheral blood glucose values are common in newborns and sick infants after cardiac surgery because of their low glycogen stores. Hypoglycemia may either cause severe cardiac dysfunction or herald early cardiac decompensation. It should be anticipated and treated promptly.

For glucose of less than 50 mg/dL, we use:

1. Dextrose 25% in water 2 mL/kg IV, then increase the concentration of the existing glucose solution by factor of 1.5 to 2 (i.e., 5% dextrose → 10% dextrose).

2. Repeat Accu-Chek, Dextrostix, or serum glucose 15 to 30 min after Step 1, repeating every hour until stable.

Fever

Fever occurs regularly in patients having open cardiac procedures. The presence of fever (up to 39.6°C) during the first 5 postoperative days has no correlation with the presence or development of infection in these patients but may indicate atelectasis, pulmonary congestion, or a low cardiac output state. Blood, urine, or sputum cultures are usually not helpful in the immediate postoperative period. White blood cell counts or differentials may be obtained during the first 5 days after the operation to follow the changes from baseline. The control of temperature to within the normal range is important because fever produces an increase in the metabolic rate, which increases the demand on the cardiopulmonary system and may adversely affect the hemodynamics. The treatment is as follows:

1. Acetaminophen 10 mg/kg q 4 h either orally or rectally. Aspirin or ibuprofen is generally not used because of platelet dysfunction.
2. A cooling blanket is not used unless the patient does not respond to acetaminophen. In general, this intervention is indicated if the temperature is greater than 39.8°C.
3. If low cardiac output is the cause, volume expansion or an increase in inotropic support is indicated.
4. If atelectasis is present, an increased frequency of chest physiotherapy and bronchodilator treatments by inhalation are necessary.
5. For fever that occurs after postoperative day 5, the patient should be evaluated with appropriate cultures, chest x-ray, and examination for a source, including the ears. Otitis is a common source of fever in children, especially after the nasopharynx has been instrumented in the perioperative period (e.g., nasogastric or endotracheal tube).

Acidosis

Acidosis is a potent myocardial depressant, and catecholamine infusions do not work well in an acidic environment. Pulmonary artery pressures also are adversely affected by low pH values, and therefore, acidosis may significantly reduce the cardiac output in patients with poor ventricular reserve. If the base deficit is greater than -5, treatment should be given according to the following formula:

1. Dose of sodium bicarbonate (in milliequivalents) = base deficit × body weight (in kilograms) × 0.3.
2. Thirty minutes after treatment, the blood gases should be remeasured, and correction of the deficit or repeat

treatment according to this formula should be documented. Any time acidosis develops, reassessment of filling pressures, cardiac output, and peripheral perfusion should be done. Abnormalities of these parameters should be treated, if possible, along with the acidosis.

BIBLIOGRAPHY

Barasch PG, Berman MA, Stansel HC, et al: Markedly improved pulmonary function after open heart surgery in infancy utilizing surface cooling, profound hypothermia and circulatory arrest. Am J Surg 1976; 131:499–503.

Berner M, Jaccard C, Oberhansli I, et al: Hemodynamic effects of amrinone in children after cardiac surgery. Intensive Care Med 1990; 16:85–88.

Burrows FA, Williams WG, Teoh KH, et al: Myocardial performance after repair of congenital cardiac defects in infants and children: Response to volume loading. J Thorac Cardiovasc Surg 1988; 96:548–556.

Epstein ML, Kiel EA, Victorica BE: Cardiac decompensation following verapamil therapy in infants with SVT. Pediatrics 1985; 75:737–740.

Fyfe DA, Buckles DS, Gillette PC, et al: Preoperative prediction of postoperative pulmonary arteriolar resistance after surgical repair of complete atrioventricular canal defect. J Thorac Cardiovasc Surg 1991; 102:784–789.

Gross MA, Keefer V, Liebman J: The platelets in cyanotic heart disease. Pediatrics 1968; 42:651–658.

Hultgren MS: Pulmonary management of children after cardiac surgery. Crit Care Nurse 1991; 11:55–69.

Lerberg DB, Bahnson HT: Coarctation of the aorta in infants and children: 25 years experience. Ann Thorac Surg 1982; 33:159–170.

Levin DL, Perkin RM: Postoperative care of the pediatric patient with congenital heart disease, in Shoemaker WC, Thompson WL, Holbrook PR (eds): Textbook of Critical Care. Philadelphia, WB Saunders, 1984, pp 395–403.

Lynn AM, Opheim KE, Tyler DC: Morphine infusion after pediatric cardiac surgery. Crit Care Med 1984; 12:863–866.

Martin TC, Smith L, Hernandez A, Weldon CS: Dysrhythmias following the Senning operation for dextrotransposition of the great arteries. J Thorac Cardiovasc Surg 1983; 85:928–932.

Norwood WI Jr: Hypoplastic left heart syndrome. Ann Thorac Surg 1991; 52:688–695.

Oka Y, Lin T: Postoperative management: Complications. Int Anesthesiol Clin 1980; 18:217–231.

Overhold ED, Rheuban KS, Gutgesell HP, et al: Usefulness of adenosine for arrhythmias in infants and children. Am J Cardiol 1988; 61:336–340.

Penny DJ, Redington AN: Doppler echocardiographic evaluation of pulmonary blood flow after the Fontan operation: The role of the lungs. Br Heart J 1991; 66:372–374.

Pfenninger J, Shaw S, Ferrari P, et al: Atrial natriuretic factor after cardiac surgery with cardiopulmonary bypass in children. *Crit Care Med* 1991; 19:1497–1502.

Radford D: Side effects of verapamil in infants. *Arch Dis Child* 1983; 58:465–466.

Rea HH, Hanes EA, Seelye ER, et al: The effects of cardiopulmonary bypass upon pulmonary gas exchange. *J Thorac Cardiovasc Surg* 1978; 75:104–120.

Rossi AF, Burton DA: Adenosine in altering short and long term treatment of supraventricular tachycardia in infants. *Am J Cardiol* 1989; 64:685–686.

Ryan CA, Soder CM: Hemodynamic responses to $PaCO_2$ in children after open heart surgery. *Crit Care Med* 1989; 17:874–878.

Sealy WC: Coarctation of the aorta and hypertension. *Ann Thorac Surg* 1967; 3:15–28.

Till J, Shinebourne EA, Rigby ML, et al: Efficacy and safety of adenosine in the treatment of supraventricular tachycardia in infants and children. *Br Heart J* 1989; 62:204–211.

Weil MH, Houle DB, Brown DB, et al: Vasopressor agents: Influence of acidosis on cardio and vascular responsiveness. *Calif Med* 1958; 88:437–440.

Wheller J, George BL, Mulder DG, et al: Diagnosis and management of postoperative pulmonary hypertensive crisis. *Circulation* 1979; 60:1640–1643.

Wilkinson C, Clark H: Refractory hypertension during coarctectomy. *Anesthesiology* 1982; 57:540–542.

CHAPTER 28

Pediatric Neuroanesthesia

Ralph F. Erian
Deborah K. Rasch

In considering neuroanesthesia for the pediatric patient, this chapter will first review basic neurophysiology and then, second, discuss the effects of anesthetic agents on cerebral dynamics. Particularities of the pediatric central nervous system (CNS) will also be discussed, and the anesthetic considerations for the most common pathologic disorders dealt with in our practice (hydrocephalus, myelomeningocele, intracranial disease, neuroradiologic procedures, and head trauma) will be reviewed.

BASIC NEUROPHYSIOLOGY

Cerebral Blood Flow (CBF) and Cerebral Metabolic Rate for Oxygen (CMRO$_2$)

The factor that determines blood flow in the intact brain is the cerebral metabolic rate. The CMRO$_2$ and CBF vary according to the region of the brain and the age group. The CBF ranges from 20 mL/100 g/min for white matter to 100 mL/100 g/min for gray matter. In adults, the total CBF is maintained at 50 mL/100 g/min, whereas it is 40 mL/100 g/min in neonates and 100 mL/100 g/min in children (Fig. 28-1). The critical blood flow at which ischemia develops and is associated with electroencephalographic (EEG) flattening seems to be 20 mL/100 g/min in the adult. In the infant, this threshold is lower by 5 to 10 mL/100 g/min.

Autoregulation allows for a constant total CBF within a certain range of mean arterial blood pressure (MABP). In the adult, the total CBF is maintained constant for a MABP of 50 to 150 mmHg, whereas in the pediatric population, animal data suggest that the range is shifted to the left. Autoregulation is impaired by cerebral hypoxia, ischemia, trauma, and edema. Volatile anesthetics will also impair autoregulation (Fig. 28-2). When autoregulation is impaired, cerebral ischemia and peri-

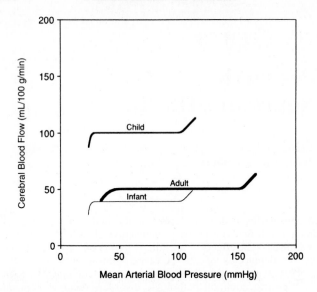

Figure 28-1 Cerebral blood flow is 50 mL/100 g/min in adults, 40 mL/100 g/min in neonates, and 100 mL/100 g/min in children. This graph is a hypothetical extrapolation of current data. The curves have not been delineated in children.

ventricular hemorrhage are more likely at the lower and higher ends of the blood pressure range, respectively.

The $PaCO_2$, despite autoregulation, will greatly affect the CBF in all age groups (Fig. 28-3). Typically, a twofold change in $PaCO_2$ will be accompanied by a twofold change in blood flow within the physiologic range of $PaCO_2$ of 20 to 80 mmHg. The effect of $PaCO_2$ seems to be related to a direct effect of the cerebrospinal fluid (CSF) pH on the arterial walls of the cerebral circulation. Prolonged hyperventilation (> 12 h) allows time for readjustment of the CSF pH through bicarbonate transfer across the blood–brain barrier and is therefore much less effective at reducing CBF. However, allowing $PaCO_2$ to return to normal should be done slowly in a stepwise fashion, monitoring intracranial pressure (ICP) whenever possible because CBF will increase with each increase in $PaCO_2$. Note that spontaneously ventilating preterm infants are more susceptible to the effects of hypercarbia because they will not increase their minute ventilation in response to elevated $PaCO_2$.

The PaO_2 will also affect the CBF (Fig. 28-3) because a reduction in PaO_2 will be accompanied by a concomitant reduction in the oxygen supply to the brain. Because the oxygen-

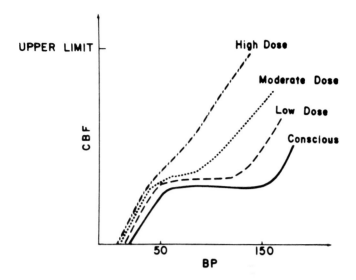

Figure 28-2 Cerebral blood flow (CBF) autoregulation is impaired by volatile anesthetics in a dose-dependent fashion. BP = blood pressure. (Reproduced with permission from Miller RD: *Anesthesia.* vol. 1. New York, Churchill Livingstone, 1990, p 808.)

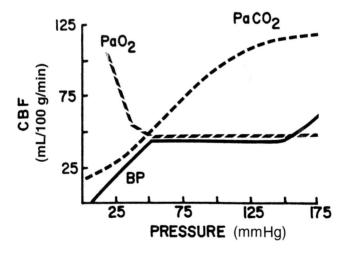

Figure 28-3 Cerebral blood flow (CBF) is affected by mean arterial pressure, PaO_2, and $PaCO_2$. (Reproduced with permission from Shapiro HM: Intracranial hypertension: therapeutic and anesthetic considerations. *Anesthesiology* 1975; 43.)

carrying capacity of hemoglobin at a given PO_2 is higher in infants than in adults, the CBF will increase significantly at PO_2 less than 50 mmHg in the adult and a PO_2 less than 25 mmHg in the neonate. However, the infant who is older than 3 months old should be considered an adult in this respect.

CSF

The CSF is produced in all four ventricles of the brain, although the majority originates in the lateral ventricles where there is a greater amount of choroid plexus tissue compared with the midline ventricles. It is formed at a rate of 0.5 mL/min through active secretion by the choroid plexus. It has a higher Na^+ and PCO_2 concentration than plasma but lower K^+, Ca^{++}, glucose, and protein concentrations. Several factors can decrease its secretion:

1. Decreased MAP.
2. Decreased CBF.
3. Increased intraventricular hydrostatic pressure (hydrocephalus).
4. Increased serum osmolality (as in diabetic ketoacidosis).

Acetazolamide, spironolactone, furosemide, vasopressin, and steroids have been shown to decrease CSF formation. The mechanisms of action for most of them are still unclear. The CSF flows from its site of secretion within the ventricles through the medial foramen of Magendie and the lateral foramina of Luschka into the cisterna magna and then into the subarachnoid space surrounding the brain and the spinal cord. Most of the absorption of CSF occurs at the arachnoid villi that protrude into the cerebral venous sinuses.

ICP

The ICP is the supratentorial CSF pressure and is normally less than 15 mmHg. It is pulsatile because of respiration and the cardiac pulse. The combined respiratory and cardiac variation is 3 mmHg. As the ICP increases, the pulse pressure increases.

An increase in intracranial volume can be the result of several factors:

1. Intracranial brain volume (tumor).
2. Blood flow (usually reflects an increase in blood volume but not necessarily).
3. CSF volume.

This increase in intracranial volume will not necessarily increase ICP because increases in ICP depend on how a specific quantity of intracranial volume relates to the intracranial compliance curve and how much compensatory ability remains (Fig. 28-4). At Point 1, the ICP is low with a large compensatory ability available. An increase in intracranial volume at that point will not be associated with an increase in ICP. At Point 2, the ICP is still almost the same, but very little accommodation for increased volume is available. A small increase in volume will cause a moderate rise in ICP. Finally, at Point 3, no compensating ability is left. Pressure increases precipitously with any change in intracranial volume.

Cerebral Perfusion Pressure (CPP)

The CPP is determined by the difference between the mean arterial pressure (MAP) and the intracranial pressure.

$$CPP = MAP - ICP$$

The normal range in the adult is 80 to 100 mmHg. At a CPP below 20 mmHg, irreversible cellular damage occurs. In the neonate and infant, the range is shifted to the left because of the lower MAP. The accepted lower limit for CPP clinically is

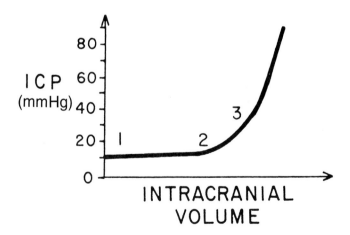

Figure 28-4 The intracranial compliance curve. 1. Compliant portion of curve: large volume shifts may occur with almost no change in ICP. 2. Critical volume where small changes in content result in more dramatic rises in ICP. 3. Steep area of compliance curve where miniscule changes in volume result in tremendous elevations in ICP. (Reproduced with permission from Shapiro HM: Intracranial hypertension: therapeutic and anesthetic considerations. *Anesthesiology* 1975; 43.)

50 mmHg in the intact brain of a nonhypertensive patient outside of the newborn period.

ANESTHETIC AGENTS

The ideal anesthetic agent from a neurosurgical point of view is one that is going to reduce CBF and cerebral blood volume (CBV) and at the same time equally reduce cerebral oxygen consumption. From a practical point of view, it should also be easily reversible. A reduction in CBF will decrease cerebral edema formation, a decrease in CBV will decrease ICP, and a reduction in cerebral oxygen consumption will maintain a balance between supply and demand, preventing the development of anaerobic metabolism, which in the brain, is poorly tolerated. Let us, therefore, look at the effects of intravenous and volatile anesthetics on CBF and $CMRO_2$.

Anesthetic drugs, laryngoscopy, intubation, positive-pressure ventilation, and positioning will all affect CPP through either an effect on MAP or on ICP. Most of the drugs we use will also affect the $CMRO_2$ and CBF.

Volatile Anesthetics

All the volatile anesthetic agents are cerebrovascular dilators and will therefore increase CBF, CBV, and potentially, ICP (see Fig. 28-2). Nevertheless, they all also reduce $CMRO_2$ and have cerebral protective effects. Of those used clinically, isoflurane at minimum alveolar concentrations less than two percent accompanied by hyperventilation or N_2O with fentanyl and hyperventilation seem to cause the least increase in CBF.

Intravenous Agents

Barbiturates

Thiopental, the most commonly used intravenous induction agent, produces the greatest decrease in CBF and $CMRO_2$. The depression of metabolic requirements is limited to that necessary for neuronal function and not for cellular integrity and is attained with an isoelectric EEG (usually a 50 percent reduction of both) during barbiturate coma. A further reduction could be produced by hypothermia, and this would affect the oxygen requirements necessary for maintaining cellular integrity. Although barbiturates would seem to possess the ideal properties for neurosurgical anesthesia, when used in higher amounts (as in a barbiturate anesthetic), the apparent half-life increases 10-fold to 50 to 60 h. This increase is the result of a change from first-order to zero-order kinetics. This naturally will defer neurologic examination from 24 to 96 h postoperatively, which is unacceptable for most neurosurgical procedures. Furthermore, with moderate- to high-dose barbiturates, there is a dose-dependent cardiovascular depression, which has to be pharmacologically counteracted.

Droperidol
An antiemetic and neuroleptic drug, droperidol produces a moderate reduction in CBF and ICP and a slight reduction in $CMRO_2$, which is potentiated by the addition of fentanyl.

Etomidate
An intravenous anesthetic induction agent, this drug decreases both CBF and $CMRO_2$ (up to 50 percent) although, unlike thiopental, the $CMRO_2$ reduction is nonuniform, being greater in the cerebral cortex than the brainstem. This effect is advantageous in patients who may present with hemodynamic instability because it causes minimal changes in cardiac index and systemic vascular resistance. There are some reports of seizures when used in patients with a history of epilepsy, and therefore, etomidate is not recommended in this group of patients.

Fentanyl
The most widely used narcotic in neuroanesthesia, fentanyl causes small reductions in CBF and $CMRO_2$ at normocapnia in adults. The CPP seems better preserved than with sufentanil or alfentanil.

Ketamine
This is the only intravenous anesthetic that raises CBF, ICP, and $CMRO_2$. It should be avoided in any patient with a potential for increasing ICP.

Midazolam
This is benzodiazepine with greater potency and faster onset and recovery than diazepam. It will reduce CBF and $CMRO_2$ by 40 percent. When used as an induction agent, it can cause a severe drop in blood pressure in the face of hypovolemia.

Muscle Relaxants
Devoid of their hemodynamic effects as a result of histamine release or their vagolytic properties, nondepolarizing muscle relaxants (NDMR) have no effect on CBF and ICP. For that reason, vecuronium and pipecuronium would be the ideal NDMR when the prevention of ICP elevation and of CPP reduction is imperative. However, when a primary narcotic anesthetic technique is chosen for children, pancuronium is preferable to offset the vagotonic effects of the narcotics. Otherwise, particularly if the child is bradycardic preinduction, laryngoscopy and intu-

bation may precipitate severe bradycardias or sinus arrest. Atracurium given slowly and in lower doses is also acceptable for the maintenance of muscle relaxation. The only depolarizing muscle relaxant in use, succinylcholine, can cause an increase in ICP as a result of cerebral vasodilatation. This increase in ICP can be prevented by pretreatment with a NDMR, hyperventilation, and a thiopental induction. Note that succinylcholine is contraindicated in patients with chronic neurologic and neuromuscular disease because of the potential for severe hyperkalemia. However, for rapid-sequence induction, where "full stomach" considerations prevail, succinylcholine is still considered the agent of choice for providing rapid intubating conditions.

Propofol

This is a newer intravenous anesthetic useful for both induction and maintenance of anesthesia. It decreases both CBF and $CMRO_2$ by 30 percent. Although it lowers ICP, it will also lower CPP because of a pronounced effect on MAP with induction doses. The hemodynamic effects seem less important during maintenance.

ANESTHETIC MANAGEMENT

When considering the CNS of a neonate or infant, it is imperative to remember the differences from those of an older child or an adult. The infant has an immature CNS, with incompletely myelinated nerve fibers and an incompletely developed cerebral cortex. The skull is somewhat compliant, accommodating increased intracranial volume by expansion of the fontanelles and separation of suture lines. Autoregulation is impaired, which causes flow to be pressure dependent. Therefore, a greater risk of ischemia exists at low pressures. Hyperemia and intraventricular bleeding are more likely with high arterial pressures. Neuroanesthetic management of these patients must take into account these differences.

Premedication

In patients with symptoms of increased ICP, do not give any drug that can depress respiration, prolong recovery, or hamper postoperative assessment. In most cases, no sedative premedication should be given to neurosurgical patients before arrival in the operating room (OR) or induction area. If, on arrival to the OR, the child is frightened or anxious, incremental doses of midazolam (0.025 mg/kg), droperidol (50 μg/kg), or diphenhydramine (1 mg/kg) may be useful to help make the transition to the OR go more smoothly. Never leave the patient after a medication has been given because delayed respiratory depression may occur!

Monitoring

In addition to routine pediatric monitors, the following may be needed: an esophageal stethoscope, arterial line (24 or 22 gauge), a urinary catheter for major surgery, a precordial Doppler, and a central venous pressure line if the risk of venous air embolism exists.

Induction

As discussed previously, many induction sequences are acceptable; however, an intravenous induction is usually preferred. One example of an induction regimen for a hemodynamically stable infant or child that may be useful in preventing increases in ICP includes:

1. Head elevation in neutral position and hyperventilation with oxygen.
2. Atropine 10 μg/kg.
3. Lidocaine 1 mg/kg 3 min before laryngoscopy.
4. Thiopental 4 to 6 mg/kg.
5. Vecuronium 0.1 mg/kg.
6. Fentanyl 3 to 5 μg/kg.

For the hemodynamically unstable infant, the following sequence might be a better choice:

1. Head elevation in neutral position and hyperventilation with oxygen.
2. Fentanyl 10 to 20 μg/kg.
3. Pancuronium 0.15 mg/kg.

Intubation

Nasal tubes are easier to secure in neonates and infants, especially in the sitting or prone position. It is imperative to recheck endotracheal tube placement after final positioning of the child.

Maintenance

In our institution, the most frequent maintenance regimen for prolonged neurosurgical cases is either a nitrous narcotic or isoflurane technique with controlled ventilation. Nitrous oxide is avoided by many clinicians when the risk for venous air embolus is present, and an air–oxygen mixture is substituted.

Emergence

The patient should be fully reversed (neostigmine, 0.05 to 0.08 mg/kg plus atropine 0.02 mg/kg) and awake before leaving the OR.

Intravenous Therapy

A good reliable intravenous line is essential for pediatric neurosurgery before induction. Dextrose 5% in to normal saline is used as maintenance fluid at a rate of 2 to 4 mL/kg/h for infants under 5 kg of weight or younger than 2 months of age. For other fluid administration and for older infants and children, glucose-free balanced electrolyte solutions should be used as required, keeping in mind the effect of overhydration on cerebral edema. The 5% glucose solution is replaced by a glucose-free balanced electrolyte solution in all children older than 2 to 3 months of age (unless hypoglycemia is present), obviating the need for two separate solutions and decreasing the risk of hyperglycemia, which is known to exacerbate ischemic neurologic injury.

Blood loss less than 20 percent of estimated blood volume (EBV) is replaced milliliter for milliliter with colloid (unless the patient is anemic at the onset). Blood loss more than 20 percent of the EBV is generally replaced with blood. See Chap. 9 for guidelines to calculate the EBV and acceptable blood loss for each patient. The blood loss during neurosurgery must be gauged clinically from observation of the in-line suction traps, sponge weights, and the amount of blood visible in the field. This may not always be easily accomplished because draping for neurosurgical procedures often isolates the anesthesiologist. The cooperation of nursing personnel and the surgeon is essential, especially when acute blood loss occurs, to alert the anesthesiologist regarding the severity of the situation. In pediatric patients, hemodynamic variables, especially blood pressure, will be maintained until 20 to 25 percent of the circulating volume is lost.

SPECIFIC PROCEDURES

Hydrocephalus

Hydrocephalus means excess water in the cranial vault. It is frequently subdivided into communicating and noncommunicating hydrocephalus. In communicating hydrocephalus, CSF flows readily from the ventricular system into the subarachnoid space. The accumulation of CSF is caused either by overdevelopment of the choroid plexuses (oversecretion) in the newborn infant or by mechanical obstruction of the surface pathways outside the brain as a result of inflammatory meningeal changes (decreased absorption) after hemorrhage or infection.

In noncommunicating or obstructive hydrocephalus, the block to fluid flow is present in the pathways within the brain. This interferes with the flow of CSF into the subarachnoid space where it is reabsorbed. It may be congenital, such as the Arnold Chiari malformation, aqueductal stenosis, and Dandy-Walker syndrome (occlusion outlet of fourth ventricle), which are more common in the newborn or acquired (as in posterior fossa tumors, which are more common in children).

Children with obstructive hydrocephalus may be seriously ill because of raised ICP, and urgent treatment may be required. The surgical treatment consists of either excision, if the lesion is resectable, or a variety of shunting procedures, using catheters with one-way valves to provide a pathway from the cerebral ventricles into a site where it can be absorbed. The more common distal sites are the peritoneal cavity and the right atrium.

Anesthetic Considerations
The precautions are standard in patients with increased ICP:

1. Head neutral position.
2. Head elevation 30° to 45°.
3. Good oxygenation.
4. Hyperventilation.
5. Adequate MABP.
6. Pharmacologic interventions to reduce CBV and CSF volume.

Hydrocephalic children may have CSF drainage for several days before surgery. Fluid and electrolytes may be depleted and should be adequately replaced before surgery.

Intubation can be difficult because of a large head and frontal bossing. Special positioning may be required to facilitate intubation. In this situation, a shoulder roll may be useful to help align the intubation axes for easier visualization of the larynx. As in all neurosurgical cases, ventilation should be controlled.

When the blood pressure is elevated secondary to an elevated ICP, decompression of the ventricles may result in hypotension. The anesthetic depth should be reduced before drainage, and volatile anesthetics should be discontinued if hypotension does occur.

Air embolism is possible during ventriculoatrial shunt insertion in the internal jugular vein. The risk can be minimized by positive-pressure ventilation and the use of a Valsalva maneuver immediately before insertion. Also the shunt tubing should be primed with saline or CSF.

The ideal midatrial position of the catheter can be verified by connecting the left arm lead to the distal shunt filled with hypertonic saline and obtaining a biphasic P wave on lead III. X-ray confirmation is mandatory.

Multiple procedures are frequently required to relieve blockage, treat shunt infections, and provide elective lengthening of shunt tubes during growth. Postoperatively, the patient should be nursed in a 30° head-up position and kept supine or on the left side (for right-sided shunts) to ensure proper functioning of the valve.

Myelomeningocele

Myelomeningocele is a condition that results from failure of the neural tube to close in the fetus. Failure of closure of the caudal end results in either spina bifida, characterized by defects of the vertebral bodies; meningocele, characterized by a sac containing the meninges; or myelomeningocele, characterized by a sac containing neural elements. The incidence of myelomeningocele is 1 per 4000 live births. Hydrocephalus with Arnold-Chiari malformation and aqueductal stenosis occur in 80 percent of infants with myelomeningocele. Surgery is usually undertaken within hours after birth to reduce the risk of infection and further neurologic damage.

Anesthetic Considerations

If airway difficulty is anticipated, awake intubation in the left lateral decubitus position or supine with the defect lying in the center of a soft round support material is recommended. For hemodynamically stable infants, where difficult intubation is not expected, an intravenous induction followed by intubation, as discussed previously may proceed.

Minimize heat loss by warming the OR to 25°C and using warming blankets, radiant heat lamps, a heated humidifier, and a thermal cap over the head.

Considerable blood loss can occur; therefore, blood should be available in the OR. A drop in systolic blood pressure indicates significant intravascular volume reduction.

The operation is performed in the prone position, and therefore, several considerations specific to positioning are important:

1. Endotracheal tube taped securely; consider nasal tube.
2. Bolsters placed under the lateral aspects of the chest and abdomen to allow free excursion of chest. We should realize that pressure on the abdomen can compress the vena cava causing increased hydrostatic pressure in the epidural veins and increased bleeding. Bolsters should

run from the clavicle to the anterior superior iliac spine. Ascertain that there is no pressure on the eyes, nose, ears, and genitalia. The arms should not be extended more than 90° to prevent traction on the brachial plexus, and the bony prominences should be padded.

Occasionally, surgeons request that neuromuscular blocking agents be withheld if they plan to use a nerve stimulator to localize the nerve roots. In most cases, however, these patients can be safely paralyzed—which may be preferable because the patient is prone and movement may result in extubation. In addition, it is often difficult to anesthetize neonates deeply to prevent movement because they are sensitive to the cardiovascular effects of the volatile anesthetics and hypotension may result, despite movement.

Craniotomy for Tumor Resection

Intracerebral tumors are seen with relative frequency in pediatric patients, with 60 percent of these occurring within the posterior fossa. Increased ICP is a common finding, which may result in any of the following symptoms: loss of consciousness, bradycardia, hypertension, pupillary dilation, and respiratory center abnormalities. This group of patients requires aggressive preoperative preparation, which may include ventriculostomy placement under local anesthesia to decrease CBV by draining the CSF if obstructive hydrocephalus is present. Diuretics and steroids may also be necessary.

Anesthetic Management

Induction of general anesthesia can be accomplished with a variety of agents, as discussed previously. For the sitting position, for the prone position, or in small infants, a nasotracheal intubation will provide greater stability for the tube. After the child is anesthetized, arterial, central venous, and additional peripheral venous catheters may be inserted while the head is being prepared for surgery.

The positioning of the patient may be quite involved for the prone or sitting cases. For supine operations, care must be taken to prevent jugular venous obstruction when the head is turned to the side because this may produce acute elevations in ICP. A pad placed under the contralateral shoulder will help prevent venous obstruction. For the sitting position, hemodynamic changes can be very difficult to control because many patients are hypovolemic from fluid restriction and diuretic use. All anesthetic agents tend to reduce compensatory mechanisms that would otherwise maintain blood pressure when placed in a sitting position. For an accurate measure of CPP, the transducer for the arterial line should be kept at head level to prevent over-estimation of MAP because the arterial pressure will be lower at the head than at the heart. Venous air embolism is much more likely with the sitting position, and correct placement of a central venous catheter for air aspiration should be confirmed by x-ray. Signs of venous air embolism include:

1. "Mill wheel" murmur in esophageal stethoscope or precordial Doppler.
2. Acute decrease in end-tidal PCO_2.
3. Increase in central venous and pulmonary artery pressures.
4. Hypotension.
5. Arrhythmias and ST segment changes.

If any of these symptoms occur, the surgeons should be notified immediately because their cooperation is essential, especially if hemodynamic changes have occurred.

Immediately treat the patient as follows:

1. Place the patient on 100% fraction of inspired oxygen.
2. Ask the surgeon to flood the field with saline if they cannot immediately identify the source of the air entrainment.
3. Aspirate using a 35- to 60-mL syringe on the central venous pressure catheter.
4. May need the head of the bed lowered so that the intracranial venous pressure will no longer be subatmospheric.
5. Compression of the jugular veins will acutely increase cerebral venous pressure, which may stop air uptake and cause venous bleeding that will assist the surgeon to identify the source of air entry. Practically speaking, this maneuver is difficult because of patient position and requires one extra person whose only job it is to maintain compression until the offending vein is ligated.

The removal of posterior fossa tumors frequently produces cardiovascular changes intraoperatively caused by stimulation of the brainstem or cranial nerves. A sudden onset of tachycardia, bradycardia, hypotension, or hypertension is a result of surgical impingement, and the surgeon must be notified immediately to prevent damage to these structures. Patients who have extensive dissection in close proximity to the brainstem should be considered at risk for postoperative pulmonary compromise, including an impaired CO_2 response curve, abnormalities in the respiratory pattern, and aspiration risks secondary to vocal cord dysfunction and impaired gag reflex and swallowing. Postoperative ventilation should therefore be planned for these patients.

Arteriovenous Malformations

Pediatric patients with aneurysms or arteriovenous malformations are at significant risk for bleeding perioperatively; therefore, this group of patients should receive sedative premedication unless they are obtunded secondary to a recent bleed. Massive blood loss and venous air embolism are prominent risks of this procedure.

Blood products should be checked and available in the OR before anesthetic induction. After the child is anesthetized, intraarterial and central venous lines can be inserted. Hypertension or wide swings in intracranial volume (increased cardiac output, hypercarbia, or hypoxemia) may trigger bleeding from the vascular malformation. Therefore, the patient should be deeply anesthetized for endotracheal intubation and surgical incision. After the skull is open, the anesthetic requirements decrease significantly.

With large malformations or vein of Galen aneurysms (Fig. 28-5), the infant may be in severe congestive heart failure preoperatively. In this group of patients, insertion of a pulmonary artery catheter will help guide hemodynamic interventions, and a high-dose narcotic technique (fentanyl, 40 to 60 μg/kg) is preferable because of better hemodynamic stability. The mortality rates are high in these infants as a result of cardiac arrest secondary to myocardial ischemia and acute massive blood loss. Induced hypotension is contraindicated, and diastolic blood pressure must remain stable because decreases in diastolic and MAP lead to cardiac ischemia, arrhythmias, and cardiovascular collapse. When ligation of a vein of Galen aneurysm is completed, left ventricular afterload suddenly increases, and myocardial decompensation may occur. Inotropic agents and vasodilators should be prepared, calculated, and ready to be infused should this complication occur.

Arteriography and Myelography

General anesthesia with controlled ventilation is usually necessary. The patient may require repositioning after induction; so, extra attention to the security of the endotracheal tube and lines is very important. Be prepared for reactions to the contrast material, especially in children with a history of asthma and allergies. Remember that anaphylaxis and anaphylactoid reactions are treated with boluses of epinephrine (5 to 10 μg/kg), steroids, and isotonic fluids until blood pressure returns to

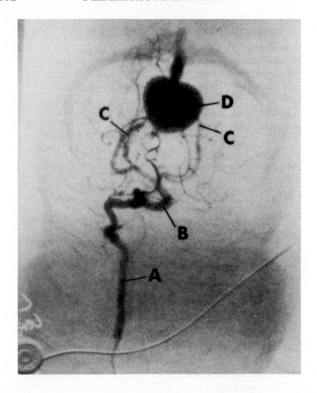

Figure 28-5 Aneurysm of the vein of Galen. These patients are often in congestive heart failure preoperatively and benefit from invasive monitoring. (A) Left vertebral artery. (B) Posterior cerebral artery. (C) Large aberrant vessel feeding the arteriovenous malformation. (D) Vein of Galen aneurysm. (Reproduced with permission from Rasch DK, Webster DE, Hutyra J, et al: Hemodynamic changes during vein of Galen aneurysm clipping. *Anesthesiology* 1988; 69:994.

normal. A detailed discussion of the treatment of anaphylaxis is contained in Chap. 3.

Head Trauma

In children, cervical spinal injuries without radiologic evidence of fracture may be present. Intubation and positioning should be done with great care.

The outcome for children with severe head injury is much better than in adults because of the plasticity of their CNS. We should, therefore, be very aggressive in treating them. Please see Chap. 12 for a discussion of this subject.

DRUGS USED IN NEUROSURGERY

Acetazolamide

This is a carbonic-anhydrase inhibitor. It can reduce CSF formation by 50 percent and transiently increase the CBF, thereby outweighing the previous benefit. The dose is 5 mg/kg/day either orally or intravenously.

Dexamethasone

This is a corticosteroid. It reduces edema around tumors but has no advantage in global edema. It can cause hyperglycemia. The dose is 0.2 mg/kg/dose orally or intravenously up to 10 mg (maximal dose).

Furosemide

This is a loop diuretic. It reduces ICP by afterload reduction, general diuresis, and a decreased rate of CSF production. The dose is 0.25 to 0.5 mg/kg intravenously.

Mannitol

This is an osmotic diuretic. It pulls interstitial water out of the brain across an intact blood–brain barrier. It causes general diuresis and can cause transient increases in CBF by increasing the intravascular volume and decreasing the viscosity. The decrease in viscosity and increase in CBF is associated with a decrease in CBV, one of the rare instances where there is a dissociation between CBF and CBV. Withhold this drug if the serum osmolality is more than 320 mosm/L. The dose is 0.25 to 0.50 g/kg intravenously.

Phenytoin

This is an anticonvulsant. Possibly it reduces CBV and $CMRO_2$. The dose is 10 to 20 mg/kg intravenously to be given slowly (1 mg/kg/min) or it can cause hypotension and arrhythmias. Maintain a plasma level of 10 to 20 μg/mL.

Thiopental

This is a barbiturate. It can be used for long-term control of ICP, but its benefits are very controversial. Hemodynamic monitoring is imperative to maintain an adequate MAP. Intravascular volume and myocardial contractility will need manipulations. The dose is ideally titrated to a flat EEG. A typical loading dose is 15 mg/kg slowly with maintenance of 12 to 15 mg/kg/h.

SUMMARY

Although there are several procedures performed in pediatric neuroanesthesia, only a few were described. The principles remain the same. With an understanding of pediatric anatomy and physiology, cerebral physiology, and the effects produced by anesthetic interventions, the management becomes straightforward. Discussing the procedure and positioning with the neurosurgeon ahead of time will allow you to plan the anesthetic management more precisely. This is best done after having seen the patient so that indications and contraindications to a specific position (e.g., sitting position) for that particular patient can be discussed.

BIBLIOGRAPHY

Albin MS, Babinski M, Marion J, et al: Anesthetic management of posterior fossa surgery in the sitting position. *Acta Anaesth Scand* 1976; 20:117–119.

Bedford RF, Berry FA: Pediatric neuroanesthesia, in Berry FA (ed): *Anesthetic Management of Difficult and Routine Pediatric Patients*. New York, Churchill Livingstone, 1986, pp 369–387.

Cucchiara RF, Bowes B: Air embolism in children undergoing suboccipital craniotomy. *Anesthesiology* 1982; 57:338–339.

Frost EAQ: Anesthesia for elective intracranial procedures. *Anesthesiol Rev* 1980; 7:13–18.

Harris MM, Yumen TA, Davidson A, et al: Venous air embolism during craniectomy in supine infants. *Anesthesiology* 1987; 67: 816–819.

Lassen NA, Christensen MS: Physiology of cerebral blood flow. *Br J Anaesth* 1976; 48:719–734.

McLeod EM, Creighton RE, Humphreys RP: Anesthesia for cerebral arteriovenous malformations of the vein of Galen. *Can J Anaesth* 1982; 29:299–306.

McLeod EM, Creighton RE, Humphreys RP: Anesthesia for cerebral arteriovenous malformations in children. *Can J Anesthesia* 1982; 29:299–306.

Newfield P, Cottrell JE: *Handbook of Neuroanesthesia: Clinical and Physiologic Essentials*. Boston, Little, Brown, 1983.

Rasch DK, Webster DE, Hutyra J, et al. Anesthetic management of hemodynamic changes during vein of Galen aneurysm clipping. *Anesthesiology* 1988; 69:993–995.

Rockoff MA: Anesthesia for children with hydrocephalus. *Anesthesiol Rev* 1979; 6:28–34.

Shapiro AM, Aidnis SJ: Neurosurgical anesthesia. *Surg Clin North Am* 1975; 55:913–928.

Shapiro HM: Intracranial hypertension therapeutic and anesthetic considerations. *Anesthesiology* 1975; 43:445–471.

Sperry RJ, Stirt JA, Stone DJ: *Manual of Neuroanesthesia.* Toronto, BC Decker, 1989.

Youmans JR: *Neurological Surgery.* Philadelphia, WB Saunders, 1990.

Part V

Pediatric Transplantation (Anesthetic and Surgical Concerns)

CHAPTER 29

Pediatric Renal Transplantation

Mary Ann Gurkowski
Deborah K. Rasch

The incidence of end-stage renal disease (ESRD) in children younger than age 16 years ranges from 1.5 to 4.5 per million per year, and the frequency varies with the geographic area. Approximately 50 percent of these children will be between the ages of 11 and 16 years. The ability to provide adequate nutrition and maximize growth potential is difficult in a child with uremia. Because normal infants achieve 30 percent of their entire growth potential in the first 2 years of life, it is understandable that children younger than age 2 years with ESRD may be severely affected. Dialysis and eventually renal transplant as a means of maintaining near normal body homeostasis become important.

The two commonly used forms of dialysis are continuous ambulatory peritoneal dialysis (CAPD) and hemodialysis. CAPD is more commonly used in children than hemodialysis. Hemodialysis in children younger than age 2 years is technically difficult although it has been successfully done in large centers. There will also be some children who are in need of a transplant who have never been dialyzed.

Most children with ESRD will be evaluated for renal transplantation. The size of the child and not their age is important when considering the optimal time for transplantation. The survival rates for the transplanted kidney are lower in children who weigh less than 10 kg. Survival rates of a cadaveric versus a living related-donor (LRD) kidney become nearly equal as the very young patients grow older. In children weighing under 5 kg, cadaveric kidneys from child donors are a necessity, but over this weight, LRD kidneys may be used. In a child younger than age 5 years, it appears that a LRD kidney does better than a cadaveric kidney, but after age 5 years, the two types of transplants are equal in outcome.

PRETRANSPLANT EVALUATION

A complete history and physical examination, a comprehensive psychiatric evaluation, blood typing, a renal biopsy, and an arteriogram must be done before a recipient can be scheduled for an LRD transplant or before the child can be placed on the computerized international cadaver organ waiting list. If the LRD's ABO matches that of the recipient, then a cross match, tissue typing, and mixed leukocyte culture assay are performed. The donor must also lack other physical barriers, such as hypertension, diabetes, or malignancy, and be well psychologically. If donors pass these tests, then they must undergo an arteriogram to look for any renovascular abnormalities and define the renal artery anatomy. The presence of more than two donor renal arteries is incompatible with surgery. Unlike cadaveric kidneys with multiple arteries that can be taken with a common patch of aorta, the LRD kidney must have each artery sewn in individually. The more arteries present, the longer the ischemic time is for the donor kidney. The smaller of the two kidneys of the LRD is usually harvested because it provides a size advantage for a small child. Otherwise, the left kidney is preferred because of its long left renal vein.

The recipient is not a candidate for transplantation if there is evidence of untreated septic foci or malignancy. In the past, splenectomies were performed as an adjunct to conventional immunosuppression. Today, only if the recipient has a leukocytopenia secondary to hypersplenism is a splenectomy performed. Liver functions must be checked pretransplant, and if there are any abnormalities, then transplantation is delayed until the problem is treated, if possible, and any infections or inflammatory diseases are resolved. If the recipient's kidneys are a source of continued infection or the cause of uncontrolled renin-dependent hypertension or massive proteinuria, which impairs nutrition and growth, then nephrectomies are performed. All urologic abnormalities must be corrected pretransplant. If the child has an ileal loop, colostomy, or ureterostomy, then these must be repaired before the transplant operation to minimize the risk of posttransplant infection. If these repairs are done at the time of actual transplantation, the surgical and anesthesia time will be significantly lengthened. In children weighing less than 20 kg, when removal of the kidneys is necessary, it can be done simultaneously with the transabdominal transplant if the kidneys are not infected. If the child weighs over 20 kg, the native kidneys are usually removed before the transplantation surgery. In larger children, the new kidney is placed extraperitoneally in the pelvis, and the peritoneal cavity is not invaded.

**Table 29-1 Dosing Table for Preoperative Preparation
and Sedation**

Midazolam 0.5 mg/kg PO, pentobarbital 2 to 4 mg/kg PO (ages,
1 to 8 yrs), or diazepam 0.25 mg/kg PO (maximum, 10 mg)

Shohl's solution or Na citrate 1 mL/kg PO

Methylprednisolone 15 mg/kg IV

Azathioprine 3 mg/kg IV

Living related-donor kidney, cefamandole 15 mg/kg IV

Cadaveric kidney, ceftazidime 25 to 50 mg/kg IV before skin
incision.

PO = orally; IV = intravenous

PREMEDICATION

Many of these children have had multiple hospital visits and
have had to undergo many procedures before the actual transplantation. For this reason, these children are often very fearful
of needle sticks. Oral agents such as pentobarbital, diazepam,
or midazolam should be used for preoperative sedation whenever possible (Table 29-1). The children with an elevated blood
urea nitrogen or abdominal distention from CAPD also have delayed gastric emptying; so aspiration prophylaxis with metoclopramide, ranitidine, and a nonparticulate antacid would be
prudent.

PREOPERATIVE PREPARATION

A complete history and physical examination should be performed. The laboratory tests that should be ordered include
electrolytes, creatinine, complete blood count, platelet count,
prothrombin time, partial thromboplastin time, and a type and
cross. These children may have low hematocrits (18 to 25 percent), but they are usually hemodynamically compensated.
Many children in renal failure now receive parenteral erythropoietin, which tends to normalize their hematocrit preoperatively.

It is also important to note the potassium value. If this value
is high normal, it is acceptable to proceed with the anesthetic,
but avoidance of succinylcholine is recommended. If the potassium value is greater than normal (5.5 to 6.0 mEq/L), preoperative dialysis should be performed. Many of these children will
have either a peritoneal dialysis catheter or a hemodialysis
catheter already in place.

If the child has just been peritoneally dialyzed, there may be
an increase in intraabdominal pressure secondary to the dialy-

**Table 29-2   Equipment and Supplies for Pediatric
Renal Transplantation**

Room temperature 28° to 32°C. Blood warmer 32° to 35°C
Warming blanket for bed and small warming pad for vascular
    access
Equipment and supplies for CVP (triple-lumen) or PA catheter
    and arterial line
Sterile ET tube
Standard monitors, including train-of-four
IV fluids without K^+ (e.g., D5 ½ NS, colloid)*
Dressing for CVP, IVs, arterial line: clear bioclusive dressing
    (Use sterile technique)
Blood, check to see if surgeons want "CMV negative"
Enhancement of GFR: mannitol 0.25 to 1 g/kg/IV*, furosemide
    1 mg/kg/IV, albumin 1 g/kg IV, and NaHCO₃ 1 mEq/kg/IV

CVP = central venous pressure; PA = pulmonary artery; ET = endotracheal; IV = intravenous; D5 = 5% dextrose; ½ NS = half-
normal saline; CMV = cytomegalovirus; GFR = glomerular filtration rate
*Doses may be modified as directed by CVP catheter estimates of
circulating volume. More mannitol may be requested for kidneys preserved for more than 24 h.

---

sate, which could further increase the risks associated with a
full stomach. Therefore, the dialysate should be allowed to
drain before proceeding with anesthetic induction.

The operating room should be prewarmed to a temperature
of 28° to 32°C. A blood warmer should be used for all intravenous (IV) fluids and blood products. The irrigation fluid should
be prewarmed. At least 10 mL/kg of packed red blood cells
should be in the room at the time of the incision. A heated humidifier and a warming blanket are essential to help maintain
body temperature. The equipment for insertion of arterial central venous pressure, and peripheral IV lines should be readily
available. If the child has an arteriovenous fistula, a warm blanket should be placed over the fistula to help maintain flow. In
addition to the routine drugs used for induction and maintenance, there are five others that need to be drawn into labeled
syringes. These include: mannitol, 0.5 to 1 g/kg; furosemide, 1
mg/kg; albumin, 1 g/kg; NaHCO₃, 1 mEq/kg; and methylprednisolone, 15 mg/kg. See Table 29-2 for a summary of equipment
and supply needs.

INDUCTION AND INTUBATION

Induction of anesthesia by the inhalation of halothane or by an
IV route have both been successfully performed. It is the
younger child who usually receives an inhalational induction.

The IV induction can safely be performed with a combination of narcotic, thiopental sodium (providing the intravascular volume is not decreased), or etomidate plus a nondepolarizing muscle relaxant, such as atracurium or vecuronium. Succinylcholine is usually avoided because of the risk for hyperkalemia, but if the child has a normal preoperative potassium value, succinylcholine can be used. Gentle cricoid pressure should be applied before and during intubation to decrease the risk of gastric reflux and aspiration. Careful handling of the endotracheal tube to keep it as sterile as possible should be done because all these patients are immunosuppressed.

MAINTENANCE ANESTHESIA

Anesthesia can be maintained using narcotics, an inhalational agent, and a nondepolarizing muscle relaxant. The most commonly used narcotic is fentanyl, and the inhalational agent is isoflurane. Halothane is often used for induction, but because of its ability to sensitize the myocardium to catecholamines and to decrease both urine output and urine sodium excretion, it is usually discontinued after intubation. Enflurane is not recommended for anesthesia during renal transplantation because of the accumulation of fluoride ions that result from its metabolism. Fluoride ions can cause nephrotoxicity. Nitrous oxide is also not recommended because of its ability to distend the bowel and, therefore, make closure much more difficult. Vecuronium, atracurium, pancuronium, and tubocurarine have all been successfully used for maintenance muscle relaxation. Both pancuronium and tubocurarine have a significantly prolonged duration of action in patients with impaired renal function, whereas vecuronium is only slightly prolonged and the duration of atracurium is not affected at all. Therefore, the most commonly used nondepolarizing muscle relaxants are atracurium and vecuronium.

The placement of a continuous caudal or epidural catheter after intubation can help reduce anesthetic requirements and also provide excellent postoperative analgesia. Intraoperatively, a local anesthetic is most commonly used, whereas postoperatively, narcotics are used. The child will wake up comfortably if the epidural narcotic is given approximately 30 min before the end of the case (see Chap. 10 for a more detailed discussion of techniques and doses).

INTRAOPERATIVE MANAGEMENT
AND SURGICAL TECHNIQUE

After induction and intubation, arterial and central lines should be placed either percutaneously by the anesthesiologist or by cut down by the surgeon. Strict sterile technique should be followed because these patients will be immunosuppressed. The central line is used for monitoring central venous pressure, for rapid infusion of fluids, and for blood sampling. It will be important to have the child's central venous pressure 8 to 12 mmHg before revascularization of the kidney to promote renal blood flow and to prevent hypotension. If the child is receiving an adult kidney, it may sequester as much as 300 mL of blood acutely on revascularization, thus decreasing the central venous pressure by several points. It is important to keep the child warm during the surgery and maintain hemostasis, acid–base balance, and cardiovascular stability. This is accomplished by monitoring the central venous pressure; warming all irrigation fluids, blood products, and crystalloid to 32°C; and monitoring blood electrolytes, pH, and arterial oxygenation every 30 min or as indicated by the case. If the child has an arteriovenous fistula, it must be kept warm, and the thrill must be closely monitored.

In children weighing over 20 kg, the procedure is performed similar to an adult transplantation. The donor kidney is placed retroperitoneally, and the donor renal artery is anastomosed to the common iliac artery of the recipient. The renal vein is an-

Table 29-3 Intraoperative Management

---

1. *Check thrill* of vascular access every 15 to 30 min intraoperatively; if it decreases, may need higher blood pressure.
2. *CVP catheter* (Broviac or Hickman catheters) placed by surgeon in small children and percutaneously in older children. Use sterile technique.
3. *NG tube:* aspirate to decompress stomach.
4. *Laboratory values:* ABG, Na^+, K^+, Hct, glucose every 30 min or prn. After revascularization, every 1 h plasma and urinary electrolytes, osmolarity, and glucose.
5. *Before vascular clamps are removed* (i.e., kidney gets perfused in recipient), give the appropriate doses of mannitol and furosemide (see Table 29-2), guided by CVP or PA catheter estimates of circulating volume.
6. *After revascularization:*
    A. D5 with 100 mEq NaCl, 15 mEq/L $NaHCO_3$, 10 mEq/L KCl, milliliter for urine output.
    B. If urine > 8 mL/kg/h, use glucose-free solution.
7. *Extubation criteria:* train-of-four, sustained tetanus; adequate tidal volume; awake, pharyngeal reflex present; head and leg lift, normothermia.

CVP = central venous pressure; NG = nasogastric; ABG = arterial blood gases; Hct = hematocrit; prn = as needed; PA = pulmonary artery; D5 = dextrose 5%.

astomosed to the common or external iliac vein. In the child weighing under 20 kg, the usual method is to place the donor kidney intraabdominally, anastomosing the donor renal artery to the recipient's aorta and the donor renal vein to the recipient's vena cava or common iliac vein. Small kidneys from pediatric donors may be placed in the extraperitoneal position.

The cadaveric kidney is transported in cold Collins solution, which is an intracellular electrolyte solution containing very high concentrations of potassium. It is mandatory that the kidney be flushed with ice-cold Ringer's lactate before being brought to the operating table for anastomosis because, if not, fatal hyperkalemia may occur in the recipient during reperfusion of the kidney. After anastomosis of the kidney, but before unclamping, the patient is volume loaded to a central venous pressure of 8 to 12 mmHg and mannitol, 0.25 to 1 g/kg, and furosemide, 1 mg/kg, should be given IV. Acidosis, even if mild, should be treated with $NaHCO_3$ before unclamping the renal vessels. These interventions are designed to promote good urinary flow and counteract the lactic acid return from the lower extremities caused by the cross clamping of the iliac vessels or the aorta. Table 29-3 summarizes several important points of intraoperative management.

EXTUBATION

Extubation can usually be performed in the operating room, provided the child's temperature is normal and that adequate muscle relaxant reversal has been achieved. The child must be able to maintain a tidal volume of 5 to 10 mL/kg and be awake with intact airway reflexes. If the child does not meet these criteria, then they should be taken to the recovery room, placed on oxygen by ventilator or T-piece, and monitored closely. When these parameters are met, then extubation may be performed.

POSTOPERATIVE CONCERNS

During the postoperative period, assuming adequate diuresis, the urine output should be replaced at 15 min intervals on a milliliter per milliliter basis. This is done to prevent hypotension secondary to hypovolemia. Either a standard crystalloid solution may be used or, in our institution, a solution made up of the following: glucose, 5 g/dL; NaCl, 100 mEq/L; $NaHCO_3$, 15 mEq/L; plus KCl, 10 mEq/L. If the urine output exceeds 8 mL/kg/h, it is suggested that a lower glucose concentration (1 g/dL) or a sugar-free solution be used. To adjust the crystalloid electrolyte composition appropriately, urine osmolality and sodium, potassium, and glucose values should be checked every hour initially, then every 2 h when stable. If glycosuria or hyperglycemia occurs, then a nonglucose-containing electrolyte solution is substituted. If this does not correct the hyperglycemia, then insulin may be administered.

These children are also given antibiotics and immunosuppressive drugs. Antibiotics are used as prophylaxis to decrease the risk of urinary sepsis and *Pneumocystis carinii* and *Nocardia* infections. The two most commonly given antibiotics are cefamandole (15 mg/kg) or ceftazidime (25 to 50 mg/kg/dose). Trimethoprim plus sulfamethoxazole is given for prophylaxis against *Pneumocystis*. Ketoconazole is often administered to prevent *Candida* overgrowth in the gastrointestinal tract. Children who have undergone splenectomy for any reason should also receive daily oral penicillin as well as receiving pneumococcal and *Haemophilus* vaccines intraoperatively.

Immunosuppressive therapy is important to prevent rejection of the kidney. Conventional immunosuppression consists of azathioprine, cyclophosphamide, prednisone, or methylprednisolone and antilymphoblast globulin. Controversy results when cyclosporine is discussed.

Cyclosporine first became available to transplant centers in 1983. The advantages of the drug include a decreased infection rate and the potential for a lower dose of steroids, which would be important in terms of the child's long-term growth and development. The disadvantages are that it is extremely expensive (approximately, $200/mo), it may cause an elevation in serum creatinine, and long-term studies on its effect on growth have not been performed. Because of this controversy, the use of cyclosporine varies between institutions. The doses and dosing interval of all immunosuppressive drugs varies among transplant programs, but usually methylprednisolone, azathioprine, prednisone, and cyclosporine are started the morning of surgery or just after induction. Only antilymphoblast globulin is begun postoperatively.

BIBLIOGRAPHY

Broyer M, Gagnadoux MF, Beurton D: Transplantation in children: Technical aspects, drug therapy and problems related to primary renal disease. *Proceedings of the European Dialysis and Transplant Association* 1981; 18:313–321.

Fine RN, Salusky IB, Ettenger RB: The therapeutic approach to the infant, child, and adolescent with end-stage renal disease. *Pediatr Clin North Am* 1987; 34:789–801.

Graybar BG, Bready LL: *Anesthesia for Renal Transplantation.* Boston, Martinus Nijhoff, 1987, pp 139–176.

Lum, CT, Wassner SJ, Martin DE: Current thinking in transplantation in infants and children. *Pediatr Clin North Am* 1985; 32:1203–1232.

McHugh MJ: Intensive care aspects of organ transplantation in children. *Pediatr Clin North Am* 1987; 34:187–201.

Sheldon CA, McLoire GA, Churchill BM: Renal transplantation in children. *Pediatr Clin North Am* 1987; 34:1209–1232.

Weimar W, Geerlings W, Bijnen AB: A controlled study on the effect of mannitol on immediate renal function after cadaver donor kidney transplantation. *Transplantation* 1983; 35:99–101.

CHAPTER 30

Pediatric Cardiac Transplantation

Christopher A. Bracken

In a landmark operation, Dr. Christiaan Barnard ushered in the age of cardiac transplantation when he performed his historic first human allograft heart transplantation in South Africa in 1967. Between 1967 and the early 1980s, progress was slow, mostly because of problems with immunosuppression and rejection. Since the introduction and acceptance of cyclosporine as an effective immunosuppression agent, cardiac transplantation has achieved widespread acceptance and remains one of the preeminent "public awareness" operations. The registry of the International Society for Heart Transplantation (ISHT) listed 12,600 heart transplantations by the end of 1989, with 85 percent occurring between 1985 and 1989. At the beginning of 1990, there were 148 centers in the United States and 88 centers in the rest of the world performing heart and heart–lung transplantations (Kriett & Kaye, 1990).

THE HISTORY OF PEDIATRIC CARDIAC TRANSPLANTATION

The first pediatric heart transplant was performed in 1967, only days after Dr. Barnard's first allograft operation, by Kantrowitz in a 1-month-old infant. In 1968, Cooley performed the first heart–lung transplant in a 2-month-old infant. Currently, 10 percent of all heart transplants are performed in pediatric patients.

INDICATIONS FOR TRANSPLANTATION

Transplants are being performed in children and teen-agers as a means to treat end-stage disease that is not responsive to medical treatment and for which no other surgical treatment is available or justified. It is estimated that 10 percent of patients with congenital heart disease, or 3000 cases per year in North America, have anomalies too complex for surgical repair (Boldt, 1991). In general, congenital disease responds best to transplantation early in life. This fact is reflected in the marked shift in the average age of the pediatric heart transplant recipient over the past 8 years. There is a bimodal age distribution pattern for the pediatric heart transplantation group, with a large group younger than 1-year of age and a second peak in the early teenage years. A potential benefit to early transplantation (0 to 30 days of life) is the apparently blunted incidence of rejection, thus requiring lesser levels of immunosuppression with a resultant increased quality of life (Bailey, 1988). Additionally, delaying transplantation in congenital lesions with high QP/QS ratios (e.g., hypoplastic left heart syndrome [HLHS] or large ventricular septal defect [VSD]) may increase the risk of developing reactive pulmonary hypertension, which may make eventual transplantation no longer feasible.

Older children undergoing heart transplantation are most often suffering from acquired cardiomyopathies. These children frequently have less clear indications for transplantation and require more extensive evaluation. Historically, cardiomyopathy was the leading indication for transplantation, both in adults and children, accounting for more than 60 percent of the total transplants in children by 1990. However, the percentage of pediatric heart transplantations occurring as a result of cardiomyopathy has been steadily decreasing, secondary to the rapid expansion in transplantations for severe congenital defects.

Another indication for transplantation is in children with cystic fibrosis. These children undergo heart–lung block transplants, occasionally utilizing the cystic fibrosis candidate's good heart for subsequent transplantation into another recipient with a simpler cardiac defect (de Leval, 1991).

PATIENT SELECTION

An excellent review article by Martin and Allard from Loma Linda was published as a Society of Cardiovascular Anesthesiologists monograph in 1992. They emphasize that the most important factor in a successful outcome seems to be the original patient selection, and various statistics confirm this observation. The primary determinant is a cardiac evaluation consistent with a limited life expectancy with no other accepted means of surgical correction, either because of a complex congenital anomaly or severe acquired heart disease. Table 30-1 lists examples of the preoperative cardiac conditions most frequently associated with cardiac transplantation in children.

Each center has developed it own list of required medical and social criteria that must be met before accepting a patient

Table 30-1   Conditions Associated with Pediatric Heart Transplantation

---

Congenital cardiac conditions
  Hypoplastic left ventricle
  Severe Ebstein's anomaly with normal pulmonary arteries
  Multiple obstructive rhabdomyoma
  Pulmonary atresia with intact ventricular septum
  Hypoplastic left heart equivalent:
    D-transposition with hypoplastic right ventricle
    Single ventricle with hypoplastic aorta
    Left transposition with single ventricle and heart block
  Atrioventricular canal with hypoplastic left ventricle
  Single ventricle with subaortic obstruction
  Complex truncus arteriosus

Acquired cardiac conditions
  Irreversible dilated cardiomyopathy of unknown cause
  Hypertrophic cardiomyopathy
  Severe nonmalignant cardiac tumors

---

as a transplant candidate. In general, social requirements include the need for the patient's family to reside within 45-min travel from the transplant center for up to 6 months after the transplant and to demonstrate adequate long-term support structures to meet the exceptional long-term needs. Neonatal candidates have special considerations, as outlined from Loma Linda. The potential candidate must be older than 36 weeks' gestational age, and the birth weight should be greater than 2200 g to allow adequate pulmonary development, especially to the pulmonary arteries. Tables 30-2 and 30-3 contain lists of exclusion factors and relative exclusion factors, respectively. Not all centers rigidly enforce all the exclusion factors listed in these

Table 30-2   Pediatric Cardiac Transplantation Exclusion Factors

---

Marked prematurity and low birth weight
Unclear cardiac diagnosis
Persistent acidosis below pH 7.10
Active sepsis
Abnormal neurologic evaluation
Markedly elevated pulmonary vascular resistance (Woods units [varies among centers], 5 to 8)
Irreversible and progressive renal or hepatic disease
Positive drug screen
Significant dysmorphy or genetic problems
Other coexisting life-threatening disease

Table 30-3   **Pediatric Cardiac Transplantation
Relative Exclusion Factors**

Vascular anomalies
Infection, subacute
Elevated pulmonary vascular resistance
Recent pulmonary infarction
Insulin-dependent diabetes mellitus
Active duodenal ulcer
Renal or hepatic dysfunction
Limited family support structure
Financial constraints

two tables, but they modify these lists to suit their own transplantation philosophy. Some centers are very rigid in their acceptance criteria, citing the relative lack of donor organ availability and seeking to maximize the utilization of the available organs. Other centers, notably Pittsburgh, admit they rarely exclude a potential candidate.

DONOR ACQUISITION

The process of donor acquisition begins with the identification of a potential donor. There are 72 licensed regional organ procurement organizations (OPO) in the United States. A local doctor would notify a transplant coordinator from the nearest OPO that a patient in the hospital was a potential organ donor candidate. Screening of the donor candidate would include certification of brain death, according to the statutes outlined in the Uniform Determination of Death Act. The donor would also be screened for compatible ABO blood typing, organ size determination, absence of sepsis, intravenous drug abuse, and assurance of grossly normal organ function. For example, heart function would require left ventricular shortening of greater than 28 percent (Travitsky, 1988). After consulting with the next of kin to obtain approval, the regional coordinator would notify United Network for Organ Sharing (UNOS) of the potential donor. UNOS maintains computer files and would institute a computer search for an appropriate candidate within the geographic proximity necessary to keep the ischemic time less than 4 h. Screening for human leukocyte antigen typing is controversial at this time and does not seem to correlate well with survival or rejection statistics. Frequent causes of death for neonatal and pediatric heart donors are asphyxia at birth, sudden infant death syndrome, intracranial hemorrhage, child abuse, tumor or central nervous system abnormalities, and anoxic injuries (smoke or drowning). The use of anencephalic babies as organ donors remains controversial, although Loma Linda University

Table 30-4 Anesthetic Management of the Donor

Monitors:	Electrocardiography, pulse oximeter, blood pressure cuff, arterial line (easy access to blood for frequent laboratory work), and central venous pressure (monitor fluid balance, administer fluids)

Administer colloid or crystalloid to obtain satisfactory (normal for age) systolic and central venous pressures

Administer fluids to match urine output milliliter for milliliter. (ideal urine output, 1 to 2 mL/kg/h)

Low-dose dopamine for further blood pressure maintenance (may also respond to calcium or other inotropes)

Monitor electrolytes and maintain normal laboratory values

Monitor arterial blood gases; keep $PO_2 \geq 100$ mmHg

Use sterile technique
Maintain hematocrit > 30 percent
Maintain body temperature > 34°C
Desmopressin or pitressin as needed

Centers vary. In some circumstances, you may be asked to give:

    Prophylactic antibiotics
    Steroids
    Prostaglandin infusions
    Other medications
Discuss these needs with the organ procurement team you will be working with.

---

has reversed its earlier position, and now believes that it is not practical to harvest organs from these unfortunate babies (Shewmon, 1989).

There are several problems associated with donor management in the preharvest time period. The donor is often subjected to periods of hemodynamic instability secondary to loss of neurologic function. Frequently, maneuvers designed to minimize intracranial pressure (hyperventilation, diuretics, and fluid restriction) further impair hemodynamic autoregulation. Alternatively, the loss of sympathetic tone associated with vasodilation and fluid resuscitation may result in a grossly overhydrated patient. These patients are often subject to infection, either from trauma or from loss of immunologic competence. Primary neurologic injury may cause neurogenic diuresis from diabetes insipidus in about 50 percent of the patients. This is often treated with vasopressin (100 μU/kg/h) or desmopressin (5 to 20 μg). Donors younger than 6 months of age are frequently transported to the recipient's hospital before the har-

vest because neonatal hearts appear to be particularly sensitive
to cold ischemia. Optimal management of the donor is an intrinsic part of a successful transplantation. The goal of anesthetic
management of the donor is to optimize the stability and function of vital organs to be donated, by normalizing the donor's
blood pressure, oxygenation, urine output, and fluid and electrolyte balance. Table 30-4 describes a brief basic protocol for
these cases.

PRETRANSPLANTATION
PATIENT MANAGEMENT

As pointed out by Boldt and associates (1991), transplant candidates often require intensive care unit management before
transplantation. Of the 10 cases in their institution, 5 were performed for HLHS and 5 for cardiomyopathy. Preoperatively,
five children required mechanical ventilation, eight required
inotropic support, and six required either prostaglandin or nitroglycerin infusion to maintain pulmonary blood flow. Clearly,
the majority of these patients required intensive care admis-
sions. An extreme measure utilized by Delius and coworkers
(1990) at the University of Michigan demonstrated the feasibil-
ity of maintaining the transplant candidate on extracorporeal
membrane oxygenation (their term was extracorporeal life support). Further work in this field was demonstrated by Galantowicz and Stolar (1991).

ANESTHESIA PROTOCOLS

The anesthetic management for pediatric heart transplant is
very similar to that of cardiac surgery for any life-threatening
congenital defect. The anesthesia is accompanied by profound
hypothermic cardiac arrest in infants or smaller children or by
standard cooling in children large enough to maintain cannulation and perfusion during the actual transplantation. Most anesthesia protocols include the use of a high-dose narcotic and
muscle relaxant technique (e.g., fentanyl 50 to 100 μg/kg and
pancuronium) with intubation and controlled ventilation accomplished before placement of invasive monitoring. Vascular access is often problematic in these infants and may require surgical cut down. Volume lines most often are saphenous or left
external jugular in location. A double-lumen central venous line
is instituted for vasoactive infusions (right internal jugular if en-
domyocardial biopsy is not standard postoperative protocol;
otherwise, left subclavian). Percutaneous radial arterial catheterization is preferentially on the left because the aortic cannulation may distort the pressure readings taken from a right
radial line. Percutaneous cannulation is preferred, when possible, to minimize trauma and postoperative infection. At least

one institution (Loma Linda) employs the left groin approach for arterial and central venous access in infants. The surgeon will often provide a left atrial line and possibly a pulmonary artery line for hemodynamic measurement and vasoactive infusion before the discontinuation of bypass, especially if other central venous access is marginal.

Before the bypass, the hallmark of the anesthetic is to maintain an optimal heart rate, preload, contractility, and afterload because most patients have little cardiovascular reserve. "Optimal" frequently means "preoperative," or the best the child was able to obtain before the anesthetic induction. The children often respond poorly to increased preload or afterload. This is especially true in the case of patients with dilated cardiomyopathy. Their response to inotropic drugs may be blunted secondary to receptor downregulation and receptor uncoupling. They may respond better to a non-β_1-agonist (digoxin, glucagon, amrinone, or a β_2-agonist). These patients are also more prone to dysrhythmias than normal children, especially if they have elevated inotropic levels. It is especially important to understand the pulmonary hemodynamics. In patients with elevated pulmonary vascular resistance or cyanosis, the anesthesiologist must avoid increases in right ventricular afterload by maintaining adequate alveolar oxygen levels and avoiding hypoxemia, hypothermia, hypercarbia, or acidemia. Abrupt decreases in afterload during induction may destabilize these patients and should be aggressively treated. In patients with large QP/QS shunt fraction (e.g., large VSD or HLHS), it may be beneficial to minimize inspired oxygen by titrating to appropriate peripheral saturations and to avoid hyperventilation to minimize any increase in the pulmonary shunt fraction. Ideally, the QP/QS ratios and the degree of response to inspired oxygen will be determined at cardiac catheterization. Appropriate peripheral saturation may be mid-90s in a child with minimal QP/QS ratios to the low 80s with a high ratio. Rarely, paradoxic peripheral desaturation may be observed with increased inspired oxygen as the pulmonary vasculature dilates and QP/QS worsens. These children do especially poorly with increases in afterload caused by anxiety or pain. In general, the anesthetic should be approached with the expectation of instability between induction and the institution of cardiopulmonary bypass. Most require some support before bypass. In general, isoproterenol is utilized for maintaining heart rate and contractility, whereas dopamine is utilized for maintaining pressure and contractility. In cases of elevated preoperative pulmonary artery pressures, some centers choose to use dobutamine in place of dopamine, although other centers believe the synthetic agent is not effective in the face of the receptor downregulation and catecholamine exhaustion.

Because all these procedures are accomplished in a cooled patient, warming lights should be removed, and peripheral cooling should be initiated at the time of skin preparation. Especially for cases involving circulatory arrest, the head should be surrounded in ice before draping the patient. Care should be taken to ensure access to all invasive monitors and intravascular lines because relocation after draping is often nearly impossible. These patients require at least two temperature monitors: one to monitor the core temperature (urinary bladder in larger children and rectal in infants) and a second to monitor the brain temperature (nasopharyngeal or tympanic). Esophageal temperatures are often misleading during bypass or arrest because they are closest to the aortic cannulation site or behind the pericardial operative site. The core temperature should be allowed to drift down to 33° to 35°C before instituting cardiopulmonary bypass. The perfusion machine prime should be calculated to provide a hematocrit between 18 and 22 percent during the cooling phase. Many centers add phentolamine (2- to 5-mg bolus) into the pump prime to help vasodilate during cooling. Other medications added include narcotics, benzodiazepines, antibiotics, bicarbonate, and steroids, depending on the institutional protocol. The core temperature ideally is lowered to 16°C to 18°C, with nasopharyngeal temperatures approaching 18°C before initiating circulatory arrest.

POSTBYPASS MANAGEMENT

The transplanted heart is totally and permanently denervated, has been subjected to global ischemia, and often has to contend with an elevated pulmonary vascular resistance (Lowe, 1990). The denervation often results in an abnormal electrocardiogram, resulting in two p waves. The residual recipient sinoatrial (SA) node remains innervated but is not in electrical continuity with the transplanted heart. The donor SA nodal segment is denervated and, thus, freed from the usual predominant parasympathetic (vagal) tone. The resultant heart rate is commonly 90 to 120 beats/min. Because of the denervated state, tachyarrhythmias will not respond to carotid massage. The patients also lack the ability to respond appropriately with baroreceptor-mediated reflex responses to hypovolemia or vasodilation. They do not respond to autonomic neurotransmission initiated by pain, fear, or surgical stimulus. They must wait for circulating humoral transmitters (catecholamines). The inotropic response is limited to direct-acting agents and may display β-receptor up-regulation. On resuming function, the transplanted heart demonstrates a decrease in diastolic compliance and ventricular contractility. This results in a heart rate-dependent cardiac output secondary to a fixed stroke volume (Novitsky, 1985). This decrease in compliance also causes increased measured preload, resulting in a perceived decrease in contractility. Therefore, the postbypass period is characterized by the necessity to maintain a high preload to compensate for the decreased diastolic compliance (central venous pressure, 10 to 16 mmHg; left atrial pressure 12 to 18 mmHg). Additionally, the right ventricle is often forced to contend with elevated pulmonary artery pressures. This is thought to be the most frequent cause of intraoperative death (Curling, 1987). It is often advantageous to have pulmonary artery and left atrial catheters placed by the surgeon to maximize the ability to monitor and adjust pulmonary vascular resistance.

Before weaning from bypass, the patient must be fully rewarmed, must have a good rhythm (fast sinus or paced) and a good hematocrit (25 to 30 percent), and should be fully paralyzed, adequately ventilated on 100% oxygen, and hyperventilated to achieve alkalemia (pH 7.45 to 7.55). Some centers add morphine sulfate to ensure anesthesia and promote pulmonary vasodilation; other centers avoid narcotics until after separation from the bypass. Hyperventilation is maintained to ensure maximum pulmonary vasodilation. Although inotropic support is almost always required, preferences vary. Original protocols used isoproterenol (0.02 to 5.0 μg/kg/min) almost exclusively. Many institutions, including ours, now use dopamine (5 to 10 μg/kg/min), occasionally supplemented with dobutamine (5 to 15 μg/kg/min), epinephrine (0.05 to 1 μg/kg/min), and/or amrinone (0.75 to 1.5 mg/kg bolus, followed by 5 to 10 μg/kg/min infusion) in various combinations. Afterload reduction with nitroglycerin, nitroprusside, or prostaglandin E_1 (30 to 150 ng/kg/min) is also frequently employed as necessary. In cases that are refractory to weaning, Novitsky and coworkers reported a good response to triiodothyronine administration. Controlled trials are pending, but clinical use of this drug in difficult situations of poor myocardial function may be justified.

Posttransplantation patients all have impaired gas exchange. All patients are returned to the intensive care unit intubated. The usual protocol has the patients intubated and ventilated for 24 to 48 h before extubation. Patients with marginally high pulmonary vascular resistance may require pulmonary vasodilation (nitroglycerin, hyperventilation, increased inspired oxygen, prostaglandin E_1, or amrinone) for a time to allow equilibration between the new right ventricle and the pulmonary vasculature. Fluid shifts occasioned by the bypass may result in fluid-overloaded lungs for a time, and extubation should be delayed until the fluid status is stable. Table 30-5 summarizes the special anesthetic concerns in these patients.

Table 30-5   Cardiac Transplantation: Special Considerations

Prebypass
 Poor response to increased preload and afterload
 Possible blunted response to inotropic drugs
 More prone to dysrhythmia
 Deteriorate easily in the face of sudden changes in right or
   left ventricular afterload and changing shunt fractions
 More likely to need inotropic support prebypass

Characteristics of the newly transplanted heart (caused by loss
   of baroreceptor-mediated reflex and response to pain, fear,
   and surgical stimulus)
 Decreased diastolic compliance and ventricular contractility
   (the stroke volume is relatively fixed, and the cardiac
   output is independent. There is a necessity to maintain a
   high preload.)
 Pulmonary artery pressures are often elevated, resulting in
   right ventricular dysfunction.

Weaning from bypass: Criteria
 Warm
 Good rhythm (fast sinus, paced)
 Hematocrit, 25 to 30 percent
 Muscle relaxant adequate
 Well ventilated, 100% O_2
 Hyperventilated pH 7.45 to 7.55 (pulmonary vasodilation)
 Narcotics (morphine sulfate may help produce pulmonary
   vasodilation) either pre- or postweaning
 Inotropic support (per institution)
 Afterload reduction as needed

Postoperative care
 Postoperative ventilation is the norm
 Pulmonary vasodilation and inotropic support frequently
   needed

MORTALITY

Operative mortality is defined statistically as deaths occurring
within 30 days of the operation. There has been a gradual improvement in operative mortality as experience grows, but the
operative mortality rate for pediatric heart transplants remains
higher than the comparable statistics in adult heart transplant
patients. The operative mortality rate is highest in the youngest
recipient age group (ages, 0 to 4 years). Within this age group,
the operative mortality rate is highest for the congenital disease
subgroup. As this group is, by definition, also the youngest age
group, it is unclear whether the age, the disease process, or a
combination of the two is primarily responsible for the in-

creased rate. The incidence of pulmonary hypertension is higher in the congenital disease subgroup and has previously been implicated as the greatest single contributor to operative mortality. Kriett and Kaye (1990) documented right-sided heart failure as the primary cause accounting for up to 59 percent of the operative mortality in the pediatric age group transplant patients. There is room for optimism. Perhaps, as the age for congenital transplants falls, more operations will occur before pulmonary hypertension develops, and the statistics will improve. In 1990, Loma Linda reported 33 of 35 patients (96 percent) survived 30 days.

Other causes of mortality include the twin terrors of all transplantations: infection and rejection. Infection has been implicated in up to two thirds of all hospital deaths, with most occurring in the first 6-month period. Infection is also the most common cause of prolonged hospitalization. Two thirds of the patients experience at least one significant episode of infection within the first 3 months. Opportunistic infections cause the greatest problems. One of the chief clinical problems is discriminating infection from rejection episodes. Rejection is thought to be nearly a universal phenomenon of heart transplantation in the first 3 months. At Pittsburgh, only three children (18 percent) could be documented free of rejection in the first 3 months, and all three belonged to a group that received prophylactic immunosuppression with antithymocyte globulin (Fricker 1990). Stanford also quotes a 75 percent incidence of at least one rejection episode in the first 3 months. Bailey points out that there is no entirely reliable surveillance tool to diagnose rejection, which contributes to the problem.

Over the long term, coronary artery disease is a major problem for these patients. The development of coronary artery disease appears to be about 23 percent at 1 year (compared with 36 percent in adults at 1 year) and is unrelated to the recipient's (or donor's) age, sex, or preoperative cardiac diagnosis, recipient serum lipid profile, number of rejection episodes, dose of corticosteroid, or degree of cross-match (Baum and associates, 1990; Gao and colleagues, 1987). The detection of a compromised circulation is difficult because denervation eliminates angina and diagnostic tests are often insufficiently sensitive to detect the disease. As a consequence, these patients often undergo annual coronary angiography. (This is of particular interest to the anesthesiologist who may be called on to anesthetize posttransplant patients for noncardiac surgery).

Finally, cancer seems to be much more prevalent in the immunosuppressed patient. Some studies indicate a 100-fold increase, especially in the incidence of non-Hodgkin's lymphoma. Approximately 10 percent of Stanford's patients developed malignancies, all but one of which was lymphoma.

CONCLUSION

The survival statistics for pediatric heart transplantation have been improved since Stanford began accumulating statistics in 1974. All institutions seem to have a brief learning curve, during which the survival statistics are about 10 points lower than the long-term statistics. Pediatric survival is still statistically less than adult cardiac transplant survival, apparently as a result of the neonatal rate. The ISHT actuarial rates for the 118 total patients reported in the United States showed the average 1-year survival rate in children younger than 1 year of age to be 76 percent and for children older than 1 year old, 66 percent. The 5-year survival rate across the board was 62 percent. It seems clear that, as improvements in organ-preservation techniques, patient selection criteria, immunosuppression techniques, and infection control are implemented, the survival of seriously ill children is medically feasible. It remains up to the larger segment of society to address the issues of improved organ procurement and determining how society will finance this highly technical (and expensive) medical therapy.

BIBLIOGRAPHY

Anderson TM: Indications and candidacy for heart transplantation in children, in Dunn JM, Donner RM (eds): *Heart Transplantation in Children*. Mount Kisco, NY, Futura, 1990, pp 7–16.

Armitage JM, Hardesty RL, Griffith BP: Prostaglandin E_1: An effective treatment of right heart failure after orthotopic heart transplantation. *J Heart Transplant* 1987; 6:348–351.

Bailey LL, Assadd AN, Trimm RF, et al: Orthotopic transplantation during early infancy as therapy for incurable congenital heart disease. *Ann Surg* 1988; 208:279–286.

Baum D, Bernstein D, Starnes V: Assessing the results of heart transplantation in children: Morbidity, mortality and quality of life, in Dunn JM, Donner RM (eds): *Heart Transplantation in Children*. Mount Kisco, NY, Futura, 1990, pp 223–232.

Boldt J, Zickmann B, Netz H, et al: Heart transplantation in children: Anesthetic considerations. *Paediatr Anaesth* 1991; 1:119–124.

Clark NJ, Martin RD: Anesthetic considerations for patients undergoing cardiac transplantation. *J Cardiothorac Vasc Anesth* 1988; 2:519–542.

Cooley DA, Bloodwell RD, Hallman GL, et al. Organ transplantation for advanced cardiopulmonary disease. *Ann Thorac Surg* 1969; 8:30–46.

Curling PE, Zaidan JR, Murphy DA, et al: Treatment of pulmonary artery hypertension after human orthotopic heart transplantation. *Anesth Analg* 1987; 66:537.

DeBegona JA, Kawauchi M, Fullerton D, et al: Heart transplantation in children. *Compr Ther* 1990; 16:61–64.

de Leval MR, Smyth R, White B, et al: Heart and lung transplantation for terminal cystic fibrosis. *J Thorac Cardiovasc Surg* 1991; 101:633–642.

Delius RE, Zwischenberger JB, Cilley R, et al: Prolonged extracorporeal life support of pediatric and adolescent cardiac transplant patients. *Ann Thorac Surg* 1990; 50:791–795.

Fricker FJ, Trento A, Griffith B, et al: Experience with heart transplantation in children at the University of Pittsburgh and Children's Hospital, in Dunn JM, Donner RM (eds): *Heart Transplantation in Children*. Mount Kisco, NY, Futura, 1990, pp 233–241.

Galantowicz ME, Stolar CHJ: Extracorporeal membrane oxygenation for perioperative support in pediatric heart transplantation. *J Thorac Cardiovas Surg* 1991; 102:148–152.

Gao SZ, Schroeder JS, Alderman EL, et al: Clinical and laboratory correlates of accelerated coronary artery disease in the cardiac transplant patient. *Circulation* 1987; 76(suppl 5,pt 2):56–61.

Hutchings SM, Monett ZJ: Caring for the cardiac transplant patient. *Crit Care Nurs Clin North Am* 1989; 1:245–261.

Jones S: Care of children after transplants. *Nursing* 1991; 4:35–38.

Kantrowitz A, Haller JD, Joos H, et al: Transplantation of the heart in an infant and an adult. *Am J Cardiol* 1968; 22:782–790.

Kriett JM, Kaye MP: The registry of the International Society for Heart Transplantation: Seventh official report. *J Heart Transplant* 1990; 9:323–330.

Lowe DA: Anesthetic considerations in pediatric cardiac transplantation, in Dunn JM, Donner RM (eds): *Heart Transplantation in Children*. Mount Kisco, NY, Futura, 1990, pp 39–69.

Martin RD, Allard MW: Pediatric cardiac transplantation, in Fabian JA (ed): *Anesthesia for Organ Transplantation*. Philadelphia: JB Lippincott, 1992, pp 21–42.

Novitzky D, Cooper D, Boniaszcuk J, et al: The significance of left ventricular volume measurement after heart transplantation using radionuclide techniques. *Heart Transplant* 1985; 4:206–209.

Novitzky D, Cooper DK, Zuhdi N: Triiodothyronine therapy in the cardiac transplant recipient. *Transplant Proc* 1988; 20(5 suppl 7): 65–68.

Shewmon DA, Capron AM, Peacock WJ, et al: The use of anencephalic infants as organ sources: A critique. *JAMA* 1989; 261:1773–1781.

Starnes VA, Bernstein D, Oyer PE, et al: Heart transplantation in children. *J Heart Transplant* 1989; 8:20–26.

Taylor SR, Yunis EJ, Fricker FJ: Cardiac transplantation in children. *Perspect Pediatr Pathol* 1991; 14:60–93.

Travitsky VA, Cooney CA, Nathan HM: Organ procurement process, in Dunn JM, Donner RM (eds): *Heart Transplantation in Children*. Mount Kisco, NY, Futura, 1990, pp 23–38.

CHAPTER 31

Pediatric Liver Transplantation

Scott E. LeBard

The past 10 to 15 years has seen a marked improvement in the success of orthotopic liver transplantation because of a combination of factors. The utilization of cyclosporine and OKT-3, which have improved immunosuppressive abilities; the development of newer surgical techniques; the improved intraoperative anesthetic care that comes with increasing experience; and the improved postoperative management account for this success. Because of these factors, 5-year survival rates for pediatric liver transplantation currently approach 70 to 80 percent.[1] The following is intended to be a general review of the anesthetic management for the pediatric patients in this population.

PREOPERATIVE EVALUATION

As in any patient, it is important to know the exact disease process because it might affect the urgency of the transplant and the preoperative evaluation. The nature of the disease may also have a significant impact on the ability to "fine tune" the patient before surgery. Two extremes of hepatic disease that exemplify the differences in terms of onset and possible urgency are acute fulminant hepatitis and congenital biliary atresia. Different classifications of liver disease have been proposed. A general classification of the indications for liver transplantation in children could be as follows: (1) obstructive primary liver disease, (2) acute and chronic hepatitis, (3) metabolic disease, (4) primary malignancy, and (5) retransplantation. Table 31-1 represents a general list of the most common disease processes for which liver transplantations occur in children.

In addition to knowing the diagnosis, a routine preoperative history with a complete review of systems should be performed. Table 31-2 summarizes the general information that should be obtained. Other specific aspects of this patient population deserve further comment.

Table 31-1 Indications for Liver Transplantation

Obstructive biliary disease
  Biliary atresia
  Choledochal cyst
  Sclerosing cholangitis
  Biliary hypoplasia
  Familial intrahepatic fibrosis
  Postsurgical and other traumatic biliary tract diseases

Acute and chronic hepatitis
  Fulminant hepatic failure
    Acute viral hepatitis
    Toxin- or drug-induced hepatitis
  Chronic hepatitis
    Hepatitis B
    Hepatitis C (non-A, non-B)
    Autoimmune
    Idiopathic
    Neonatal
    Hyperalimentation-induced

Metabolic disease
  α_1-antitrypsin deficiency
  Tyrosinemia
  Wilson's disease
  Glycogen storage disorders

Primary malignancy
  Hepatoblastoma
  Hepatocellular carcinoma

Retransplantation

A general review of the cardiopulmonary system probably is the most important aspect to review in light of the intraoperative hemodynamic stresses that occur. Whereas the presence of intrinsic cardiac disease is rare in children, the transplant candidate may be a child who has received chemotherapy for a primary hepatic malignancy. Doxorubicin is a common chemotherapeutic medication used for treatment of hepatic tumors, and it is noted to result in a dose-dependent cardiotoxicity. When the total dose exceeds 550 mg/m$_2$, irreversible cardiomyopathy may result. For this patient, the anesthesiologist may find it helpful to have a baseline electrocardiogram (ECG), chest x-ray, and echocardiogram to evaluate the cardiac reserve, the results of which may influence intraoperative monitoring.

Pulmonary function may be affected by the presence of extensive abdominal ascites and the development of diffuse arteriovenous shunting, both of which can develop with portal hypertension. This may be important to note for the following

Table 31-2   Preoperative Information

General information
  Age
  Weight (in kilograms)
  Diagnosis
  Drug allergies
  Current medications
  Anesthesia and surgical history
  Medical history
  Oral intake status
Laboratory information
  Chest x-ray
  Electrocardiogram
  Echocardiogram (+/−)
  Head CT (+/−)
  Electrolytes
  Blood urea nitrogen and creatinine
  Serum glucose
  Serum ionized calcium
  Serum albumin and protein levels
  Prothrombin and partial thromboplastin times
  Thromboelastogram (if available)
  Hemoglobin and hematocrit
  Platelet level
  Arterial blood gas

reasons. First, with extensive ascites, there is an upward compressive effect on the diaphragm that can result in a restrictive lung defect. Not only can this have an effect on ventilation techniques, but also because of the decreased functional residual capacity in this state, there is an increased propensity toward hypoxemia. Second, if diffuse arteriovenous shunting is present, the risk of hypoxemia is even greater. This is important to know because both of these factors can influence induction techniques (especially in the patient with a difficult airway) and maintenance of fraction of inspired oxygen concentrations. Finally, because the occurrence of systemic air embolization has been reported during the vascular anastomosis, knowledge of the presence of arteriovenous shunts is even more important.

The gastrointestinal system should be reviewed for the presence of portal hypertension with associated esophageal varices. A history consistent with delayed gastric emptying and any recent gastrointestinal bleeding should also be noted because this may affect induction methods. Although placement of a nasogastric tube and esophageal stethoscope have not been noted to be associated with esophageal hemorrhage in one patient population,[2] care must be taken with their placement.

The existence of clotting abnormalities is to be expected in the patient with liver failure as a result of the impaired synthetic function of the liver. The extent of the recipient's impairment is important to know for two reason. First, during any surgery and in any patient, the presence of a coagulopathy may result in a greater need for blood component therapy. Second, because liver transplantation is associated with transfusion of multiple units of blood, which in itself can result in a coagulopathy, it is useful to know the baseline status. Hence, before embarking on the procedure, a knowledge of the current coagulation status is needed and should include the prothrombin and partial thromboplastin times or thromboelastography measurements and the platelet level. A baseline hemoglobin concentration should also be noted. Finally, as part of the preoperative preparation, there should be communication with the blood bank to ensure an adequate supply of blood products.

The evaluation of the renal system should include a review for the presence of hepatorenal syndrome or inadequate renal preload and serum electrolyte values. Diuretic therapy may be in place to aid in the management of ascites, which is usually present. This may result in mild electrolyte disturbances and mild intravascular depletion. Whereas electrolyte abnormalities infrequently added to any morbidity in the perioperative period in one patient population,[3] the presence of renal insufficiency has been associated with worse mortality rates.[4] Hence, there is a need to ensure adequate intravascular volume in the perioperative period, thus hopefully, optimizing the environment of the kidneys.

Finally, a knowledge of current intracranial pathophysiology should be noted. It is well recognized that diffuse cerebral edema can develop in the final stages of hepatic failure. Knowing that the anesthetic technique can affect the intracranial pressure and that there are hemodynamic events intraoperatively that can affect the cerebral perfusion pressure, consideration might be given to the placement of an intracranial pressure monitoring device preoperatively.[5] If this monitor is not in place in the patient with probable elevated intracranial pressure, then the anesthesiologist should always attempt to respond to hemodynamic events, keeping in mind the concerns for maintaining the cerebral perfusion pressure.

ANESTHETIC MANAGEMENT

Little has been written regarding premedication for the pediatric liver transplant candidate. Because coagulopathies are frequently present, the option of intramuscular administration may be limited. This leaves the anesthesiologist with the choice of no premedication versus premedication by the oral, rectal, or nasal route. Although some may consider the oral route undesirable for a patient who may be at increased risk for aspiration because of a "full stomach," this must be determined at the discretion of the responsible anesthesiologist. If coagulopathy is not an issue, one reported intramuscular premedication regimen is atropine (10 to 20 μg/kg), morphine (0.1 mg/kg), and pentobarbital (3 to 5 mg/kg).[6] On many occasions, the patient will present to the operating room with an intravenous catheter in place, in which case a parenteral premedication, such as midazolam, can be given. In general, the medications and their doses should be chosen based on the desired effect, an estimate of the hepatic reserve of the patient and its effect on drug metabolism pretransplant, and the patient's current neurologic status.

On arrival of the patient in the operating suite, the monitors are applied. These should routinely include placement of ECG leads, a blood pressure cuff, pulse oximetry, and a precordial stethoscope. If patients are considered at risk because of a full stomach, they should be preoxygenated first with application of cricoid pressure during a rapid-sequence induction. Possible induction medications are thiopental (3 to 5 mg/kg) or ketamine (1 to 2 mg/kg) and succinylcholine (1 to 2 mg/kg). Narcotics, such as fentanyl, have also been successfully used as the primary induction agent. However, if this choice is made, the anesthesiologist must tailor the technique to ensure amnesia for the intubation process. If the risk of aspiration is not considered to be an issue, then a routine inhalation induction can be performed, with only a pulse oximeter and precordial stethoscope first placed, followed readily by placement of the monitors noted previously after the patient is induced.

General anesthesia can be maintained by a variety of techniques. Currently, there are no controlled clinical studies to prove conclusively which technique preserves hepatic blood flow and function. The most commonly utilized method is maintenance with isoflurane and an air–oxygen mixture. Halothane is usually avoided to minimize questions regarding its potential toxic effects on the transplanted liver, although it has been successfully used for both induction and maintenance. Nitrous oxide is frequently avoided to minimize the potential bowel distention and potential risk if an air embolism occurred. When nitrous oxide is avoided, concern about patient recall is perhaps an issue, and steps to prevent this must be considered, taking into account the potential for intravenous agent washout with the frequent blood losses. Alternatively, a combined nitrous oxide–narcotic technique can be used with fentanyl (20 to 50 μg/kg). Because these patients routinely return to the intensive care unit while receiving assisted ventilation, the use of high-dose narcotics for maintenance is not contraindicated. If the narcotic is chosen as the primary agent, supplementation with a benzodiazepine is recommended to ensure amnesia. In addition, the dosing of intravenous agents must take into account the washout effect that will occur during massive blood loss and transfusion.

Muscle relaxation is usually maintained with long-acting agents, pancuronium being the most common. The arguments made for pancuronium include its perceived beneficial vagolytic effects in the infant and toddler, the decreased cost because less relaxant is needed overall, and the expected postoperative return to the intensive care unit for mechanical ventilation. Alternatively, some anesthesiologists have chosen to use either atracurium or vecuronium. For those patients in renal failure preoperatively, arguments have been made that atracurium is the better choice because it does not require renal excretion. It is also possibly important to note that the dose requirements for vecuronium and pancuronium have been found to be significantly decreased during the anhepatic phase in one study,[7] another potential argument for the use of atracurium. The requirements did return to normal, however, in the postreperfusion period for these patients. Finally, the use of succinylcholine is not contraindicated. Although liver transplant candidates may have a relative pseudocholinesterase deficiency from inadequate synthetic function of their liver, the prolonged duration of action of atracurium does not appear to be a problem because of the duration of the surgery and the dilutional effect of multiple-unit blood product transfusions. Whatever agent is chosen, as long as appropriate monitoring of neuromuscular blockade is maintained, there should be no clinically significant problems with prolonged blockade.

After anesthesia is induced, the airway is secured, and controlled ventilation is in place, additional monitors should be placed. Recommended monitors are listed in Table 31-3. The placement of 2 to 4 large-bore intravenous catheters should also be given high priority at this time. At least two of the venous lines should be large bore and placed in reliable large vessels, the placement of which may influence the insertion site for the central venous catheter. The placement of other venous catheters should be above the diaphragm to allow for volume administration during the time of venous cross-clamping. The ability to utilize a rapid transfusion system through one of these lines should also be planned ahead of time. Internal or external jugular sites are usually chosen for the central venous catheter, although occasionally, the antecubital site is chosen in the older child. The arterial catheter is typically placed in the radial artery because the aorta is occasionally cross-clamped during the hepatic artery anastomosis. A decision to place a pulmonary artery catheter may be influenced by a history of marginal myocardial reserve, such as in a child who has received chemo-

Table 31-3   Intraoperative Monitoring

Electrocardiography
Pulse oximeter
Blood pressure cuff
Precordial stethoscope
Esophageal stethoscope
Temperature probe (esophageal and rectal)
Urinary catheter
End-tidal CO_2 monitor
Mass spectroscopy
Arterial catheter (radial)
Central venous catheter
Pulmonary artery catheter ($+/-$)
Neuromuscular blockade monitor

---

therapy for a primary hepatic tumor. As a whole, however, a pulmonary artery catheter is of questionable overall benefit intraoperatively in the common pediatric liver transplant candidate.

Additional monitoring with mass spectroscopy is ideal because it allows for monitoring of, not only end-tidal CO_2, but also for nitrogen if air is not being used. It is the practice of some anesthesiologists to administer 100% oxygen before reperfusion of the liver with the intention of increasing oxygen delivery to the previously ischemic donor liver. A further benefit of this practice, however, is that it will also aid in the detection of air embolism if nitrogen is subsequently measured. Mass spectroscopy will also allow determination of the anesthetic gas concentration, which can be useful at the completion of a prolonged anesthetic if there is a desire to attain a patient who will be readily arousable.

There are other generalized care measures that should be considered before initiating the surgery. First, efforts should be made to pad the extremities and any potential pressure points to prevent neuropathies and compromise of perfusion to the skin. Second, because hypothermia to some degree is frequently a problem and can potentiate other problems, every effort should be made to maintain thermoneutrality. This can be accomplished by the addition of any or all of the following: warming blanket, wrapped extremities, head stocking or plastic cap, heated humidified gas system, room temperature to 75° to 80°F, and warming devices for all fluids delivered.

SURGICAL PERIODS

The surgical procedure is, in essence, broken down into three different stages: preanhepatic (or dissection) phase, Stage I; anhepatic phase, Stage II; and postanhepatic (or reperfusion) phase, Stage III. Stage I, the preanhepatic stage, involves entering the abdominal cavity through a wide bilateral subcostal incision with cephalad extension to the xiphoid process, followed by dissection of the liver to its vascular pedicle. Usually, this is a relatively uneventful time period for the average patient. There are two possible exceptions to this, however. One might be the child who has previously undergone a Kasai procedure and has significant adhesions that most likely will result in increased blood loss and duration of the procedure. The other might be the child with severe ascites who might require volume administration when the abdominal cavity is entered.

The anhepatic phase (Stage II) is the time period in which the suprahepatic inferior vena cava, infrahepatic inferior vena cava, portal vein, and the hepatic artery are cross-clamped and the liver is removed. The donor liver is then implanted with revascularization of the suprahepatic inferior vena cava and partial anastomosis of the infrahepatic inferior vena cava. After this, the portal vein is flushed with 200 to 300 mL of lactated Ringer's solution to aid in removing the perfusate, thus minimizing a potential large potassium load and eliminating potential air uptake. Drainage for this solution is through the open portal vein. After the surgeon is satisfied with the flushing of the donor liver, the final anastomosis of the infrahepatic inferior vena cava and portal vein is accomplished.

The final stage, the reperfusion phase (Stage III) is accomplished by a sequence of events. This typically involves releasing, in sequence, the clamps on the portal vein, the infrahepatic inferior vena cava, and the suprahepatic inferior vena cava. The hepatic artery is then anastomosed, and after hemostasis is adequate, the biliary system is reanastomosed or reconstructed. If the extrahepatic biliary system is normal, a primary anastomosis is performed with placement of either a stent or T-tube. If this repair is not possible, then a Roux-en-Y choledochojejunostomy is performed. Finally, the biliary system is evaluated by an intraoperative cholangiogram and, if acceptable, is followed by abdominal closure.

INTRAOPERATIVE CONCERNS

There are a variety of concerns that the anesthesiologist must be aware of during a liver transplant. Some of these have previously been mentioned and might be considered relatively minor. There are others that might be considered more major, however, and they deserve highlighting. These include cardiovascular instability, metabolic derangements, and coagulopathies. However the anesthesiologist is inclined to perceive these issues, they become relatively easy to manage when the practitioner anticipates and mentally prepares for them.

Cardiovascular Instability

The maintenance of intravascular volume and cardiovascular stability in the pediatric patient may be one of the more challenging aspects of these cases. The reasons for and the intraoperative times of this challenge are multiple, hence, underscoring the priority given to good venous access. First, in patients with chronic progressive liver failure, the presence of ascites, with or without hepatorenal syndrome, may be managed by chronic diuretic therapy. These patients frequently may be mildly intravascularly depleted, thereby potentiating the risk of hypotension during induction or on opening of the abdominal cavity. Second, the younger pediatric patient's cardiac output, and hence blood pressure, is more heart rate dependent because of a decreased ventricular compliance compared with that of an adult. In addition, the baroreceptor reflexes in this age group are more sensitive in a dose-dependent manner, making these patients more readily prone to have bradycardia. Hence, if hypotension occurs, the ability to respond by an increase in stroke volume and heart rate is diminished, and the ability to compensate may be compromised.

The most frequent periods of hypotension occur around the times of cross-clamping and unclamping. When the inferior vena cava is cross-clamped, there is an acute decrease in preload to the heart, which can result in hypotension. Some of this decrease in preload may be modulated by the presence of the collateral blood flow that might have developed from existing portal hypertension. Although hypotension occurs less frequently in children than in adults during this period, the anesthesiologists cannot assume this transition to have no hemodynamic effects. Therefore, to minimize a decrease in blood pressure, the central venous pressure should be maintained at a high normal to slightly above normal range before cross-clamping. Despite the presence of collateral flow and a presumably adequate preload, however, some patients may still become relatively hypotensive and require further volume after clamping. Venovenous bypass has been used at this time in adult patients to minimize the usual hypotension. Although the successful use of this technology has been somewhat limited to children weighing over 20 kg, advancements are being made to allow its use in the 10- to 20-kg child. Another therapy to consider for managing hypotension besides volume administration is initiating dopamine at a dose of 3 to 5 μg/kg/min before cross-clamping. This may help minimize or prevent the drop in blood pressure that can occur and has the potential to benefit renal perfusion, which is always somewhat compromised.

At the end of the anhepatic phase, during revascularization, hypotension always occurs to some degree. A brief (5- to 10-min) drop in systolic and diastolic blood pressure measurements up to 30 to 50 mmHg is commonly experienced, despite seemingly adequate volume preloading. A few reasons for this occurrence are as follows. First, when the clamps are removed, the intravascular volume expands to include the donor liver. The exact magnitude of this effect is influenced by the size of the liver and, hence, venous pool, which is transplanted. Second, with the restoration of normal venous return, there is the release of acidotic blood from the lower half of the body, reported to decrease the pH by an average of 0.15.[8] This acidotic load may affect myocardial contractility and, hence, cardiac output. Third, despite diligent efforts to flush the donor liver before completing the reanastomosis, there may be a large potassium load released from the remaining "potassium cardioplegia" after unclamping. This has resulted in life-threatening arrhythmias and cardiac arrest. Management of this may include hyperventilation, administration of sodium bicarbonate, calcium chloride, glucose and insulin, and cardiac compressions. Finally, because of the magnitude of blood products transfused during the average case (approximately 3.5 to 4 blood volumes[6,9]), cardiac dysfunction may occur as a result of decreased serum ionized calcium levels from citrate intoxication. The preferred management of symptomatic hypocalcemia is the administration of 10 to 20 mg/kg of intravenous calcium chloride, the management being guided by the serum ionized calcium levels.

There are other causes of hypotension to be considered that were not mentioned and can occur at any time during the operation. These include: (1) surgical manipulation affecting venous return during the dissection phase; (2) inadequate replacement of volume from blood, evaporative, or third-space losses; (3) hypothermia; (4) preexisting cardiac disease, possibly as a result of previous chemotherapy; and (5) air embolism.

Metabolic Derangements

Metabolic derangements are also to be expected. In addition to those already mentioned, two other conditions commonly are present. Although hypoglycemia has been noted, hyperglycemia is more the norm. The extent of the hyperglycemia appears to be related more to the amount of blood administered than to the amount of glucose-containing crystalloid solutions. Whereas some anesthesiologists are inclined to administer insulin to correct this state, it appears this state persists during the anhepatic stage regardless of management, peaking within 1 h after completion of this phase and spontaneously decreasing thereafter.[6] If the anesthesiologist chooses to administer insulin, the dosing guidelines are 0.05 to 0.1 U/kg by intravenous bolus or 0.05 to 0.1 U/kg/h by continuous infusion.

A second metabolic derangement, which is not necessarily obvious intraoperatively but is important to be aware of, is the development of a metabolic alkalosis. Primarily, the alkalosis is the result of the large citrate load that is usually accumulated from blood product transfusion and is metabolized into buffer. In addition, because of the frequent use of furosemide near the end of the procedure and in the postoperative period, there is an obligatory concomitant loss of chloride ion, which exacerbates the alkalosis. Because of the potential effects of alkalosis on ionized calcium, the oxyhemoglobin dissociation curve, and neuronal hyperexcitability, it is best to try to minimize this. If the anesthesiologist is overly aggressive in correcting the metabolic acidosis that presents after unclamping with sodium bicarbonate, then this state is exacerbated. Hypernatremia may also be created if treatment is too vigorous.

Coagulopathy

Finally, the liver transplant candidate almost always has a coagulopathy. Hence, it is important to recognize when the disorder becomes significant and to know how to manage it. First, because the mean blood loss in at least two studies was approximately 3.5 to 4 blood volumes[6,9] and dilutional thrombocytopenia may be an issue at 1.5 to 2 blood volumes, it is likely that transfusion of platelets will be necessary. After a period of significant blood loss, platelet levels should be checked every 1 to 2 h during the procedure and therapy given as indicated. One guideline for calculating the amount of platelets to transfuse is: 1 U per 6 to 8 kg will result in a 50,000 to 100,000 increase in platelet level. The absence of adequate clotting factors, as a result of the compromised hepatic synthetic function and the dilutional effects, makes it the norm to transfuse fresh-frozen plasma and sometimes cryoprecipitate. Based on preoperative and intraoperative prothrombin and partial thromboplastin times or thromboelastography, decisions can be guided for transfusion therapy. A common practice, or even necessity, may be the administration of 1 mL of fresh-frozen plasma for every milliliter of packed red blood cells transfused to manage the dilutional effects of massive transfusion.

However the anesthesiologist monitors and decides to manage the coagulopathies, the general principle of evaluating the surgical field for oozing to guide decisions should be maintained for two main reasons. First, overly aggressive transfusion (or more appropriately, fluid administration) may potentiate the general tendency for volume overload at the end of the procedure. Prevention of volume overload helps minimize the problem of intraoperative and postoperative pulmonary edema. Second, hepatic artery thrombosis occurs in approximately 10 percent of pediatric patients,[10] and it has been suggested that overtransfusion of clotting factors may be a contributing factor.[11] Because of this, maintenance of prothrombin and partial thromboplastin times to 1.5 to 2 times normal has been proposed in an attempt to minimize this complication.[12]

SUMMARY

The evolution of pediatric liver transplantation has seen much progress since its inception in the 1960s. Not only has the success rate improved, but it is now readily accepted as a standard procedure, having somewhat moved out of the experimental stages. Although anesthesiologists have learned how to monitor these patients better and are more aware of intraoperative issues, undoubtedly there is more to learn. The future will likely see technologic improvements for pediatric patients that might allow for more hemodynamic stability intraoperatively (along the lines of venovenous bypass), an improved understanding and ability to manipulate the coagulation pathways, and controlled studies to help identify anesthetic techniques that result in improved hepatic function postoperatively. It, therefore, will be important for anesthesiologists to be aware of these developments so they may be added to the knowledge that has already been attained.

REFERENCES

1. Whitington PF, Balistreri WF: Liver transplantation in pediatrics: Indications, contraindications, and pretransplant management. *J Pediatr* 1991; 118:169–177.
2. Ritter DM, Rettke SR, Hughes RW Jr, et al: Placement of nasogastric tubes and esophageal stethoscopes in patients with documented esophageal varices. *Anesth Analg* 1988; 67:283–285.
3. Khoury GF, Foster S, Raybould D, et al: Anesthetic management of severely hypokalemic patients for liver transplantation. *Anesthesiology* 1990; 73:337–340.
4. Ellis D, Avner DA, Starzl TE: Renal failure in children with hepatic failure undergoing liver transplantation. *J Pediatr* 1986; 108:393–398.
5. Brajtbord D, Parks RI, Ramsay MA, et al: Management of acute elevation of intracranial pressure during hepatic transplantation. *Anesthesiology* 1989; 70:139–141.
6. Borland LM, Roule M, Cook DR: Anesthesia for pediatric orthotopic liver transplantation. *Anesth Analg* 1985; 64:117–124.

7. O'Kelly B, Jayais P, Veroli P, et al: Dose requirements of ve-curonium, pancuronium, and atracurium during orthotopic liver transplantation. *Anesth Analg* 1991; 73:794–798.

8. Borland LM: Anesthesia for organ transplantation in children. *Int Anesthesiol Clin* 1985; 23:173–199.

9. Lichtor JL, Emond J, Chung MR, et al: Pediatric orthotopic liver transplantation: Multifactorial predictions of blood loss. *Anesthesiology* 1988; 68:607–611.

10. Esquivel CO, Koneru B, Karrer F, et al: Liver transplantation before one year of age. *J Pediatr* 1987; 110:545–548.

11. Massaferro V, Esquivel CO, Makowka L, et al: Hepatic artery thrombosis after pediatric liver transplantation: Medical or sur-gical event? *Transplantation* 1989; 47:971–977.

12. Davis PJ, Cook DR: Anesthetic problems in pediatric liver transplantation. *Transplant Proc* 1989; 21:3493–3496.

BIBLIOGRAPHY

Carlier M, Veyckemans R, Scholtes JL, et al: Anesthesia for pediat-ric hepatic transplantation: Experience of 33 cases. *Transplant Proc* 1987; 19:3333–3337.

Everts EA Jr: Aneshesia for organ transplantation, in Cote CJ, Ryan JF, Todres ID, et al (eds): *A Practice of Anesthesia for Infants and Children*. ed.2 Philadelphia, WB Saunders, 1993, pp 377–400.

Rettke SR, Chantigian RC, Janossy TA, et al: Anesthesia approach to hepatic transplantation. *Mayo Clin Proc* 1989; 64:224–231.

Robertson K, Borland LM: Anesthesia for organ transplantation, in Motoyama EK, Davis PJ (eds): *Smith's Anesthesia for Infants and Children*. ed 5. St. Louis, CV Mosby, 1990, pp 689–722.

Appendix A

Pediatric Syndromes and Their Anesthetic Implications

NAME	DESCRIPTION	ANESTHETIC IMPLICATIONS
Adrenogenital syndrome	Inability to synthesize hydrocortisone and/or aldosterone. Virilization of girls.	All need hydrocortisone even if not salt-losing type. Check electrolytes. Recommended dose of steroids for operation is 1.5 to 3 times their maintenance dose.
Albers-Schönberg disease (marble bone disease or osteopetrosis)	Brittle bones, pathologic fractures.	Anemia from marrow sclerosis. Hepatosplenomegaly. Care in positioning and restraint.
Albright-Butler syndrome	Renal tubular acidosis, hypokalemia, renal calculi.	Correct electrolytes to within normal limits. Renal impairment.
Albright's osteodystrophy (pseudohypoparathyroidism)	Ectopic bone formation, mental retardation.	Hypocalcemia (possible ECG conduction defects), neuromuscular problems, convulsions.
Alport's syndrome	Nephritis and nerve deafness. Renal pathology, variable.	Renal failure in 2nd to 3rd decade. Care with renally excreted drugs. Communication may be a problem because of deafness.
Alström syndrome	Obesity, blindness, hearing loss, diabetes after puberty, glomerulosclerosis.	Renal impairment. Management of diabetes and obesity (delayed gastric emptying). Care should be taken with renally excreted drugs.
Amyotonia congenita (infantile atrophy)	Anterior horn cell degeneration	Sensitive to thiopental (reduced muscle mass) and respiratory depressants. Care with neuromuscular blocking agents. Use narcotics with care.

Amyotrophic lateral sclerosis	Degeneration of motor neurons	Avoid succinylcholine. Possible K^+ release and cardiac arrest. Minimal thiopental and curare. Avoid respiratory depressants.
Analbuminemia	Almost absent albumin (4 to 100 mg/dL).	Very sensitive to protein-bound drugs including thiopental and warfarin-type anticoagulants.
Andersen's disease (glycogen storage disease IV)	Debrancher enzyme deficiency.	Possibility of hypoglycemia under anesthesia. Coagulopathy possible due to early hepatic cirrhosis.
Apert syndrome (acrocephalosyndactyly)	Craniosynostosis.	Difficult intubation. Possibly raised intracranial pressure. Associated congenital heart disease.
Arthrogryposis multiplex	Multiple congenital contractures.	Ten percent have congenital heart disease. Minimal thiopental required. Muscles replaced by fat. Possible airway problem with mandible. May have associated CNS malformations and seizures. Very sensitive to respiratory depressants.
Asplenia syndrome	Absent spleen, midline liver (situs ambiguous).	Very complex cardiovascular anomalies. Present with cyanosis and heart failure.
Ataxia-telangiectasia	Cerebellar ataxia, skin and conjunctival telangiectasia, decreased serum IgA and IgE. Ten percent develop reticuloendothelial malignancy.	Defective immunity (recurrent chest and sinus infections). Bronchiectasis. Because of high probability of chronic lung disease, CXR, ABG, and possibly PFT will help in preoperative evaluation.

(Continued)

NAME	DESCRIPTION	ANESTHETIC IMPLICATIONS
Beckwith-Wiedemann syndrome (infantile gigantism)	Birth weight > 4000 g, macroglossia, and exomphalos.	Persistent severe neonatal hypoglcemia. Airway problems. May have associated omphalocele. Increased incidence of Wilms' tumor, adrenal cysts, and nesidioblastosis (hyperplasia of insulin-producing cells of pancreas) follow glucose intraoperatively. May require cardiac evaluation for associated cardiomyopathy.
Blackfan-Diamond anemia syndrome	Congenital idiopathic red cell aplasia	Liver and spleen enlarged. Hypersplenism. Thrombocytopenia. Steroid therapy required.
Bowen syndrome (cerebrohepatorenal syndrome)	Hepatomegaly and neonatal jaundice, polycystic kidneys, associated congenital heart disease, muscular hypotonia.	Hypoprothrombinemia. Care with renally excreted drugs and muscle relaxants. Check liver function and evaluate for associated cardiac disease.
Carpenter's syndrome	Cranial synostosis, associated congenital heart disease (CHD).	Hypoplastic mandible. Possibly difficult intubation. May have increased intracranial pressure. Evaluate for associated CHD.
Central core disease	Muscular dystrophy.	See amyotonia congenita.
Chédiak-Higashi syndrome	Partial albinism, immunodeficiency, hepatosplenomegaly.	Steroid therapy. Use sterile technique. Recurrent chest infection. Thrombocytopenia may require platelets.
Cherubism	Tumorous lesion of mandibles and maxillae with intraoral masses. May cause respiratory distress.	Intubation may be extremely difficult. May require tracheostomy for acute respiratory distress. Profuse bleeding at surgery.

Chotzen's syndrome	Craniosynostosis, possible renal anomalies.	May be difficult intubation. Associated renal anomalies and possible impaired renal excretion of drugs. Blood loss may be considerable because of vascularity of skull and scalp.
Christ-Siemens-Touraine syndrome (anhidrotic ectodermal dysplasia)	Hypotrichosis (absent hair), absent sweating, heat intolerance, sex-linked with full expression only in males.	Cannot control temperature by sweating. Persistent upper respiratory and chest infection because of poor mucus formation. May have underdeveloped maxilla and mandible, which may make ventilation with bag and mask or intubation difficult. Lacrimal production is decreased; therefore, eyes should be lubricated and taped closed.
Chronic granulomatous disease	Inherited disorder of leukocyte function, recurrent infection with nonpathogenic organisms.	Hepatomegaly in 95 percent. Poor pulmonary function. Avoid infection—use strict aseptic technique.
Collagen diseases: dermatomyositis, rheumatoid arthritis, systemic lupus erythematosus, polyarteritis nodosa	Systemic connective diseases frequently treated with steroids, osteoporosis and fatty infiltration of muscle, variable systemic involvement.	Often have pulmonary infiltration or fibrosis. May have temporomandibular or cricoarytenoid arthritis, causing airway and intubation difficulties. Anemia common. Risk of fat embolism after osteotomy, fracture, or minor trauma. May have renal involvement and cardiomyopathy. Check electrolytes, renal function, and in selected cases, ECG, CXR. May need more detailed cardiac workup.

(Continued)

549

NAME	DESCRIPTION	ANESTHETIC IMPLICATIONS
Conradi's syndrome	Chondrodystrophy with contractures, saddle nose, mental retardation, associated congenital heart disease and renal anomalies.	Problems are those of associated renal and cardiac disease.
Cretinism (congenital hypothyroidism, large tongue	Absent thyroid tissue or defective synthesis of thyroxine and goiter. If untreated, infants suffer neurologic sequelae.	Airway problems (large tongue and goiter). Respiratory center very sensitive to depression. CO_2 retention common. Hypoglycemia, hyponatremia, hypotension. Adrenal insufficiency with an impaired ACTH response to stress. Low cardiac output. Transfusion poorly tolerated. Hypothyroidism should be corrected before a planned surgical procedure because sudden cardiac death may occur and the patients are difficult to resuscitate. Thyroxine and thyroid-stimulating hormone will be normal in adequately treated patients.
Cri du chat syndrome	Chromosome 5p abnormal, abnormal cry, microcephaly, micrognathia, congenital heart disease.	Airway problems (stridor and laryngomalacia). Possibly difficult intubation. Evaluate cardiovascular system completely.
Crouzon's disease	Craniosynostosis.	Possibly difficult intubation. Severe blood loss with cranial operation and possibly increased intracranial pressure.

Cutis laxa	Elastic fiber degeneration, pendulous skin, frequent hernias, emphysema, cor pulmonale, arterial fragility.	Pulmonary infection, emphysema, and cor pulmonale. Poor tissues; IV difficult to maintain. Excess of soft tissues around larynx may lead to respiratory obstruction.
DiGeorge syndrome (3rd and 4th brachial arch syndrome)	Absent thymus and parathyroids, immune deficiency, susceptibility to fungal and viral infections, hypocalcemia.	Recurrent chest infections. Hypoparathyroidism. Low Ca^{++} and tetany. Stridor. Aortic arch abnormalities and congenital heart disease. Evaluate cardiac anomaly. Donor blood must be irradiated with 3000 rad to prevent graft-versus-host reaction.
Down's syndrome (monogolism)	Microcephaly, small nasopharynx, hypotonia. Sixty percent have congenital heart disease. Duodenal atresia in some. Cervical spinal abnormalities.	Difficult airway (large tongue and small mouth). Risk of laryngeal spasm, especially on extubation. Problems related to specific cardiac anomalies. Evaluate for atlantooccipital dislocation with flexion–extension views of cervical spine.
Duchenne type muscular dystrophy	Muscular dystrophy with frequent cardiac muscle involvement, usually die in 2nd decade.	As for amyotonia congenita plus cardiac involvement. Minimal drug doses. Avoid respiratory depressants, muscle relaxants. Postoperative IPPV may be required. Increased risk for development of malignant hyperthermia.
Edwards's syndrome (trisomy 18(E))	Congenital heart disease in 95 percent, micrognathia in 80 percent, renal malformations 50 to 80 percent. Usually die in infancy.	Possible difficult intubation. Care with renally excreted drugs. Evaluate for cardiac disease.

(Continued)

NAME	DESCRIPTION	ANESTHETIC IMPLICATIONS
Ehlers-Danlos syndrome	Collagen abnormality with hyperelasticity and fragile tissues, dissecting aneurysm of aorta, fragility of other blood vessels, bleeding diathesis possible.	Cardiovascular system, spontaneous rupture of vessels. Angiogram carries one percent mortality rate because of bleeding from aneurysm of femoral artery puncture site. ECG conduction abnormalities. IV difficult to maintain (hematoma). Poor tissues and clotting defect lead to hemorrhage, especially GI tract. Spontaneous pneumothorax is common.
Ellis-van Creveld syndrome (chondroectodermal dysplasia)	Ectodermal defects, skeletal anomalies. Fifty percent have congenital heart disease, usually septal.	Chest wall anomalies lead to poor lung function. May have abnormal maxilla and upper lip, making airway management difficult. Evaluate cardiopulmonary system preoperatively for associated anomalies. Hepatosplenomegaly.
Epidermolysis bullosa	Erosions and blisters from minor skin trauma.	Airway (oral lesions and adhesions of tongue). Ketamine is recommended or use small oral tube to avoid laryngeal trauma. Avoid skin trauma from tapes. History of steroid therapy. Check for porphyria (similar skin lesions).
Fabry's disease (angiokeratoma corporis diffusum universal)	Lipid storage disease with deposits of glycolipids in blood vessels of mucous membranes, eyes, heart, kidneys, liver, and nervous system.	Cardiovascular system, hypertension, myocardial ischemia, mitral insufficiency (before 2nd or 3rd decade). Renal failure (care with renally excreted drugs). May have limited mouth opening because of TMJ involvement. Neurologic complications include seizures, mental retardation, and cerebrovascular accidents.

Familial periodic paralysis	Periodic muscle weakness (hyperkalemic or hypokalemic types), attacks of quadriplegia.	Monitor serum K^+. Limit use of dextrose because weakness may be exacerbated by carbohydrate loading. Spironolactone or acetazolamide may be given to maintain serum K^+. Monitor ECG. Avoid relaxants.
Fanconi's syndrome (renal tubular acidosis)	Usually secondary to other disease, proximal tubular defect, acidosis, K^+ loss, dehydration.	Impaired renal function. Treat electrolyte and acid-base abnormalities. Look for primary disease (e.g., galactosemia or cystinosis).
Farber disease (lipogranulomatosis)	Sphingomyelin deposition, widespread visceral lipogranulomas, especially in the CNS.	Granuloma formation on epiglottis and in larynx (careful intubation with an endotracheal tube that is a size smaller than predicted to avoid laryngeal trauma). Macroglossia may cause airway compromise. Generalized systemic involvement leading to cardiac and renal failure.
Favism	Glucose-6-phosphate dehydrogenase deficiency, hemolytic anemia (transfuse if necessary).	Hemolysis after oxidant drugs, (e.g., aspirin, methylene blue, and sulfonamides). Anemia.
Friedreich's ataxia	Degeneration of cerebellum, lateral and posterior column of spinal cord, scoliosis, myocardial degeneration and fibrosis.	Heart failure and arrhythmias. Care with cardiac depressant drugs. Positioning under anesthesia may be a problem because of scoliosis.
Gardner's syndrome	Multiple polyposis, bony tumors, sebaceous cysts, fibromas.	No anesthetic problems described.

(Continued)

553

NAME	DESCRIPTION	ANESTHETIC IMPLICATIONS
Gaucher's disease	Cerebroside accumulation in CNS, liver, and spleen. Classic triad of trismus, strabismus, and opisthotonos.	May be difficult to intubate because of neuromuscular rigidity and trismus. Pulmonary disease from aspiration (pseudobulbar palsy). Hepatosplenomegaly, hypersplenism may cause platelet deficiency. Aseptic necrosis of femoral head and vertebral fractures are common.
Glanzmann's disease (thrombasthenia)	Platelet adenosine diphosphate (ADP) reduced, abnormal function.	No specific therapy for bleeding. Platelet transfusion disappointing. History of steroids.
Goldenhar's syndrome (oculoauriculovertebral syndrome)	Unilateral facial hypoplasia, congenital heart disease in 20 to 60 percent, mandibular hypoplasia.	Difficult airway and intubation. Problems of associated cardiac disease.
Gorlin-Goltz syndrome (focal dermal hypoplasia)	Hernia, prolapse, congenital heart disease, renal anomalies.	Asymmetry of head (difficult airway). Evaluate for cardiac and renal anomalies.
Gorlin's syndrome	Basal cell nevi, skeletal anomalies.	No anesthetic problem described.
Grönblad-Strandberg syndrome (pseudoxanthoma elasticum)	Degeneration of elastic tissue in skin, eye, and cardiovascular system.	Rupture of arteries, especially in GI tract, hypertension, arterial calcification. Occlusion of cerebral and coronary arteries. Difficult maintenance of IV cannula.

Guillain-Barré syndrome (acute [idiopathic] polyneuritis)	Acute polyneuropathy, progressive ascending peripheral neuritis, often involving cranial nerves. Hypotension may occur. Autonomic dysfunction with bulbar palsy with hypoventilation.	Avoid succinylcholine because of K$^+$ release. May require tracheostomy, IPPV, and support of blood pressure.
Hand-Schüller-Christian syndrome (histiocytosis X)	Histiocytic granulomata in bones, viscera, larynx, lungs, liver, and spleen.	Laryngeal fibrosis. Pulmonary, diffuse or hilar infiltration. Respiratory failure. Cor pulmonale. Hypersplenism and pancytopenia. Liver involvement. Diabetes insipidus if sella tucica involved. History of steroids.
Hermansky-Pudlak syndrome	Albinism, bleeding diathesis caused by morphologic, chemical, and functional defects in platelets.	Restrictive lung disease, ulcerative colitis, and renal dysfunction. Platelet abnormality. No specific treatment. Consultation with hematologist may be needed to evaluate most effective blood product therapy.
Holt-Oram syndrome	Upper limb abnormalities, congenital heart disease (normally ASD, possibly sudden death from pulmonary embolus, coronary occlusion.	Problems of cardiac defect. May have rhythm disturbance of both atrial or ventricular origin or conduction abnormalities. No other anesthetic problem.

(Continued)

555

NAME	DESCRIPTION	ANESTHETIC IMPLICATIONS
Homocystinuria	Inborn error of metabolism, thromboembolic phenomena from intimal thickening, ectopia lentis, osteoporosis, kyphoscoliosis.	Dextran 40 to reduce viscosity and platelet adhesiveness and increase peripheral perfusion. Angiography may precipitate thrombosis, especially cerebral.
Hunter's syndrome (mucopolysaccharidosis II)	Stiff joints, dwarfing, hepatosplenomegaly, pectus excavatum, kyphoscoliosis, valvular and coronary heart disease.	Upper airway obstruction caused by infiltration of lymphoid tissue in pharynx, tongue, and larynx. Pneumonias. Possible hypersplenism. Cardiac failure.
Hurler syndrome (mucopolysaccharidosis I)	Pulmonary hypertension. Usually die before 10 years of age from respiratory and cardiac failure.	Similar to Hunter syndrome but more severe. Frequent upper respiratory infection. Abnormal tracheobronchial cartilages. Severe coronary artery disease at early age. Valvular and myocardial involvement.
Jervell and Lange-Nielsen syndrome (cardioauditory syndrome)	Cardiac conduction defects, deafness.	Syncope, arrhythmias. ECG has large T waves, prolonged QT. May need digoxin, propranolol, or pacemaker.
Kartagener's syndrome (immotile cilia syndrome)	Dextrocardia, sinusitis, bronchiectasis, abnormal immunity because of polymorpholeukocyte motility problem, asplenia syndrome.	Chronic respiratory infection. Bronchospasm. Optimize pulmonary function before surgery (physiotherapy, bronchodilators, and possibly antibiotics). With otitis media, nitrous oxide is contraindicated. Asepsis during IV insertion and intubation.

Kasabach-Merritt syndrome	Hemangioma and thrombocytopenia. Average age at death, 5 weeks.	Hemangioma suddenly increases in size with associated severe thrombocytopenia and hemorrhage. Replace blood loss; transfuse platelets. Splenectomy. Steroids.
Klinefelter's syndrome (gonosomal aneuploidy)	Tall stature, reduced intelligence, vertebral collapse from osteoporosis.	No described anesthetic problem. Care in positioning. Evaluate for vertebral osteoporosis.
Klippel-Feil syndrome	Congenital fusion of two or more cervical vertebrae, leading to neck rigidity.	Difficult airway and intubation.
Klippel-Trenaunay syndrome (angioosteohypertrophy)	Usually unilateral, arteriovenous fistulae, thrombocytopenia.	Arteriovenous fistulae and anemia lead to high cardiac output state. Thrombocytopenia in visceral hemangiomas. Evaluate cardiac function and optimize failure symptoms before surgery.
Larsen's syndrome	Multiple congenital dislocations, connective tissue defect, poor cartilage in rib cage, epiglottis, arytenoids. May have hydrocephalus.	Possible difficult intubation. Chronic respiratory problems. Evaluate for evidence of increased ICP.
Laurence-Moon-Biedl syndrome	Obesity, retinitis pigmentosa, polydactyly, mental retardation.	May be associated with cardiac defects. Renal disease and, occasionally, diabetes insipidus.
Leopard syndrome	Multiple large freckles, congenital heart disease, ECG anomalies (aberrant conduction).	Ninety-five percent have pulmonary stenosis. Evaluate cardiac anomaly. ECG and CXR, minimally. Intubation may be difficult.

(Continued)

557

NAME	DESCRIPTION	ANESTHETIC IMPLICATIONS
Leprechaunism	Failure to thrive, endocrine disorders, severe mental retardation.	Hypoglycemia caused by hyperinsulinism from hyperplastic islets of Langerhans. Renal tubular defects impair renal function.
Lesch-Nyhan syndrome	Hyperuricemia and mental retardation. Renal failure by age 10 years.	High serum uric acid leads to red cell damage and renal stones. Care with renally excreted drugs. Delayed gastric emptying, so at risk for aspiration.
Letterer-Siwe disease (histiocytosis X)	Histiocytic granulomas in viscera and bones, clinical course similar to acute leukemia, gingival necrosis, loss of teeth.	Pancytopenia with anemia and thrombocytopenic purpura hemorrhage. Pulmonary infiltration. Hepatic involvement. Gingival inflammation and necrosis, loss of teeth. May have history of steroids.
Lipodystrophy (total lipoatrophy)	Generalized loss of all body fat, fatty fibrotic liver, portal hypertension, splenomegaly, nephropathy, diabetes.	Liver failure (avoid halothane and drugs metabolized by liver). Check clotting factors. Hypersplenism (anemia and thrombocytopenia). Possible renal failure. Usual diabetic precautions.
Lowe syndrome (oculocerebrorenal syndrome)	Boys only. Cataract, glaucoma, mental retardation, hypotonia, renal acidosis, proteinuria, osteoporosis, and rickets.	Check electrolyte and acid–base balance. Check serum Ca^{++} (treated with vitamin D and Ca^{++}). Care with renally excreted drugs. May be difficult to communicate with patient because of mental retardation.
Maffucci's syndrome	Enchondromatosis and hemangiomas with malignant change.	Pathologic fractures. GI bleeding from hemangiomas. Orthostatic hypotension. May be sensitive to vasodilator drugs.

Maple syrup urine disease (branched-chain ketonuria)	Amino acid disturbance treated by diet only, severe neurologic damage, respiratory disturbances.	General supportive measures. May have gastroesophageal reflux. Evaluate for aspiration pneumonitis and other pulmonary problems. Check glucose perioperatively and when placed NPO, start glucose infusion at least 10–15 mg/kg/min.
Marfan syndrome (arachnodactyly)	Connective tissue disorder, dilatation of aortic root leads to AI, aortic, thoracic, or abdominal aneurysm, pulmonary artery and mitral valve involvement, kyphoscoliosis, pectus excavatum, lung cysts, joint instability and dislocation.	Care with myocardial depressant drugs. Complete evaluation of cardiovascular system because aneurysms may be asymptomatic. Beware possible dissection of aorta. Lung function poor. Possible pneumothorax. Care in positioning because of easily dislocated joints.
Maroteaux-Lamy syndrome (mucopolysaccharidosis IV)	Myocardial involvement, kyphoscoliosis, chest infection, hepatosplenomegaly.	Heart failure by age 20 years. Care with cardiac depressant drugs. Chronic respiratory infection with poor lung reserve. Hypersplenism, anemia, thrombocytopenia.
McArdle disease	Glycogen storage disease V.	Muscles affected including cardiac muscle. Care with cardiac depressant drugs and evaluate and optimize cardiac function preoperatively.
Meckel's syndrome	Microcephaly, micrognathia, cleft epiglottis, congenital heart disease, renal dysplasia.	Intubation may be difficult. Cardiac problems and renal failure may be present in infancy. Care with renally excreted drugs. Evaluate and optimize cardiac performance.

(Continued)

559

NAME	DESCRIPTION	ANESTHETIC IMPLICATIONS
Median cleft face syndrome	Varying degrees of cleft face, frontal lipomas, dermoids.	Cleft nose, lip, and palate pose intubation difficulties.
Möbius syndrome (congenital facial diplegia)	Associated limb malformations, micrognathia. Congenital paralysis of CN VI and VII.	Feeding difficulties and aspiration may cause chronic pulmonary problems. May be difficult to intubate. Very sensitive to respiratory depressant drugs.
Morquio-Ullrich syndrome (mucopolysaccharidosis IV)	Severe dwarfing, aortic incompetence, thoracic deformities, unstable atlantoaxial joint.	Cardiorespiratory symptoms by 2nd decade because of severe kyphoscoliosis with poor lung function. All develop spinal cord damage from atlantooccipital subluxation. Upper airway obstruction during head flexion may occur as a result of tracheal collapse.
Moschcowitz disease (thrombotic thrombocytopenic purpura)	Hemolytic anemia and thrombocytopenia, small vessel disease, neurologic damage, renal disease, treatment with splenectomy and steroids.	History of steroid therapy. Care with renally excreted drugs if kidney affected. Check hematocrit.
Myasthenia congenita	Like adult myasthenia gravis.	Avoid respiratory depressants, muscle relaxants. May require postoperative IPPV. Problems of anticholinesterase therapy pre- and postoperatively. Possibility of cholinergic crisis.

Myositis ossificans (fibrodysplasia ossificans)	Bony infiltration of tendons, fascia, aponeuroses, and muscle.	Airway and intubation problems if neck rigid. Thoracic involvement leads to aspiration and asphyxia, lung pathology, and grossly reduced thoracic compliance.
Myotonia congenita (Thomsen disease)	Decreased ability to relax muscles after contraction, diffuse hypertrophy of muscle.	Avoid relaxants and depressants as in myotonic dystrophy, although this a more benign disease that is nonprogressive.
Myotonic dystrophy (myotonia dystrophica)	Weakness and myotonia, ptosis, cataracts, partial baldness, gonadal atrophy, cardiac conduction defects and arrhythmias, impaired ventilation.	Avoid succinylcholine, which causes myotonia in 50 percent. Nondepolarizing drugs do not relax myotonia. Neostigmine induces myotonia. Monitor ECG. Extremely sensitive to respiratory depressants. Use regional or inhalational agents. IPPV postoperatively if necessary. Halothane may cause postoperative shivering and myotonia. Pulmonary complications because of poor cough.
Neonatal hypoglycemia (idiopathic)	Symptomatic hypoglycemia in infancy (convulsions, lethargy, and mental retardation if untreated), no ketosis. Therapy is subtotal pancreatectomy.	Extreme care in monitoring blood glucose. Steroids, diazoxide, and glucagon as required. After pancreatectomy may need insulin and glucose to maintain blood sugar in normal limits.
Niemann-Pick disease	Sphingomyelin and cholesterol accumulation in CNS, marrow, liver, and spleen, diffuse infiltration of lungs, epilepsy, ataxia, mental retardation.	Anemia and thrombocytopenia because of marrow and spleen involvement. Pulmonary insufficiency and pneumonia.

(Continued)

NAME	DESCRIPTION	ANESTHETIC IMPLICATIONS
Noack's syndrome	Craniosynostosis, digital anomalies, obesity.	May be difficult to intubate because of skull deformity. Obese patients may have upper airway obstruction and delayed gastric emptying.
Noonan's syndrome (male Turner's syndrome)	Short stature, mental retardation, congenital heart disease, micrognathia, hydronephrosis or hypoplasia of kidneys.	Usually pulmonary stenosis or PDA, tetralogy of Fallot, ASD. Evaluation of cardiovascular system preoperatively and specific heart lesions may deter anesthetic management. Care with renally excreted drugs if kidneys affected.
Ollier's disease (enchondromatosis)	Multiple chondromas within bones, usually unilateral, pathologic fractures.	With cavernous hemangioma is described as Maffucci syndrome. Care with positioning.
Orofacio digital syndrome	Cleft lip and palate, lobed tongue, hypoplasia of mandible and maxilla, digital anomalies, hydrocephalus, polycystic kidneys.	Difficult airway and intubation. Possible renal failure (care with renally excreted drugs).
Osteogenesis imperfecta (fragilitas ossium)	I. Congenita (stillborn or rapidly fatal). II. Tarda (pathologic fractures, osteoporosis leads to kyphoscoliosis).	Chest deformity leads to lung pathology. Fragile vessels lead to subcutaneous hemorrhage. Carious and easily broken teeth. Extreme care in positioning.
Paramyotonia congenita (Eulenburg's disease)	Myotonia on exposure to cold, paroxysmal weakness, serum K^+ may be high or low level.	Anesthesia as in myotonic dystrophy. Also care with K^+ level.

Patau's syndrome (trisomy 13)	Mental retardation in 100 percent of patients, microcephaly, micrognathia, and/or dextrocardia CHD (usually VSD), cleft lip or palate, congenital heart disease. Usually fatal by 3 years of age.	Difficult intubation. Cardiac defect is usually VSD.
Pendred's syndrome	Deafness and goiter, incomplete block of thyroxine production.	May be euthyroid or hypothyroid. Make sure euthyroid preoperatively. Otherwise as for cretinism.
Phenylketonuria (PKU)	Phenylalanine hydroxylase deficiency, vomiting, irritability, mental retardation. hypertonia, convulsions, very sensitive to narcotics and other CNS depressants.	Inhalation induction and maintenance. Continue antiepileptic drugs. Tendency to hypoglycemia. Dextrose infusion and close monitoring of blood sugars intraoperatively are necessary.
Pierre Robin syndrome	Cleft palate, micrognathia, glossoptosis, associated congenital heart disease.	Newborn may asphyxiate (nurse prone in a slightly head down position to cause tongue to fall forward out of the airway). May require tongue suture, intubation, or tracheostomy. May be very difficult to intubate. Awake intubation often preferred.
Polycystic kidneys	One third have associated cysts in liver, pancreas, spleen, lungs, bladder, thyroid, cerebral aneurysm in 15 percent.	Care with renally excreted drugs. Beware of lung cysts (may lead to pneumothorax). Avoid hypertension because of possible cerebral aneurysm.

(Continued)

563

NAME	DESCRIPTION	ANESTHETIC IMPLICATIONS
Polycystic liver	Familial. Sixty percent have polycystic kidneys, lung, and pancreas.	Usually liver function not impaired until late (fibrosis, splenomegaly, and esophageal varices). Beware possible renal failure, lung cysts.
Polysplenia	Bilateral visceral left sidedness (see also asplenia).	Complex cardiac anomalies common (ASD and endocardial cushion defects). Usually not as complex as in asplenia.
Pompe's disease (glycogen storage II)	Muscle deposits, severe hypotonicity, massive cardiomegaly. Death before 2 years of age.	Extreme care. Avoidance of respiratory depressants, muscle relaxants, cardiac depressants. Large tongue may cause airway problem.
Porphyria	Paralysis, psychiatric disorder, autonomic imbalance, hypertension, tachycardia, abdominal pain precipitated by drugs and infections.	Avoid barbiturates (including thiopental), sedatives (meprobamate, chlordiazepoxide, glutethimide, carbromal, hydantoin derivatives, sulfonamides, antipyretics, hypoglycemia agents). Have been used safely: chlorpromazine, promazine, promethazine, chloral hydrate, morphine, procaine, N_2O, succinylcholine, tubocurarine, gallamine, atropine, neostigmine, atracurium.
Prader-Willi syndrome	In neonates, hypotonia, poor feeding, absent reflexes. Second phase, hyperactive, uncontrollable polyphagia, mental retardation.	Obesity of extreme proportions leading to cardiopulmonary failure. May be difficult intubation.

Progeria (Hutchinson-Gilford syndrome)	Premature aging starts at 6 months to 3 years. Cardiac disease includes ischemia, hypertension, cardiomegaly.	Anesthesia as for adults with myocardial ischemia.
Prune-belly syndrome	Agenesis of abdominal musculature with renal anomalies.	Poor cough, respiratory infections. Respiration requires use of muscles. Treat as full stomach. Intubate and assist or control ventilation. Avoid muscle relaxants. Beware possible renal failure.
Pyle's disease (metaphyseal dysplasia)	Craniofacial abnormalities, enlarged mandible, cranial nerve paralyses.	No decribed anesthetic problem. Carefully assess airway.
Rendu-Osler-Weber syndrome (hemorrhagic telangiectasia)	No coagulation abnormalities, but multiple capillary and venous hemangiomas, pulmonary and hepatic arteriovenous fistulae common.	Blood loss may be impossible to control. IV may be difficult to maintain because of poor tissues. More than 90 percent have recurrent chest infection, dyspnea, cyanosis, clubbing by age 60 years.
Rieger's syndrome	Myotonic dystrophy and other myopathies, maxilla, abnormal teeth, mental retardation, occasional imperforate anus, glaucoma.	Anesthetic requirements dictated by associated muscle disease (see amyotonia congenita, myontonic dystrophy). May be receiving β-blocker eye drops for glaucoma.

(Continued)

565

NAME	DESCRIPTION	ANESTHETIC IMPLICATIONS
Riley-Day syndrome (familial dysautonomia)	Deficiency of dopamine hydroxylase, hyper- and hypotensive attacks, absent lacrimation, abnormal sweating, poor suckling and swallowing.	Emotional liability. Recurrent aspiration, pneumonia, and chronic lung disease. Labile blood pressure (care with halothane and cardiodepressant drugs). Hypovolemia is not well tolerated. Insensitivity to pain may reduce anesthetic requirements, yet absence of cardiovascular signs makes assessment of anesthetic depth difficult. Hypersensitivity to adrenergic and cholinergic drugs. Premedication (atropine, diazepam, and H_2-blocker). Respiratory center insensitive to CO_2, may need IPPV. Avoid respiratory depressants.
Rubinstein's syndrome	Mental retardation, microcephaly, frequent chest infections, swallowing abnormality, congenital heart disease.	Repeated aspiration leads to pneumonia and chronic lung disease. Assess cardiovascular system for congenital defects.
Sanfilippo's syndrome (mucopolysaccharidosis type III)	CNS malfunction in childhood progresses to mental retardation and dementia, no hepatosplenomegaly or cardiac problems.	No anesthetic problems described. Emotional disturbance, agitation, and dementia.
Scheie's syndrome (mucopolysaccharidosis type I)	Corneal clouding, glaucoma, hernias, joint stiffness (especially hands and feet), aortic valve involvement, sleep apnea.	May be difficult intubation because of large tongue. Aortic incompetence by third decade. Joint stiffness (care in positioning). CXR to assess cardiac size and pulmonary disease and ECG. IV access may be difficult because of contractures and thick skin.

Scleroderma	Diffuse cutaneous stiffening. Plastic surgery required for contractures.	Diffuse cutaneous stiffening. Plastic surgery required for contractures. Scarring face and mouth (difficult airway and intubation). Chest restriction, decreased compliance. Diffuse pulmonary fibrosis, hypoxia. Veins often invisible and impalpable. Cardiac fibrosis or cor pulmonale. History of steroid therapy.
Sebaceous nevus (linear)	Linear nevii from forehead to nose, hydrocephalus, mental retardation, associated with coarctation and hypoplasia of aorta.	Cardiovascular complications.
Shy-Drager syndrome	Orthostatic hypotension, diffuse degeneration of CNS and autonomic nervous system, decreased sweating, hypersensitive to angiotensin and epinephrine.	Labile pulse and blood pressure, possibly as a result of defective baroreceptor response. Cautious use of halothane and isoflurane. Treat hypotension with infusion of phenylephrine.
Silver's syndrome (Russell-Silver dwarf)	Short stature, skeletal asymmetry, micrognathia, abnormal sexual development.	Possibly difficult intubation.
Sipple's syndrome (multiple endocrine adenomatosis type II)	Pheochromocytoma and medullary thyroid carcinoma, parathyroid adenoma, CNS tumors, schwannoma of mediastinum associated with Cushing's disease.	Management of pheochromocytoma (75 percent bilateral). Problems of multiple endocrine disorders. Beware of possibility of mediastinal mass, which may compromise ventilation after patient anesthetized.

(Continued)

567

NAME	DESCRIPTION	ANESTHETIC IMPLICATIONS
Smith-Lemli-Opitz syndrome	Mental retardation, genital and skeletal anomalies, micrognathia, thymic hypoplasia.	Airway and intubation problems. Pneumonia possible. Increased susceptibility to infection.
Sotos' syndrome (cerebral gigantism)	Acromegalic features, dilated ventricles but normal intracranial pressure.	All features nonprogressive. Possible airway problems because of acromegalic skull. No other described problems.
Stevens-Johnson syndrome	Erythema multiforme, urticarial lesions, erosions of mouth, eyes, genitalia, possible hypersensitivity to exogenous agents (e.g., drugs and infections).	Oral lesions (avoid intubation and esophageal stethoscope). Monitoring difficult because of skin lesions but essential. ECG (fibrillation, myocarditis, and pericarditis occur). Temperature control for febrile episodes. Intravenous infusion essential but avoid cut down because of infection. Ketamine anesthetic. Pleural blebs and pneumothorax may occur.
Sturge-Weber syndrome	Cavernous angioma over one to three divisions of cranial nerve V, intracranial calcification, convulsions, may have progressive neurologic deficit.	No specific anesthetic problems. Be aware that angiomas may also be present in brain. Forty to fifty percent have congenital glaucoma.
Supravalvular aortic stenosis syndrome (idiopathic infantile hypercalcemia or Williams syndrome)	Hypercalcemia and mental retardation, abnormal facies, cardiac angina, therapy with low-calcium diet and steroids, cardiac surgery.	Fixed cardiac output and ischemia. History of steroids. Monitor serum Ca^{++}.

Tangier disease (α-lipoprotein deficiency)	Elevated cholesterol ester and triglicerides, orange tonsils and rectal mucosa, splenomegaly, 50 percent neurologic abnormality, premature coronary disease.	Anemia and thrombocytopenia because of hypersplenism. Abnormal EMG (care with muscle relaxants). Beware premature ischemic heart disease.
Tay-Sachs disease	Gangliosidosis, blindness, progressive dementia, degeneration of CNS.	No described anesthetic hazard. Progressive neurologic loss leads to respiratory complications. Supportive measures as only treatment.
Thomsen's disease	See myotonia congenita.	
Thrombocytopenia with absent radius	Episodic thrombocytopenia precipitated by stress, infection, surgery. Low platelets improve to normal by adulthood. Congenital heart disease in 30 percent.	Platelet transfusion for surgery or bleeding (35 to 40 percent die in first year of intracranial hemorrhage). Avoid elective surgery in first year.
Treacher Collins syndrome (mandibulofacial dysostosis)	Micrognathia, dysplastic zygomatic arches, microstomia, choanal atresia, congenital heart disease, deafness.	Often associated with airway and intubation difficulties. Less severe than Pierre Robin deformity.
Tuberous sclerosis	Adenoma sebaceum of skin, epilepsy, and mental retardation. Intracranial and lung calcification in 50 percent. Hamartomas in lungs, kidneys, heart.	Kidneys (pyelonephritis and renal failure). Care with renally excreted drugs. Lungs (possible rupture of cysts). Possible cardiac arrhythmias.

(Continued)

569

NAME	DESCRIPTION	ANESTHETIC IMPLICATIONS
Turner's syndrome	XO chromosome, micrognathia, coarctation, dissecting aneurysm of aorta, pulmonary stenosis, renal anomalies in more than 50 percent.	Possibly difficult intubation. Cardiovascular abnormality. Possible renal disease; care with renally excreted drugs.
Urbach-Wiethe disease (cutaneous-mucosal hyalinosis)	Type of histiocytosis (see Hand-Schüller-Christian disease), hoarseness or aphonia, hyaline deposits in larynx and pharynx.	Cautious intubation.
von Gierke's disease	Glycogen storage disease I, hepatomegaly, enlarged kidneys, severe attacks of hypoglycemia.	Monitors blood sugar and acid–base balance (IV glucose infusion). Diazoxide may help in treatment of hypoglycemia. Check clotting factors.
von Hippel-Lindau disease	Retinal or CNS hemangioblastoma (posterior fossa or spinal cord), associated with pheochromocytoma, renal, pancreatic, or hepatic cysts.	Problems those of associated pheochromocytoma. Renal and hepatic pathology.
von Recklinghausen's disease (neurofibromatosis)	Cafe-au-lait spots, tumors in all parts of CNS, peripheral tumors associated with nerve trunks, increased incidence of pheochromocytoma (50 percent), kyphoscoliosis, honeycomb cystic lung changes, renal artery dysplasia and hypertension.	Screen for pheochromocytoma (urinary vanillylmandelic acid). Should be investigated for lung function. Tumors may occur in the larynx and right ventricular outflow tract. Care with renally excreted drugs if kidneys involved.

von Willebrand's disease (pseudohemophilia)	Prolonged bleeding time (decreased factor VIII activity) because of defective platelet adhesiveness, possible capillary abnormality.	Bleeding can be controlled by fresh-frozen plasma, cryoprecipitate. Avoid salicylate therapy (effect on platelets, possible GI bleeding).
Weber-Christian disease (chronic nonsupportive panniculitis)	Necrosis of fat, in any situation, including retroperitoneal, pericardial, meningeal.	Involvement of retroperitoneal tissues may cause acute or chronic adrenal insufficiency, involvement of pericardium leads to restrictive pericarditis; of meninges, causes convulsions. Avoid trauma to fat by heat, cold, or pressure.
Welander's muscular atrophy	Initial involvement of peripheral muscles, prognosis good for life, poor for ambulation.	May require spinal fusion. Extreme care with thiopental, muscle relaxants. Avoid respiratory depressant drugs.
Werdnig-Hoffmann disease	Infantile muscular atrophy more severe than in Welander, feeding difficulties, aspiration. Usually death before puberty.	Chronic respiratory problems. Minimal anesthesia required. Avoid muscle relaxants and respiratory depressant drugs. Ventilatory support may be required, and weaning may be difficult.
Wermer's syndrome (multiple endocrine adenomatosis type I)	Hyperparathyroidism, tumors of pituitary and pancreatic islet cells, gastric ulcer, occasionally have carcinoid tumors of bronchial tree.	Renal failure because of stones. Hypoglycemia from hyperinsulinism.

(Continued)

NAME	DESCRIPTION	ANESTHETIC IMPLICATIONS
Werner syndrome	Premature aging, diabetes, early cataracts, mental retardation in 50 percent, bony lesions like osteomyelitis, cardiac infarction and failure.	Anesthesia as for adult with myocardial ischemia.
Wilson's disease (hepatolenticular degeneration)	Decreased ceruloplasmin causes abnormal copper deposits especially in liver and CNS motor nuclei, renal tubular acidosis.	Hepatic failure because of fibrosis. Thiopental may be used in small doses. Muscle relaxants (succinylcholine, apnea rare despite pseudocholinesterase reduction; tubocurarine, short action as a result of globin binding). Care with renally excreted drugs.
Wilson-Mikity syndrome	Prematurity, < 1500 g birth weight, severe chronic lung disease leading to fibrosis and cystic areas, possible oxygen cause.	Right heart failure. Repeated chest infection and aspiration. Use of steroids to prevent pulmonary fibrosis.
Wiskott-Aldrich syndrome	Immunodeficiency with thrombocytopenia, 100 percent have low platelets, absent isohemagglutins, high IgA, low IgM, eczema, asthma.	Blood transfusion and platelets may be required. Bone marrow transplantation has been used. All blood products must be irradiated with 3000 rad to prevent graft-versus-host reaction. Avoid contamination (often die from generalized herpes or infection by nonpathogenic organisms).

| Wolff-Parkinson-White syndrome | ECG has abnormally short PR, prolonged QRS with phasic variation in 40 percent, associated with many cardiac defects, anomalous conduction path between atria and ventricles. | Tachycardia because of atropine or apprehension may change ECG and suggest infarction, with ST segment depression. Paroxysmal SVT on induction of anesthesia or during cardiac surgery has been reported. Treat with countershock if unstable, adenosine, digitalis, propranolol, pacemaker if necessary. Neostigmine may accentuate pattern. |
| Wolman disease (familial xanthomatosis) | Adrenal calcification, resembles Niemann-Pick disease with hepatosplenomegaly and hypersplenism, involvement of other tissues by foam cells, including myocardium, is possible. | Anemia, thrombocytopenia. Platelet transfusion only successful postsplenectomy. |

ECG = electrocardiography; CNS = central nervous system; Ig = immunoglobulin; CXR = chest x-ray; ABG = arterial blood gases; PFT = pulmonary function test; ACTH = corticotropin; IV = intravenous; IPPV = intermittent positive-pressure ventilation; GI = gastrointestinal; TMJ = temporomandibular joint; ASD = atrial septal defect; VSD = ventricular septal defect; AI = aortic insufficiency; PDA = patent ductus arteriosus; EMG = electromyography; SVT = supraventricular tachycardia.

Reproduced with permission from Jones AE, Pelton DA: An index of syndromes and their anaesthetic implications. *Can J Anaesth* 1976; 23:207–222.

Appendix B

Bacterial Endocarditis Prophylaxis

```
┌─────────────────────────────────────────────┐
│  Name: _____      │
│           needs protection from              │
│         BACTERIAL ENDOCARDITIS               │
│          because of an existing              │
│            HEART CONDITION                   │
│  Diagnosis: _____      │
│  Prescribed by: _____      │
│  Date: _____      │
└─────────────────────────────────────────────┘
```

For Dental/Oral/Upper Respiratory Tract Procedures

I. Standard Regimen In Patients At Risk (includes those with prosthetic heart valves and other high risk patients):

Amoxicillin 3.0 g orally one hour before procedure, then 1.5 g six hours after initial dose.*

For amoxicillin/penicillin-allergic patients:

Erythromycin ethylsuccinate 800 mg or erythromycin stearate 1.0 g orally 2 hours before a procedure, then one-half the dose 6 hours after the initial administration.*

—OR—

Clindamycin 300 mg orally 1 hour before a procedure and 150 mg 6 hours after initial dose.*

II. Alternate Prophylactic Regimens For Dental/Oral/Upper Respiratory Tract Procedures In Patients At Risk:

A. For patients unable to take oral medications:

Ampicillin 2.0 g IV (or IM) 30 minutes before procedure, then ampicillin 1.0 g IV (or IM) OR amoxicillin 1.5 g orally 6 hours after initial dose.*

—OR—

For ampicillin/amoxicillin/penicillin-allergic patients unable to take oral medications:

Clindamycin 300 mg IV 30 minutes before a procedure and 150 mg IV (or orally) 6 hours after initial dose.*

B. For patients considered to be at high risk who are not candidates for the standard regimen:

Ampicillin 2.0 g IV (or IM) plus gentamicin 1.5 mg/kg IV (or IM) (not to exceed 80 mg) 30 minutes before procedure, followed by amoxicillin 1.5 g orally 6 hours after the initial dose. Alternatively, the parenteral regimen may be repeated 8 hours after the initial dose.*

For amoxicillin/ampicillin/penicillin-allergic patients considered to be at high risk:

Vancomycin 1.0 g IV administered over one hour, starting one hour before the procedure. No repeat dose is necessary.*

*Note: Initial pediatric dosages are listed below. Follow-up oral dose should be one-half the inital dose. Total pediatric dose should not exceed total adult dose.

Amoxicillin:†	50 mg/kg	Vancomycin:	20 mg/kg
Clindamycin:	10 mg/kg	Ampicillin:	50 mg/kg
Erythromycin ethylsuccinate		Gentamicin:	2.0 mg/kg
or stearate:	20 mg/kg		

† The following weight ranges may also be used for the initial pediatric dose of amoxicillin:
  <15 kg (33 lbs), 750 mg
  15–30 kg (33–66 lbs), 1500 mg
  >30 kg (66 lbs), 3000 mg (full adult dose)

Kilogram to pound conversion chart: (1 kg = 2.2 lb)

Kg	Lb
5	11.0
10	22.0
20	44.0
30	66.0
40	88.0
50	110.0

For Genitourinary/Gastrointestinal Procedures

I. Standard regimen:

Ampicillin 2.0 g IV (or IM) plus gentamicin 1.5 mg/kg IV (or IM) (not to exceed 80 mg) 30 minutes before procedure, followed by amoxicillin 1.5 g orally 6 hours after the initial dose. Alternatively, the parenteral regimen may be repeated once 8 hours after the initial dose.*

For amoxicillin/ampicillin/penicillin-allergic patients:

Vancomycin 1.0 g IV administered over 1 hour plus gentamicin 1.5 mg/kg IV (or IM) (not to exceed 80 mg) one hour before the procedure. May be repeated once 8 hours after initial dose.**

II. Alternate oral regimen for low-risk patients:

Amoxicillin 3.0 g orally one hour before the procedure, then 1.5 g 6 hours after the initial dose.**

**Note: Initial pediatric dosages are listed below. Follow-up oral dose should be one-half the initial dose. Total pediatric dose should not exceed total adult dose.

Ampicillin:	50 mg/kg	Gentamicin:	2.0 mg/kg
Amoxicillin:	50 mg/kg	Vancomycin:	20 mg/kg

Note: Antibiotic regimens used to prevent recurrences of acute rheumatic fever are inadequate for the prevention of bacterial endocarditis. In patients with markedly compromised renal function, it may be necessary to modify or omit the second dose of gentamicin or vancomycin. Intramuscular injections may be contraindicated in patients receiving anticoagulants.

Adapted from *Prevention of Bacterial Endocarditis: Recommendations by the American Heart Association* by the Committee on Rheumatic Fever, Endocarditis, and Kawasaki Disease. *JAMA* 1990;264:2919–2922, © 1990 American Medical Association (also excerpted in *J Am Dent Assoc* 1991;122:87–92).

Please refer to these joint American Heart Association–American Dental Association recommendations for more complete information as to which patients and which procedures require prophylaxis.

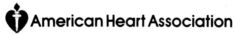 **American Heart Association**

National Center
7320 Greenville Avenue
Dallas, Texas 75231

78-1003 (CP)
90-100M
4-91-511.2M
90 06 19 B

The Council on Dental Therapeutics of the American Dental Association has approved this statement as it relates to dentistry.

Figure B-1 Bacterial endocarditis card, 1990. (Reproduced with permission from the American Heart Association. Copyright 1990 by the Association.)

Appendix C

Nomogram

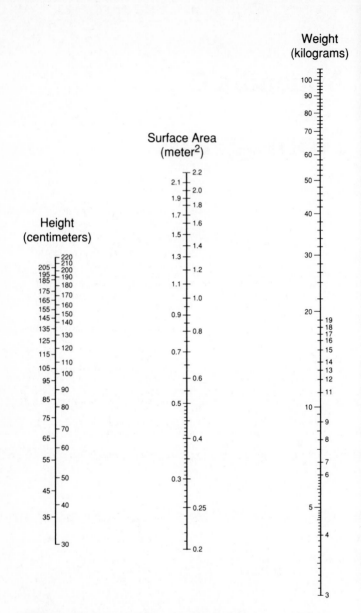

Figure C-1 Surface area is determined by lining up a straight edge with child's height and weight and then reading surface area in M² where line crosses over the scale. [Used with permission from Cole CH (ed): *The Harriet Lane Handbook,* Johns Hopkins Hospital, 10th ed. Year Book Medical Publishers, 1984.]

Index